Social Dimensions of HEALTH

Social Dimensions of HEALTH

Edited by
AJIT K. DALAL
SUBHA RAY

RAWAT PUBLICATIONS
Jaipur • New Delhi • Bangalore • Mumbai • Hyderabad • Guwahati

ISBN 81-7033-922-7

Reprinted, 2009

Published by
Prem Rawat for **Rawat Publications**
Satyam Apts., Sector 3, Jawahar Nagar, Jaipur 302 004 (India)
Phone: 0141 265 1748 / 7006 Fax: 0141 265 1748
E-mail: info@rawatbooks.com
Website: www.rawatbooks.com

New Delhi Office
4858/24, Ansari Road, Daryaganj, New Delhi 110 002
Phone: 011 2326 3290

Also at Bangalore, Mumbai, Hyderabad and Guwahati

Typeset by Rawat Computers, Jaipur
Printed at Chaman Enterprises, New Delhi

Contents

II
Indigenous Health Care Practices

III
Social Psychology of Health

IV
Indian Health Scenario

V
Community Health and Intervention

Foreword

The socio-cultural and economic variables of health are interrelated and interdependent and without comprehensive and interdisciplinary research and dialogue, the impact of social sciences on policy formulation and developmental planning will have limited impact. The discipline-bound findings have actually very little to offer in terms of finding solutions to major social problems and issues linked with health.

The challenge of improving physical and mental health status of people is an ideal meeting ground for social scientists of different backgrounds. Even physical aspect of health is rooted in socio-economic problems. Unless economists, sociologists, anthropologists, psychologists and political scientists, work in collaborative and complementary way with medical profession, their contributions will remain marginal.

The newly established (under the UGC Scheme of Potential and Excellence) Centre for Behavioural and Cognitive Sciences (CBCS), University of Allahabad has a facilitative role for interdisciplinary research and dialogue. The Centre organizes interdisciplinary seminars and supports research. This volume "Social Dimensions of Health" includes selected articles presented in the National Seminar on Social Dimensions of Health organized by the

Centre. The seminar was attended by scholars of various social science disciplines.

This volume is a good example of interdisciplinary work in the area of health and well-being. It has been meticulously edited by Prof. Ajit K. Dalal (a psychologist) and Dr Subha Ray (an anthropologist), who were the co-organizers of the seminar. The Centre highly appreciates their hard work and support for the mission of the Centre.

Janak Pandey
Professor of Psychology
Co-ordinator
Centre for Behavioural and Cognitive Sciences

Acknowledgement

The editors gratefully acknowledge the sustained support rendered by the Centre for Behavioural and Cognitive Sciences (CBCS), University of Allahabad in preparation of this manuscript. We are particularly indebted to Professor Janak Pandey, Director, CBCS, who took personal pains to see this work through all hurdles. The editors also appreciate the help rendered by Dr Asoke Saha, Dr Nishi Tripathi and Shubhra Hajela in editorial work. Dr R.N. Goyal deserves mention who did meticulous copyediting. Finally, and most importantly, we owe a great deal to our spouses and children who not only freed us to work on this manuscript but also stood by us when we were frustrated by the progress of this work

Preface

Health and well-being are the matters of concerns to all of us. These are also vital and wider issues to be confined to any one particular discipline. Though rapid advances in the field of medical science in the last century have helped in reducing mortality, the morbidity has significantly increased. There are more people suffering from various diseases today than ever in the past. Pollution, poverty, lifestyle, food habits, social and personal stresses, and many other factors have contributed to this increase in morbidity. In this sense, health and social development cannot be separated from each other, and social science research is of much significance in health care planning. Social scientists can play important role in building bridges between NGOs, communities, and government agencies working in this direction. Social scientists are indeed required to shoulder greater responsibility in improving the health status of common men.

There may be disagreement about the meaning of good health, but there is general consensus that health is much more than the absence of a disease, and that health care programmes ought to be much more than just treatment of diseases. Prevention of diseases and promotion of good health and rehabilitational aspects are integral components of health care. Health behaviour, in this sense, is a kind of social behaviour, and like any other social behaviour, it is shaped by attitudes, beliefs, customs, traditions and divisions in a society. As we know, social inequality, discrimination and prejudices are important considerations in the functioning of health institutions. These factors have to be taken into consideration, if health care programmes have to succeed. These programmes have to be compatible with the needs, aspirations and expectations of the local communities.

Social scientists in India had realized this fact long back. In fact, search for the social aspects of health is one of the most popular and productive areas of research in all social science disciplines. The failure of the present health care system has brought home the salience of social, psychological, economic and spiritual factors in prevention and treatment of diseases, as well as, in promotion of good health. Any sound health care programme has to be built on local practices, beliefs, constraints and resources. The role of social sciences in this endeavour can hardly be overemphasized.

However, health research in India is still very much confined to disciplinary boundaries. Psychology, sociology, anthropology, education, political science, economics, etc., differ not only in their approach and orientation but also in subject matter and methodology. Such compartmentalized and fragmented view of health cannot be of much use for efficient health care planning. To be relevant, all social sciences have to come together to communicate and interact from a common platform. We have to engage in a continuous dialogue in our search for viable health care models for a billion population of this country. We have to find ways to integrate rich indigenous traditions with the existing medical approach to health.

Keeping this in view, the present volume was planned to cover the whole range of issues related to improving health status. The volume contains 20 articles, which are divided into five sections. These sections are: Health, Illness and Well-being; Indigenous Health Care Practices; Social Psychology of Health; Indian Health Scenario; and Community Health and Intervention. Articles included in this volume are from varied disciplinary backgrounds but the main focus is on the theoretical and practical issues relevant to all social scientists working in the area of health. We hope that the volume will prove to be a milestone in developing interdisciplinary models of health and well-being. It is our humble view that this volume should be of use to students, researchers and practitioners working in this field.

Ajit K. Dalal
Subha Ray

Contributors

Ashish Bose is currently Honorary Professor in the Institute of Economic Growth, Delhi. He was formerly a Jawaharlal Nehru Fellow and visiting Professor at JNU. He is a member of Independent Commission on Health in India and an advisor to Voluntary Health Association of India. He has written and edited over 25 books on population and allied subjects. He is currently working on female foeticide in Punjab, Haryana and Himachal Pradesh (Address: I Block 0 1777, Chittaranjan Park, New Delhi, e-mail: ashishb@vsnl.com).

Rajat K. Das is presently a Professor of Anthropology in Vidyasagar University, Midnapore, West Bengal and Vice-President of the Indian Anthropological Society, Kolkata. He did his M.Sc. and Doctoral Research from the University of Calcutta. He has published two books and fifty research papers (Address: Department of Anthropology, Vidyasagar University, Midnapore, West Bengal).

Nisha Dhawan is a Professor, who is active in the area of women's studies. She obtained her doctorate degree from University of Allahabad. Her primary work has been in the area of motivation and psychological competence. Currently, she is conducting researches on women, their role expectations, satisfaction and conflicts, as well as violence against women (Address: Department of Psychology, University of Allahabad, Allahabad, e-mail: ndhawan@hclinfinet.com).

Shikha Dixit is Associate Professor of Psychology in the Department of Humanities and Social Sciences in the Indian Institute of Technology Kanpur. Her areas of interest are social cognition, organizational cognition, and application of cognitive psychology in armed forces. She is also working in the areas of social representations and the study of lay conceptualization of phenomena (Address: Department of Humanities and Social Sciences, Indian Institute of Technology, Kanpur, e-mail: shikha@iitk.ac.in).

S.P.K Jena is Ph.D. in clinical psychology and presently working as Reader in Applied Psychology, University of Delhi. He has published a book, *Perspectives in Mental Retardation* and several articles in national and international journals (Address: Department of Applied Psychology, University of Delhi, South Campus, New Delhi).

Nand Kishore Kannuri is a Doctoral Scholar, Department of Anthropology, University of Hyderabad, Hyderabad. He did his M.A. and M.Phil. (specialization in Medical Anthropology) from the same university (Address: 336, Doyens, Serilingampalli, Hyderabad, e-mail: nandu@geostop.com).

A.K. Kapoor holds Master's Degree and Ph.D. in Anthropology from the University of Delhi. He has carried out investigations among tribes, castes and ethnic groups in different parts of India including Andaman and Nicobar Islands. He has published seven books and 117 research papers. His interests are human population, human rights, tribal health, ageing, anthropology of NGOs and management anthropology. He was awarded UGC Research Award in 1999. Currently, he is Professor, Department of Anthropology, University of Delhi, Delhi (Address: Department of Anthropology, University of Delhi, Delhi).

Ramendra Kumar Kar is Professor in the Post-graduate Department of Anthropology, Dibugarh University, Assam. He had been the President of the Anthropology Section in the twentieth session of the Indian Social Sciences Congress in December 1997. His interest areas include health behaviour, ecology and culture, urbanization and social change, tribal development, inter-ethnic relationship and ethnicity, and anthropology of north-east India (Address: Department of Anthropology, Dibrugarh University, Assam).

Abdul Majeed Khan is Ph.D. in Psychology from the University of Allahabad and is presently Professor at the National Institute of Health and Family Welfare, New Delhi. He has widely published in the areas of inter-group relations, population studies, health systems and programme evaluation (Address: Department of Social Sciences, National Institute of Health and Family Welfare, Munirka, New Delhi).

Neena Kohli is Senior Lecturer with a doctorate from Allahabad University. She has worked on factors involved in psychological recovery following tragic life events. Her current research interests include illness cognitions, coping with chronic diseases, designing psychological interventions and stress management (Address: Department of Psychology, University of Allahabad, Allahabad, e-mail: drneenakohli@rediffmail.com).

Gautam K. Kshatriya is Reader in the Department of Anthropology, University of Delhi. He obtained his Ph.D. in population genetics and has done post-doctoral work in the same area at the University of Texas, USA. He has more than 50 research publications to his credit. Currently, he is concentrating on the study of primitive tribal groups and genctic epidemiology (Address: Department of Anthropology, University of Delhi, Delhi).

Barun Mukhopadhyay is an anthropologist who has been researching on biocultural determinants of health and health care among the tribal populations of the Sikkim-Darjeeling Himalaya. He is also engaged in studies of people and plants relationship in the Sikkim Himalaya. He is presently Associate Professor in the Anthropology and Human Genetics Unit of the Indian Statistical Institute, Kolkata (Address: Anthropology and Human Genetics Unit, Indian Statistical Institute, 203, Barrackpore Trunk Road, Kolkata, e-mail: barun@isical.ac.in).

Dinesh Nagar, Reader, Department of Psychology, Barkatullah University, Bhopal, is currently working as Associate Professor in the Department of Educational Planning and Management, Addis Ababa University, Ethiopia. He has done his post-doctoral research from the University of Texas, USA and has published a number of research papers in reputed journals and edited books (Address: Department of Psychology, Barkatullah University, Bhopal).

P. Ignatius Prabhakar has obtained his Ph.D. in 2004. He has worked in several projects including UNICEF-sponsored project on "Operational Research Project on Maternal Anaemia among Urban Poor in Tamil Nadu". He has produced jointly a documentary titled, "A Nebulous Future: The Story of Onge of Little Andaman" (2002) (Address: Department of Anthropology, University of Madras, Chennai).

Deepa Punetha is Professor with a doctorate degree from the University of Allahabad. She has worked on socialization practices for handling aggression in children and has conducted studies on values and language, inter-ethnic perception, gender issues and empowerment of women in community settings (Address: Department of Psychology, University of Allahabad, Allahabad, e-mail: deepadwujen@rediffmail.com).

K. Ramakrishna Rao has held various academic and administrative positions in India and the United States, including Professor and Head of the Department of Psychology and Parapsychology, Dean of the Faculty of Arts and Social Sciences and Vice-Chancellor of the Andhra University (Address: Department of Centre for the Study of Science and Social Anthropology, Institute of Human Science and Service, 35 Daspalla Hills, Vishakhapatnam, e-mail: IHSS_CPSS@hotmail.com).

Ashok Sharma is Lecturer in Psychology at Vaish PG College, Bhiwani (Haryana). He did his doctoral research in the field of well-being and personality. His current interests include psychological testing and health psychology (Address: Department of Psychology, Vaish PG College, Bhiwani (Haryana), e-mail: ashok_Sharma_71@yahoo.com).

A.K. Sharma is Professor of Sociology and Head of Humanities and Social Sciences Department at the Indian Institute of Technology, Kanpur. He specializes in social studies of health and family welfare, neo-social movements and studies of post-modern organizations. He has published more than seventy-five papers in national and international journals. (Address: Head, Humanities and Social Sciences Department, Indian Institute of Technology, Kanpur, e-mail: arun@iitk.ac.in).

Ashutosh Sharma is Professor, Department of Architecture in MACT, Bhopal. He has published many papers in reputed journals (Address: Department of Architecture, MACT, Bhopal).

Nov Ratan Sharma is presently Reader and Head in the Department of Psychology, M.D. University, Rohtak. He specialized in the area of personality and health psychology. He has also contributed more than thirty research articles in various reputed journals and also participated in around 35 national/international conferences and seminars (Address: Head, Department of Psychology, M.D. University, Rohtak).

V. Sudarsen obtained his Ph.D. in Anthropology from Andhra University, Vishakapatnam. Ecological anthropology and island cultures, are his two areas of interest. Presently, he is working on modes of developmental plans and implementations. He has completed about forty sponsored research projects, and has published over sixty papers in reputed journals and ten books (Address: Department of Anthropology, University of Madras, Chennai, e-mail: sudarsen@vsnal.com).

S. Sumathi obtained her Ph.D. from the Department of Anthropology, University of Madras, Chennai. She has worked in the areas of caste and communal census, biodiversity and tribal rights and their identity. She has published four papers and a book, "Is there a Creamy Layer among OBC? An Anthropology-Legal Study of Other Backward Classes" (Address: Department of Anthropology, University of Madras, Chennai).

Nishi Tripathi is a Counsellor in the Department of Psychology, University of Allahabad. She obtained her doctorate degree from the University of Allahabad. Her work is in the areas of adjustive demands, attitudes and beliefs of the physically disabled girls, role strain of their mothers and learning disability (Address: Department of Psychology, University of Allahabad, Allahabad).
e-mail: tripathi_nishi@yahoo.com

Ruchika Varma is a research scholar in the Department of Psychology, University of Allahabad. Her major areas of interest are gender and health, socialization, personal control and well-being (Address: Department of Psychology, University of Allahabad, Allahabad).

Amrita Yadava is Reader in the Department of Psychology, M.D. University, Rohtak. Her broad area of research has been experimental/comparative, environmental psychology and health issues. She has also contributed more than twenty-three research articles in various reputed journals and also participated in a large number of national/international conferences and seminars, (Address: Department of Psychology, M.D. University, Rohtak).

1

Social Dimensions of Health and Well-being: An Overview of Research Trends

AJIT K. DALAL AND SUBHA RAY

Health and well-being is a matter of concern to all strata of the society. It is a tall order to envision a society which is free from the perennial struggle against diseases. Science and technology have taken giant steps to control epidemics and to increase longevity. The success of the biomedical model lies in the fact that it has been able to control many infectious and life-threatening diseases and has given rise to a hope that one day there will be a pill for every illness. This is a very narrow view of health that only focuses on disease control and therapeutic aspect of health. Health is much larger a domain, which affects all aspects of human existence. It has wider implications for social, economic and political life of an individual and indeed cannot be fully understood within the confines of medical model. It is widely accepted that health is a social problem and well-being is still a more complex concept to be managed by medical professionals.

Social scientists have been actively engaged in empirically examining the social factors which contribute significantly in promoting good health and controlling diseases. Their persistent efforts to understand health from social perspective have firmly rooted social scientists in addressing larger issues related to causes and cures of health problems. This introductory chapter aims to highlight the place of social sciences in control, treatment and betterment of health in the context of significant research contributions. More recent annual reports of WHO and other health organizations have increasingly acknowledged the role of social and psychological factors in meeting the challenges of health in the 21st century. The chapter intends to provide an overview of the state of social science literature, particularly in reference to Indian social context, and would bring out some of the factors critical to improving health status and a sense of well-being.

This review chapter is organized along the four sectors that cover most of the areas and disciplines of social sciences. These four sectors are: socio-economic concomitants of health, health services and systems, health care practices, and health attitudes and perceptions. Schematically, this sectoral model of health is presented below:

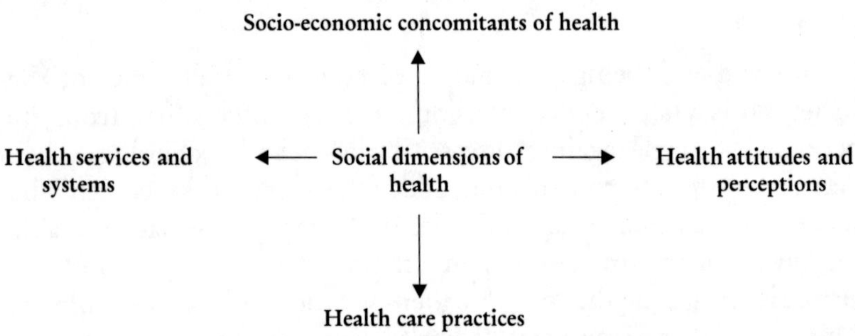

There are a number of socio-economic and socio-demographic constructs, like ethnicity, gender, age, religion, caste and social class, which affect the exposure and vulnerability to disease, shapes the perception of and responses to health problems, actuates the effectiveness of health promotion efforts and creates an impact on an individual's life and well-being. Poverty conditions, for example, create a major institutional challenge and no community health care programme can succeed unless it addresses wider issues of social and economic nature. The sector 'health services and systems' is concerned with developing the health of the people by delivering health care services which are acceptable and accessible to the people. Research in this field is concerned with developing policies and strategies keeping in view resources and requirements of the larger section of the society. The sector of health care practices deals with health behaviour and practices of the communities and the way sick people are treated by the society. It is an effort to understand health issues from the perspective of local communities, the informal health care practices and remedial measures taken by the communities. Kleinman (1978) has termed it as folk practices sector in which health care practices evolve and sustain because of their popular appeal, in contrast to professional practices, which are supported by institutional set-up. Lastly, there is research which focuses on people's attitudes and perceptions of health. It deals with people's own understanding of the cause of illness, their health behaviour, and the ways they take care of themselves when they fall ill. This micro-level approach deals with the illness experience, as well as on person's construal of health and illness. Psychological research in health area is covered within this sector.

The above four-sector approach is likely to recover the whole gamut of research conducted in social sciences. In practice, this distinction is artificial, as, a complete and meaningful understanding of health behaviour and policy formulation has to take a holistic view. However, it may be stated here that though health is an transdisciplinary field, the existing body of research is still confined to the boundaries of different social science disciplines.

The multi-sectoral approach defines health as a complex web of environmental, social, economic and individual factors, which are interrelated with each other. Moreover, health is not a commodity that is to be passed on to any community. The community should generate their own health needs, identify their solutions, mobilize their local resources and develop local organizations to meet those needs. This is essential to make health care programmes accessible and acceptable to the community. It is a non-expert social approach to health care where people from the grassroots level can take initiatives. It may be pertinent to mention here that this multi-sectoral approach and community involvement became the basis for the Alma Ata resolution of 1978 and of subsequent national and international policies and programmes to provide primary health care to all by the year 2000 (http://www.phmovement.org/charter/almaata).

As a consequence of these global efforts, the average life expectancy at birth has increased globally over the last 50 years by almost 20 years – from 46.5 years between 1950 and 1955 to 65.2 years in 2002. The child mortality rate has reduced from 17 million in the year 1970 to 10.5 million in the year 2002. Due to the global polio eradication initiative, the number of children paralyzed by this devastating disease has fallen from 35,000 in 1988 to 1,900 in the year 2003. Notwithstanding, consumption of cigarette and other tobacco products and exposure to tobacco smoke are the world's leading preventable causes of death, responsible for about 5 million deaths in the year 2003 (World Health Report, 2003). Lifestyle and eating patterns are the other major health hazards leading to millions of untimely deaths.

Socio-economic Concomitants of Health

Socio-economic conditions of the people determine their health status in terms of longevity, infant mortality and morbidity. People low on socio-economic ladder are not only more vulnerable to infection and respiratory diseases but also have lower access to health services (WHO, 1998). In general, people below poverty line, children, women, aged and displaced ones suffer more from health problems than other strata of the society.

Vulnerable Groups

According to Chambers (1989), vulnerability means not only exposure to risks, but also lack of means to overcome these risks. The people, who are most vulnerable to the environmental hazards, are those who are least able to avoid them and/or least able to cope with the illness or injury they cause. If one attempts to examine what causes people's vulnerability to environmental hazards, the interaction between environmental hazards and social, economic, political and demographic factors become much clearer. An example can be cited with the disease diarrhoea. Diarrhoea is a disease caused due to the consumption of contaminated water and the incidence is very common to individuals, particularly children living in poor living conditions. The economic underpinnings of diarrhoea become clear when the incidence of occurrence of the disease is found predominantly among the poor people, who live in unhygienic crowded conditions, have inadequate sanitation and lack piped water facilities. The incidence can also be judged to be a political problem since nearly all government agencies have the capacity to reduce the levels of morbidity and mortality related to diarrhoea by providing the basic infrastructural facilities like provision of piped water, improved living conditions and health care facilities. In the words of Stephens and Harpham (1992), "health outcomes are not only influenced by the environmental conditions but also by the inputs of health services, by the characteristics of the population and by the socio-economic conditions in which they live".

Foetuses, infants and children are particularly vulnerable to certain health-related problems. In spite of advancement in social and economic conditions, which the world has witnessed in the later part of the 20th century, about 10.5 million children under five years of age died in the year 2002, and 98 percent of the death is from the developing countries (World Health Report, 2003). An unborn child is most at risk during its foetal life. The health of a foetus is largely dependent on the nutrient intake of the mothers, morbid condition of the mother, and exposure of mother to chemical, toxic and radiation (Kalter and Warkary, 1983; UNEP and WHO, 1990; Braungart *et al.*, 1992; Barlow and Sulivan, 1982). Infants and young children are at a greater risk of dying from health problems than that of the adults because of their lower immunity level. The increasing mobility of young children as they learn to crawl and then walk increases the risk of becoming infected. The risk becomes compounded with poor living conditions (UNICEF, 1991). UNICEF (1986) has termed child refugees, working children and street children, neglected and abandoned children, abused, children caught in armed conflict as "children in especially difficult circumstances". These children are not only prone to physical health problems but also to psychosocial health problems (UNICEF, 1992; Patel, 1990).

WHO (2002) (http://www.who.int/entity/gender/en) adopted a gender policy where it acknowledges that sex – the biological facts of being male and female – and gender – the cultural norms that determine masculinity and feminity – have an important impact on health. The policy considered the fact that there are factors determining health and the burden of ill-health for men and women. In a given culture, gender norms and values give rise to gender differences and inequalities. For example, a woman cannot receive health services because her community norms do not allow her to travel alone to the medical clinic or there are societies which do not discourage males from practising promiscuity that may lead to the infection of STD or HIV; at the same time, the wives of those males become vulnerable to those infections, because the cultural norms bar them from using condom. Moreover, low status of women in most of the societies restricts them to avail the health care facilities. Again, the locations and opening hours of the health services rarely are well suited to women's need (Moser, 1993). Again, in many societies like India, girl child is more vulnerable than a boy child because her nutritional and health needs receive lower priority within the household. In many parts of the world, discrimination in women's health begins before birth and stays with them till they die. According to World Bank (1991) (cited in Satterthwaite *et al.*, 1995), "gender differentials in nutritional status are established during infancy, with discriminatory breast-feeding and supplementation practices.... Weaned earlier, they may not receive adequate supplementation foods and are given lower quality foods than boys". The Department of Gender and Women's Health, a wing of WHO (http://www.who.int/entity/gender/en), plays a role to increase the awareness of health professionals regarding the role of gender norms, values and inequality in perpetuating disease, disability death and to promote societal change with a view to eliminate gender as a barrier to good health.

Moreover, studies also show that women are more vulnerable than men to many of these health problems as they take most of the responsibilities related to bearing and rearing of child and household management (Moser, 1987; Lee-Smith and Trujillo, 1992; Sapir, 1990; Jordan and Wagner, 1993; Crewe, 1995; and Obrist *et al.*, 2003). Pregnant women are more vulnerable to certain environmental hazards. Every year, about half a million women die of causes related to pregnancy and child birth (UNICEF, 1991). As reported by WHO (1992), "the reproductive process is sensitive to adverse environmental conditions. Every stage of the multi-step process of reproduction can be disrupted by external environmental agents and this may lead to increased risk of abortion, birth defects, foetal growth retardation and perinatal deaths". Rearing of child also includes caring for the sick and handling and laundering of soiled clothes that are particularly hazardous to health. In addition to all these, a woman is exposed to a number of reproductive health problems right from her adolescent period till her death. The magnitude of reproductive and sexual health problems in South Asia is daunting (Pachuri, 1998). Most of the problems are related to child birth, abortion, sexually transmitted diseases (STDs) and gynaecological health (reproductive tract infection, infertility and menstrual irregularities) which take a heavy toll on women health (Bang *et al.*, 1989; Pachuri, 1998). The future of human health in the 21st century depends a great deal on a commitment to investing in women health in the world today. Their health largely determines the health of the children, who are the adults of tomorrow (World Health Report, 1998).

Environmental Hazards

Most of the environmental hazards that affect human health are due to human actions or human inactions. The four most pressing physical environmental problems that have direct bearing on health are biological pathogens and their vectors, chemical pollutants, a shortage of particular natural resources and physical hazards. The three other factors, though not directly but indirectly affecting health are, aspects of built environment with negative consequences on psychosocial health, natural resource degradation and national and global environmental degradation (depletion of ozone layer, concentration of green house gases, etc.) (Satterthwaite, 1995). Among these seven kinds of environmental hazards, the biological pathogen in human environment, air, water, soil, etc., takes the greatest toll on health (WHO, 1992). Water-borne diseases are the single largest category of communicable diseases of which, world wide, diarrhoea alone is the cause of large number of infant and child mortality per year (Kouray and Vasquez, 1979; WHO, 1992, 1999).

The risk factors associated with these diseases are lack of piped water, overcrowding, poor sanitation, contaminated food and hygiene (Merrick 1983;Victoria *et al.*, 1988; Rossi-Espagnet *et al.*, 1991). Moreover, diarrhoea and worm infestation, along with poor water and sanitation provisions that promote them, have complex and reciprocal relation with malnutrition in children (Rice *et al.*, 2000; Wierzba *et al.*, 2001).

Acute respiratory infections are a major cause of infant and child death and also ill-health in rural and urban areas. An estimated four to five million infants and children die each year from these infections. Tuberculosis alone is responsible for some three million deaths each year and is the single largest source of adult deaths (WHO, 1992) and accounts for a quarter of all adult deaths (cited by Satterthwaite *et al.*, 1995). Here also, the risk factors are overcrowding, ill-ventilation, nature of fuel use and dampness (Surjadi, 1993; Songsore and McGranahan, 1993; Ray, 2001). Regarding indoor air pollution, biomass fuels burnt indoors are likely to be the main chemical hazard. These certainly affect rural than the urban dwellers leading to chronic inflammation of respiratory tract (Pandey *et al.*, 1989).

The availability to any individual or household of such natural resources as food, fuel and fresh water is obviously central to health. The environmental dimension is prominent in that the ecosystem defines the limits for the availability of fresh water, soils and forests but social, economic and political factors are usually the dominant influence on who has access to them or to the land and water sources from which they can be drawn (Satterthwaite, 1993). Non-availability of fresh water is very common to people living in squatter or shanty settlements. The government considers them to have no right to public services as they live in illegal settlements (Bapat and Agarwal, 2003). According to WHO/UNICEF (2000), the standard for household water consumption is 20 litres per person per day. Lack of access to fresh water affects child health to a large extent (Bukenya and Nwokolo, 1991; WHO/UNICEF, 2000).

Among the chemical pollutants, lead remains a particular concern, especially for children since there is an increasing evidence to show that relatively low concentration of lead in the blood may have a damaging effect on their mental development that persist into adulthood (Needleman *et al.*, 1991). The four major sources from which the concentration of lead is increasing in the environment are all due to human activities. These include exhausts from the vehicles, lead water piping, industrial emissions and lead in paint.

Migration and Displacement

Migration involves a variety of health threats. Migrants or particular migrant groups are more vulnerable to certain environmental hazards than long term residents as they lack immunity to a particular disease that is common within the area where they moved (Sapir, 1990). Moreover, migrants can introduce new set of diseases to the members of their host or receiving population. Diseases like smallpox and measles were transmitted to the Native Americans after the colonization of the Europeans in America and the reciprocal effects of syphilis transmission took place from the New World to the Old World (Crosby, 1972). Migration separates families and separation has been found to correlate with both high levels of extra-marital sexual relationships and HIV/STI infection rates in other parts of the world (Mbizvo, 1996). In some cases, migrants move to the city and get settled in squatter or ghettos, characterized by unsatisfactory living conditions, which lead to high rates of epidemic diseases (McNeill, 1976; Zinsser, 1935). When migration has an economic advantage, a change in lifestyle is quite common giving rise to some new health risks, like diabetes, drug dependencies, anxiety, cardiovascular diseases (CVD) and hypertension (Kaplan, 1988; Weiss *et al.*, 1984; Zimmet *et al.*, 1977; Shaper *et al.*, 1969; Ward, 1983; Baker, 1984). In the early 1900s, cities such as New York, with migrant populations from diverse physical and cultural environments had particular difficulties because the types of disease problems varied greatly according to sub-population (Baker, 1990). Some social scientists believe that migrants develop psychosocial stress for adjusting in the new environment due to social disorganization (Levine *et al.*, 1962).

Health Systems and Services

Health systems have existed ever since people made systematic attempts to protect their health and treat diseases. Throughout the world, the traditional practices based on herbal cures and/or spiritual counselling and providing both curative and preventive care, have existed for thousands of years, and even today have survived despite the dominance of modern medicine. The modern health systems, aiming to cater to the needs of a large mass of population, existed barely a century ago. Although, in many countries, the existence of hospitals has a longer history than the organized health system. With the onset of industrial revolution, there occurred a transformation in the lives of the people, specially, in relation to health and health systems.

Most of the information available on health system refers to the provision of investment in health services, i.e., health care, including curative, preventive and palliative interventions, whether directed to individuals or populations. People come into direct contact with a health system as patients attended by the health care providers. It matters very much how the system treats people's health needs, meets their expectations, treats them with dignity, pays value to their time and anxiety and how it raises revenues from them, including how much protection it offers them from financial risk. Again, in order for an individual to utilize a service, they must believe that the service will benefit their health. Some studies that have focused on the perceptions and motivations to use health services reveal that care is often inadequate and insensitive (Thaddeus and Amine, 1994; WHO, 1991). Moreover, location of services and transportation problems in accessing services can be a barrier to the utilization of health facilities (Price, 1984; Greenwood, 1987; Sundari, 1992). Sometimes, corruption in public health services creates aversion among the care seekers. In a survey conducted in India, it was found that a quarter of all respondents had paid bribes for health services (Kumar, 2003).

"Health system includes all the activities whose primary purpose is to promote, restore or maintain health" (World Health Report, 2000). Real progress in health depends vitally on strong health systems based on primary health care. Systems should integrate health promotion and disease prevention and treatment for acute illness and chronic care on the other. This should be done across all levels of health care system, with the aim of delivering quality services equitably and efficiently to the whole population (World Health Report, 2003). Formal health services, including professional delivery of personal medical attention, are clearly within this boundary. So are actions by traditional healers, and all use of medication, whether prescribed by the provider or not and the home care for sick, which is somewhere between 70 percent and 90 percent of all sickness is managed (Kleinman, 1978). At present, enhancing interventions, like roads and environment safety improvements, improvement in sanitation, educational level in general and of girls in particular – all come under the purview of health system. The World Health Report, 2000 states that "the health systems not only have a responsibility to improve people's health but to protect them against the financial cost of illness and to treat them with dignity". Thus, it has identified three major objectives to develop the health systems: (1) improving the health of the population they serve, (2) responding to people's expectation, and (3) providing financial protection against the cost of ill-health.

Health system today represents one of the largest sectors in the world economy and the global spending on health care was about $2,985 billion in 1997 or almost 8 percent of world gross domestic product (GDP) (World Health Report, 2000). India is one of the countries of the world which has lowest health budgets (Commission for Macroeconomics and Health, 2000). The much hyped health policy of India, adopted in 2002 giving priority to revive public health system, received no budgetary allocation for 2002-03. The Government of India spends a mere 17.3 percent of its total health budget on the public health system as against England, which spends 96.9 percent, USA 44.1 percent, Srilanka 45.4 percent and China 24.9 percent (Gupta, 2003). The World Health Report (1995) identified 'poverty' as the greatest cause of suffering and showed widening gap in health status between the rich and the poor. One of the priorities given by this report is to develop Public Health Policy with its emphasis on equity, i.e., equal access to health care. However, going by the report prepared by the WHO-appointed

Commission of Macroeconomics for Health (2000), in India, in general, it has been observed that though there has been a considerable development in the health status of the people and improvement in the health system and intervention, there exist wide differentials between and within the states, between the rich and the poor and between the rural and urban populations. This report also cited a study made by NCAER that in India, 20 percent of the richest enjoy three times the share of public subsidy for health compared to the poorest quintile. In contrast, the poorest 20 percent of the Indians have more than double the mortality rates, fertility rates and undernutrition levels than the richest. On an average, a poor spends 12 percent of their incomes on health care as against 2 percent by the rich. In the rural areas, the poor who did not seek treatment because of financial reasons increased from 15 percent to 24 percent and doubled from 10 percent to 21 percent in urban areas. Treatment and hospitalization for chronic illness often means liquidification of meagre assets and indebtness (World Bank, 2001). The insufficient provision for public health facilities and the discrimination in the utilization of public health facilities can only be minimized by increasing public investment for health, accompanied by large-scale reforms at every levels with political support. The Approach Paper to the Tenth Five-Year Plan (2002-2007) (Planning Commission of India, 2001) identified improving the access to and utilization of health, family welfare and nutrition services with special focus on underserved and underprivileged segments of the population to develop the health systems. The focus has been given on reorganizing and restructuring the existing health care infrastructure at the secondary and tertiary care levels, delegating power to Panchayati Raj Institutions (PRIs) to increase the accountability of local people about the public health care providers and problems relating to poor performance and sorting out appropriate mechanisms so that the cost of severe illness and hospitalization can be borne by individual/organization. In addition to these, focus has also been laid on preservation, promotion and cultivation of medicinal plants and herbs and ensuring the availability of good quality drugs at affordable prices, horizontal integration of all aspects of the current vertical disease control programmes, including supplies, monitoring, training, administrative arrangements, etc., and continue the commitment to provide essential primary health care, emergency life saving services, services under the National Disease Control Programme and National Family Planning Welfare Programme free of cost to individuals based on their needs and not on their ability to pay.

Cooperation between governments and international institutions, the private sector and civil society spurred remarkable public health care in the 20th century. This has become possible mainly because of globalization. In an increasingly interdependent world, such collaboration across political and sectoral boundaries is more vital than ever. This interdependence of nations and the need for international cooperation are perceived clearly from the recent outbreak of the disease SARS (Severe Acute Respiratory Syndrome) and the way this disease has been controlled (World Health Report, 2003). SARS is a tale of how a new disease emerges with major international implications for health, economy and trade. Its rapid containment is one of the success stories of public in recent years and represents a major victory for public health collaboration.

Health Care Practices

Health behaviour is a kind of a social behaviour and, as such, affects and gets affected by various socio-cultural parameters. For example, understanding of a disease is not a medical issue but is largely dependent on the shared knowledge of a particular community. Traditions, social practices and role relationships – all contribute to our dealings with health and illnesses. The sick role behaviour largely depends on how a community expects its sick members to behave. These social aspects of health form the basis for informal systems of health care.

Medical anthropologist, Arthur Kleinman (1980), has classified health care practices into three sectors: popular, folk and professional. These three sectors not only differ in terms of their explanations of illness but also in the treatment regimen and the mode of social interaction. The popular sector refers to those informal health practices that primarily rely on familial and social network knowledge to deal with diseases. Home-made remedies, knowledgeable people who can be consulted, visiting spiritual centres are all part of the popular sector. These practices are the outgrowth of shared experiences and transfer of knowledge from one generation to the other. According to Kleinman, 95 percent of the health problems in a society are taken care by this popular sector. The folk sector is rather a more organized system of dealing with health and illness. These are the informal systems, which have evolved over a very long period of time, and are integrated within the community life. The folk sector comprises herbal medicine, shamans and traditional healers and time-tested indigenous medicines. These folk treatments have survived for centuries because they share the belief systems of the community and are consistent with the social and religious practices. Kakar (1982) has evidenced that, what are considered as primitive and superstitious practices have their rationality rooted in a coherent worldview and in efficacy in dealing with a wide range of health problems. Even, in this scientific age, the popularity of these folk practices has not declined. The third sector, i.e., professional sector, refers to organized professional systems, like medical system, accupuncture and ayurveda, which have a formal system of practising. These systems are based on well-laidout theoretical basis, system of education and professional bodies and code of conduct. Such professional systems compete for public patronage and their co-existence is characterized by suspicion and underlying tension.

Sick Role Behaviour

Health and illness has been a major theme within sociology since the development of Parson's theory of *The Social System* (1951). Parson, in his functionalist approach, contends that a healthy population that could undertake various tasks is required to promote the smooth functioning of a society. Sick people cannot take up their normal social roles. According to Parson, sick role behaviour is based on some rights and obligations. Sick people are exempted from the normal social role expectations and also from the responsibility of their sickness. At the time it is obligatory for a sick person to seek out treatment and get well, as soon as possible. As Parson posited, rights are contingent on obligations, and if a sick person fails to comply with treatment, he or she forfeits the privilege of the sick role.

Though Parson never conducted empirical research, his formulation of sick role behaviour has been the basis of the sociological work in this area. This sick role behaviour was considered universal, regardless of culture or social status. This approach, however, has certain limitations and cannot be applied in the case of a chronic illness. In later reformulation of sick role, Parson (1975) argued that although complete recovery was not possible for the chronically sick, it was medical practice to manage their condition in such a way that they could establish a relatively normal social role. Parson's reformulation, however, fails in the case of physical disability where the issue of recovery is often not of much relevance.

In fact, it may be argued that in such formulations of sick role, medicine becomes a mechanism of social control. Patients were conceived as powerless and at the mercy of the specialists who can dictate what a patient should do. Most of the further research on patient compliance is guided by this view of the patient. It was also presumed that once sick, a patient will always seek treatment. As we will discuss later in this section, patients vary in their understanding of the symptoms and there are large gray areas in which the patient is unclear about the implications of their physical symptoms. Most importantly, in this formulation, the patient is not given any choice to seek alternative modes of treatment. If the patient resorts to any other mode of treatment, it may be taken as non-compliance to the established medical treatment. Sick role behaviour has no meaning outside the biomedical practices. As we discuss here, in traditional societies, there are plurality of health care systems and patients have a freedom to choose anyone or more modes of treatment. Sick role, for example, has very different connotation in traditional healing.

Social Construction of Health and Illness

Health and illness are often defined in organic terms, referring to bodily conditions, as assessed by the medical professionals. This typical expert-oriented approach fails in delivering the services. In the first instance, the patient will approach health professional only when they find their symptoms threatening and realize that they need medical attention. It, thus, seems important to see health and illness from the patient's perspective (Radley, 1994).

It can be contended further, that illness is a social event and understanding of the symptoms is a collective endeavour. There is a great deal of subjectivity in the interpretation of the symptoms and social beliefs, expectations and status provides the basis for symptom interpretation. People make sense of their illness in a social interactional process; it is a joint construction in which patients, their families and social acquaintances, all play a role. This social construction of the disease and its symptoms may not necessarily match with those of the medical professional. However, patients and their families take important treatment-related decisions based on this understanding of the disease. This understanding also becomes the basis to decide which mode of treatment to pursue to recover. For example, if a disease is attributed to God's displeasure, a godman will be sought out to get healed from the disease. Dalal (2000, 2001) has found that Indian patients more frequently attribute their illness to God's will, fate and *karma*, than to germs, pollutants and lifestyle, found in most of the western studies. Accordingly, whereas in the West, people consult medical doctors for their health problems, in India and other Asian countries, they are equally likely to consult faith and spiritual healers (Joshi, 2001).

Traditional Healing Practices

All traditional societies in the world have evolved their own systems of curing and healing, and most of these systems have sustained due to their patronage by the common man. Traditional healers, which comprise family priests, gurus, ojhas, shamans, pirs, godmen, etc., are all involved in dealing with health and other personal crises. When suffering an illness, people frequently visit these healers and healing places for alternative remedies, even while they are getting medical treatment. These healers are presumed to have healing powers, or are held as medium to connect with the supernatural. Their treatment is holistic, which may combine social, spiritual and medicinal aspects to bring relief to the suffering individual. In India, there are a large number of healing centres and their popularity has not declined even with the access to western medicine.

Kleinman (1978) and Kakar (1982) have studied these healing systems as they are practised in Asian countries. A review of writings in this area suggests many common features among these traditional practices. Firstly, nowhere, it is a full-time occupation but is considered to be a social service without any expectation of payment. No fee is charged, no advance payment is made. In fact, it is often believed that if they start charging for their services, they will loose their healing powers. Of course, people who seek relief, do find some ways to make offerings to repay their gratitude. Secondly, there are only few chosen, who possess healing powers. One cannot acquire healing powers through any formal training. Mostly, these powers are transferred from one generation to the other, as some member of the family inherits it and learns to practise through apprenticeship. In other instances, these powers are transferred from guru to pupil. In this respect, much depends on the trust and faith which the believers pose in the credentials and bonafides of a healer. Thirdly, the most important aspect to be examined is patient-healer communication. The essence is not in what is communicated but how is it communicated, i.e., whether the healer succeeds in establishing a relationship and evoke the right emotions in the recipients. In this sense, healing rituals are not as important as the kind of aura which the healer is able to create. Fourthly, these healing practices are social activities in the sense that generally the whole family, including the extended social net, participates in the process of healing. People are supposed to openly share their problems, often in the presence of others and it is a collective venture, where the target is not the person but his or her own family. Thus, there is much sharing and social interaction involved in the healing process.

Health Perceptions and Attitudes

In this sectoral approach health is understood from the people's perspective. It views a person as embedded in a socio-cultural context, in which he or she imbibes certain belief system. These socio-cultural beliefs would determine the way a patient evaluates and gives meaning to his/her sickness. Kleinman (1980) has made a distinction in his research between disease and illness. Whereas disease is an organic malfunctioning as diagnosed by a medical practitioner, illness is a subjective construction of the experience of a disease by the patient. It is patient's own interpretation and perception of the disease, which is greatly influenced by the culture to which the patient belongs.

This approach to health assumes a unity of the mind and the body, and that these two in a complex interactional process determine the health status of a person. Mind is presumed to be both the cause of a disease and contributor to recovery. In a recent article published in *American Psychologist*, O. Ray (2004) reviewed the field to substantiate his argument that it is the mind which hurts and heals the body. Ray argued in favour of biopsychosocial model which will be the basis of futuristic health care programming. In this approach, patients' phenomenology, i.e., their attitudes, values and beliefs are also crucial in deciding about the type of treatment sought and the extent to which people would comply to the curative regime. According to the Health Belief Model, propounded by Rosenstock (1966, 1974), knowledge of patient's health-related beliefs is crucial in understanding the patient's psychological state of readiness to take specific action. For example, patients' compliance can be predicted considering their beliefs about severity, susceptibility and consequences of an illness, as well as, cost of a regimen and its likelihood of success (Becker and Maiman, 1975). Rosenstock originally proposed his model to predict preventive health behaviour, which was later on extended by Kasl and Cobb (1966) to explain sick role behaviour.

Social support network plays a crucial role in deciding about the course of illness an individual is experiencing, as well as, in maintaining good health and longevity. In a review of 50 recent studies, Uchino, Uno and Holt-Lunstad (1999) discovered that individuals having high level of social support have lower blood pressure and higher immunity than those having low level of social support.

Psychological Factors Shaping Health

Individual Dispositions and Temperament

Personality dispositions were found to have significant bearings on health status. Many personality traits predispose an individual to negative emotional states, such as depression, anxiety and nervousness, or lead to maladaptive coping behaviours. Mathews and Ridgeway (1981) identified a large number of personality variables associated with surgical recovery. Feeling of control and positive attitude were found to be important factors in the success of surgery (Hunt, McKenna, Backett and Pope, 1984). Also, recovery of the surgical patients was found to be contingent on patient's emotional state prior to surgery (see Cohen and Lazarus, 1979). Janis (1958) found a curvilinear relationship between anticipatory fear and post-operative recovery.

One such personality variable is Type A behaviour pattern that significantly contributes to the occurrence of coronary heart disease (Jenkins, 1978; Glass, 1976). A Type A person shows extreme competitiveness, a sense of urgency (always feels rushed or is impatient when delayed), excessive involvement in work, aggressiveness and hostility. Individuals displaying this behaviour pattern seem to be engaged in chronic, ceaseless and unnecessary struggle with themselves, with others and with circumstances. In contrast, Type B behaviour pattern is characterized by a low level of competitiveness, time urgency and hostility. They are easy-going and philosophical.

In a study of eight-and-half-year follow-up of more than five thousand people, Rosenman (1970) confirmed that Type A behaviour is strongly related to coronary heart disease incidence. The mortality from this disease was twice as high in Type A patients than in Type B patients. Their study revealed that those who exhibited competitive lifestyle were more likely to develop coronary heart disease even when biological risk factors (like smoking) were controlled. Their later work (Jenkins, Zyzanski and Rosenman, 1976) revealed that different aspects of Type A behaviour were associated with myocardial infarction, angina pretoris and silent heart attack.

A similar search for a cancer-prone personality has not been as successful. There is some evidence that those who develop cancer are unable to express positive feelings (Soloman, 1969), make an extensive use of repressive mechanism and less use of ego defenses (Bahnson, 1981). Longer survival rate among cancer patients was associated with more frequent expression of hostility and other negative feelings (Derogatis, Abeloff and Melisoratos, 1979; Pennebaker, 1990). A different personality pattern, known as Type C personality, is identified which is cancer prone. Type C people are basically nice guys who never show anger and other negative reactions in public (Scherg, 1987; Temoshok, 1987). They are helping, cooperative, smiling type, never hurting others but at the same time never expressing their true feelings. These are lonely people, even shy of seeking help when need be. Derogatis *et al.* discovered that Type C people have four times higher risk of cancer than the others.

Along similar lines, Suzanne Kobasa (1979) proposed a new personality type, called hardiness, to differentiate people who do and who do not get sick under prolonged stress. Hardiness includes three characteristics: (1) personal control – people's belief that they can influence events in their lives, (2) commitment – people's sense or purpose of involvement in events, activities and people in their lives, and (3) challenge – tendency to view changes as opportunities to growth rather than as threat to security. Hardy people are better able to deal with stressors and are less likely to fall sick. Kobasa, who studied highly stressful executives, found that those who fall sick were those who scored low on hardiness scale. However, because of the correlational nature of most of these studies, it is not yet ruled out that it is illness which could be shaping hardiness.

Cognitive and Attitudinal Factors

As stated by Lazarus (1984), people construe a stressful life event in their own idiosyncratic ways. Many studies have focused on the manner in which people appraise the severity of the events, its causal explanations and ramifications. Some people are more negative in their subjective construction of the event, view the situation as uncontrollable, and feel helpless and hopeless. Abramson, Seligman and Teasdale (1978) postulated a pessimistic explanatory style, characterized by internal (self), stable and global explanations of the negative events. In a meta analysis of 104 studies on about 15 thousand subjects, Sweeny, Anderson and Bailey (1986) found a highly stable relationship between pessimistic explanatory style and depression. In a 35-year longitudinal study, Peterson, Seligman and Valliant (1988) found that pessimistic explanatory style was not linked with poor health at the age of 25, but significantly predicted poor health above the age of 45 years. One explanation given was that at a young age people have physical resources to absorb negativity, but these get depleted as age advances.

Positive orientation or thinking about the crisis is another important cognition that has wide implications for recovery from any disease. Studies (Scheier and Carver, 1985; Scheier, Weintraub and Carver, 1986) have shown that optimism (generalized expectancy of good outcomes) is associated with problem-focused coping, seeking social support, seeing the positive side of the illness and acceptance of uncontrollable outcomes. Taylor (1983) observed that positive comparison was often used by cancer patients for self-enhancement in the event of an accident or illness. The patients who compared themselves with those who were in worse conditions recovered earlier. In a study by Agrawal, Dalal, Agrawal and Agrawal (1995) positive life orientation was found to be an important predictor of medical as well as psychological recovery of myocardial patients.

Health Impairing Behaviour

In general, behavioural factors exert their influence on health and illness status in four ways: health enhancing, health impairing, health protective and illness management. Diet, exercise and meditation are health enhancing behaviour; tobacco chewing, alcoholism will come under health impairing behaviour, which will be discussed in more detail herewith. The examples of health protective behaviour are immunization, maintaining hygiene and pollution-free environment, whereas illness management refers to taking initiatives to recover from an illness. Here, we will focus more on the behaviours which have adverse consequences for health, and may directly or indirectly become causative factors in the onset of a disease.

Much of the western literature in dealing with health impairing behaviour has focused on smoking, obesity and to a lesser extent on alcoholism. What people eat and how much they weigh are considered behavioural processes which in concert with genetic and metabolic characteristics implicate health of a person (Baum and Posluszny, 1999). An unhealthy diet appears to directly enhance risk of a disease, as low level of nutrition may contribute to pathophysiology of disease, as tobacco chewing, smoking, drug use and alcohol consumption may have direct effects on bodily systems and impair their efficiency

Consumption of tobacco in different forms is pervasive all over the world. Once tobacco use becomes a habit, it is highly resistant to change. The primary active ingredient in tobacco is nicotine, which has stimulant properties that increases SNS arousal, alertness and reduces appetite. Smoking and other forms of tobacco use are major contributors to heart diseases, hypertension, stroke, cancer and other diseases. In fact, the effect of tobacco use underlies a broad negative effect on health (e.g., Lykkesfeldt, Loft, Nielsen and Poulsen, 1997). Passive exposure to tobacco smoke is also problematic and has similar effects as that of smoking.

Alcoholism, drugs and other narcotics are no lesser evils which are much more rampant than smoking. However, there is much more concern in media and research about smoking behaviour. In the case of alcoholism, it is suggested in many studies that it is not alcohol consumption per se, which affects health but the pattern of drinking behaviour, rather its abuse. Moderate level of drinking is considered to be good for health in many western studies (*Times of India*, December 4, 2003).

Health and Well-being

The contemporary discourse on health is shifting towards positive health and well-being, moving away from sickness and treatment. The WHO's definition of health, emphasizing physical, mental and social well-being, has also contributed to this shift in the understanding of the notion of health. Health, thus, connotes an efficient functioning of the body and the mind, as well as, a capacity to participate in social activities and being able to discriminate and abide by the moral principles. It takes a holistic perspective in which nutritional status, immunity from diseases, better quality of social and family life, peace and contentment are important. Thus, good health is taken as synonymous to general well-being of a person. The concern is not with curing, i.e., treating and preventing organic malfunctioning, but with healing the person, i.e., regenerating a sense of well-being and fitness to meet life challenges.

The concept of well-being is conceived in the ayurvedic system, which defines health in terms of balance and harmony of the body, the mind, and the soul. These three are believed to be closely interrelated and the problem with anyone can affect the health status of a person. The ayurvedic system lays emphasis on the cultivation of certain positive attitudes, personality characteristics, intellectual and moral standards, freedom from anxieties and inner conflicts, and truthfulness – all considered as essential conditions for maintaining good health. According to ayurveda, only a healthy, happy and well-adjusted person can attain the state of well-being (Swoboda, 1993).

Studies on well-being have focused both on the mental and situational attributes, and have, consequently, looked into both individual and cultural aspects of well-being (Sharma, 1999). In fact, greater interest in well-being than in physical health has established the salience of social science research in contributing to improving general well-being of a person. It has highlighted psychological dimensions, i.e., attitudes, beliefs, values and expectations for a better understanding of health and well-being.

Health Scenario in India

Health policies, programmes and practices mirror the culture, society and political scenario and India is a good case in this regard. As mentioned earlier, ayurveda remained the basis of daily living and treatment of diseases for ages. After the arrival of Britishers, western medicine started dominating the scene and became the official health care practice of the country. After the independence, there was a rapid expansion of health care infrastructure and medical colleges. India has largest health care network in the world with 22 thousand primary health centres, 131 thousand sub-centres, 1,932 community health centres, and 1,500 tehsil level and 460 district level hospitals. The development was remarkable in the sense that India achieved the target of infrastructure development in nineties, almost a decade ahead of time (Chatterjee, 1993). All these developments have brought down the infant mortality rate to 85 and enhanced the life expectancy from 32 years in 1947 to 61 years by 2001.

In 1982, when the Government of India reformulated National Health Policy and officially adopted the WHO declaration of "Health for All by 2000", it made many significant changes at the policy level (Chatterjee, 1993). It brought forth the role of community and social sciences in promoting public health care. An apex committee of ICSSR and ICMR was formed to bring changes in the curriculum of medical education and to bring in more input from social science research. Many of the changes in 1982 health policy and that in Alma Ata declaration were already enunciated in the Bhore Committee Report way back in 1947. In between, the policy diverted towards high technology medicine, urban hospitals and colleges and disease-based planning. The New Health Policy was supposed to be a corrective devise to mould it in the direction of community-based services. NGOs were expected to play a major role in this endeavour (Mukhopadhyay, 1993).

Accordingly, rural health infrastructure development became a major activity in 1980s and a massive expansion of Public Health Centres (PHCs) took place with emphasis on maternal and child care, family welfare and hygiene education. Each PHC was targeted to have one doctor and one community health officer (medical doctor, of course). This expansion was so rapid that the targets of developing infrastructure by 2000 were met in 1991 itself. In terms of manpower planning, a remarkable achievement was the training of four lakh community health workers (CHW) within five years (1977-1982), almost one for each village in the country, constituting the largest health care cadre in the world (Chatterjee, 1993).

These CHWs were trained by the medical doctors to take care of common diseases and as a link between the community and medical staff. This rapid expansion did compromise in quality in many ways. Nobody knew what kind of training these CHWs should be imparted and very soon these workers began to perceive themselves as village medical practitioners. Later on, the Indian Medical Association opposed this scheme and termed these CHWs as quacks, who were indeed more popular than the medical doctors in many places. In 1981, when the Government of India transferred this scheme to the states, many states who did not commit to this scheme initially started backing out. Lack of availability of state fund made this scheme almost defunct, with CHWs demanding stipend for their work and often resorting to mass protest. These workers were rechristened as Multipurpose Health Workers, and later, as health guides. The most ambitious scheme of the government lost its direction and relevance in the present time.

In 1990s, a major shift in the policy took place in which the management of health was turned over to local self-government – *panchayati raj*. Initially, there was a lot of enthusiasm and hope that it will make health services more accountable to local communities. But, like many other schemes, it also got mired in many controversies and rarely showed the desired results. Panchayats in India are often not true representative of the people but are dominated by the power elite and power brokers, who only cater to their vested interests. In the feudal system, which still prevails in rural India, decentralization and bottom-up approach rarely succeed. It is anachronistic to the prevailing ethos and functioning of the government.

In 2001, the government announced a new health policy with the main objective of achieving an acceptable standard of good health of the general population. The policy aimed to strengthen the infrastructure, decentralize health care delivery through panchayati raj, setting up national accounting services and to regulate private practice. These were all laudable goals, as no proper mechanism was worked out to implement the provisions of this policy. In fact, this new policy was a kind of running down already depleted primary health centres. The new policy ignored earlier health policy's objectives of providing primary health care for all, specially to the underprivileged (Qadeer, 2001). The commitment of earlier policy to create a well-workedout referral system was dumped to make way for privatization and commercialization of health services. The government opened up the health sector for the private enterprises in a hope that with better monitoring and regulations the private sector will ease resource crunch in health sector.

This rampant privatization in the past two decades has indeed resulted in a total collapse of public health services. As a result, whereas in 1973, there were only 28.8 percent private hospital beds in comparison to 71.2 percent government hospital beds, by 1996, private hospitals accounted for 61 percent of the beds. Even, in the 39 percent government hospital beds, the quality of services is simply pathetic. These services have primarily catered to urban middle class, though now private sector is making inroads in rural sector as well (Baru, 2003). In a country where 35 percent of the population is below poverty line, a vast majority has nowhere to go for treatment. In sum, where Kerala has shown the way to successfully provide universal health care, the BIMARU states have witnessed a total collapse.

References

Abramson, L.Y., Seligman, M.E.P. and Teasdale, J. (1978). Learned helplessness in humans: Critique and reformulation. *Journal of Abnormal Psychology, 87*, 49-74.

Agrawal, M., Dalal, A.K., Agrawal, R.K. and Agrawal, D.K. (1994). Positive life orientation and psychological recovery of myocardial infarction patients. *Social Science and Medicine, 38*, 125-130.

Bahnson, C.B. (1981). Stress and cancer: The state of the art. *Psychometrics, 22*, 207-220.

Baker, P.T. (1984). Migrants, genetics and the degenerative disease of South Pacific islanders. In A.J. Boyce (Ed.), *Migration and Mobility: Biological Aspects of Human Movement*. Symposia of the Society for the Study of Human Biology, Vol. 23. London: Taylor and Francis.

— (1990). Modernisation and biological responses. In G.A. Harrison, J.M. Tanner, D.R. Pilbeam and P.T. Baker (Eds.), *Human Biology: An Introduction to Human Evolution, Variation, Growth and Adaptability*. Oxford: Oxford University Press.

Bang, R.A., Bang, A.T., Batule, M., Choudhury, Y., Sarmukaddam, S. and Tale, O. (1989). High prevalence of gynaecological diseases in Indian rural women. *Lancet, 8*, 85-88.

Bapat, M. and Agarwal, I. (2003). Our needs, our priorities; women and men from the slums of Mumbai and Pune talk about their needs for water and sanitation. *Environment and Urbanization, 15*, 71-86.

Barlow, S. and Sullivan, F.M. (1982). *Reproductive Hazards of Industrial Chemicals*. London: Academic Press.

Bartelett S. (2003). Water, sanitation, and urban children: the need to go beyond "improved" provision. *Environment and Urbanisation, 15*, 57-70.

Baru, R. (2003). Privatization of health services. *Economic and Political Weekly, 38(42)*, 4433-4437.

Becker, M.H. and Maiman, L.A. (1975). Sociobehavioural determinants of compliance with health and medical care recommendations. *Medical Care, 13*, 10-24.

Braungart, M. Engelfried, J. Hansen, Katja and Rosenthal J. (1992). *Impact of Lead and Agrochemicals on Children*. Hamburg: Environmental Encouragement Protection Agency.

Bukenya, G.B. and Nwokolo, N. (1991). Compound hygiene, presence of standpipe and the risk of childhood diarrhoea in an urban settlement of Papua New Guinea. *International Journal of Epidemiology, 12*, 122-131.

Chambers, R. (1989). Editorial introduction: vulnerability, coping and policy. How the poor cope. *IDS Bulletin, 20*, 1-7.

Chatterjee, M. (1993). Health for too many: India's experiments with truth. In Rohde, J., Chatterjee, M. and Morley, D. (Eds.), *Reaching Health for All*. New Delhi: Oxford University Press.

Cohen F. and Lazarus, R.S. (1979). Coping with the stresses of illness. In G.C. Stone, F. Cohen and N.E. Adler (Eds.), *Health Psychology: A Handbook*. San Francisco: Jossey-Bass.

Commission for Macroeconomics and Health (2000). *Changing the Current Health System: Current Issues, Future Directions* (www.icrier.res.in/pdf/RajivMishra.3.pdf).

Cosminski, S. and Scirmshaw, M. (1980). Medical pluralism on a Guatemalan plantation. *Social Science and Medicine, 14*, 267-278.

Crewe, E. (1995). Indoor air pollution, household health and appropriate technology; women and indoor environment in Srilanka. In B. Bradford and M.A. Gwynne (Eds.), *Down to Earth: Community Perspectives on Health, Development and Environment*. West Hartford: Kumarian Press.

Crosby, A.W. Jr. (1972). *The Columbian Exchange: Biological and Cultural Consequences of 1492*. Westport, Connecticut: Greenwood Press.

Dalal, A.K. (2000). Living with a chronic disease: Healing and psychological adjustment in Indian society. *Psychology and Developing Societies, 12*, 67-81.

— (2001). Health psychology. In J. Pandey (Ed.), *Psychology in India Revisited.* New Delhi: Sage.

Derogatis, L.R., Abeloff, M. and Melisaratos, N. (1979). Psychological coping mechanisms and survival time in metastatic breast cancer. *Journal of American Medical Association, 242*, 1504-1508.

Fifty-Fifth World Health Assembly (2002). *Ministerial Round Table: Risks to Health.* WHO document A55/DIV/5. Geneva: World Health Organization.

Gajdusek, D.C. (1977). Unconventional viruses and the origin and disappearance of Kuru. *Science, 197*, 943-960.

Glass, D.C. (1976). *Behaviour Patterns, Stress and Coronary Disease.* Hillsdale, NJ: Earlbaum.

Greenwood, A. (1987). A perspective study of pregnancy in a rural area of the Gambia, West Africa. *Bulletin of World Health Organization, 65*, 635-644.

Gupta, M. (2003). Government faces flak over meager health outlay. Calcutta: *The Telegraph*, 11th June.

Janis, I.L. (1958). *Psychological Stress.* New York: Wiley.

Jenkins, C.D. (1978). Behavioral risk factors in coronary artery disease. *Annual Review of Medicine, 29*, 543-562.

Jenkins, C.D., Zyzanski, S.J. and Rosenman, R.H. (1976). Risk of new myocardial infarction in middle-aged men with manifest coronary heart disease. *Circulation, 53*, 342-347.

Jordan, S. and Wagner, F. (1993). Meeting women's need and priorities for water and sanitation in cities. *Environment and Urbanization, 5*, 135-145.

Kakar, S. (1982). *Shamans, Mystics and Doctors.* New Delhi: Oxford University Press.

Kalter, H. and Warkary, J. (1983). Congenital malformations. *New England Medical Journal*, Vol. 308 (cited Satterthwaite *et al.* 1995).

Kasl, S.V. and Cobb, S. (1966). Health behaviour, illness behaviour and sick role behaviour. *Arch. Environmental Health, 12*, 246-66, 531-41.

Kleinman, A. (1978). Concepts and a model for the comparison of medical systems as cultural systems. *Social Science and Medicine, 12*, 85-93.

— (1980). *Patients and Healers in the Context of Culture.* Berkeley: University of California Press.

Kobasa, S.C. (1979). Stressful life events, personality, and health: An inquiry into hardiness. *Journal of Personality and Social Psychology, 37*, 1-11.

Kouray, M. and Vasquez, M.A. (1979). Housing and certain socio-environmental factors and prevalence of enteropathogenic bacteria among infants with diarrhoeal disease in Panama. *American Journal of Tropical Medicine and Hygiene, 18*, 936-941.

Kumar, S. (2003). News round up: Health care is among the most corrupt services in India. *British Medical Journal, 326*, 10.

Lazarus, R.S. (1984). On the primacy of cognition. *American Psychologist, 39*, 124-129.

Lee-Smith, D. and Trujillo, C.H. (1992). The struggle to legitimize subsistence: women and sustainable development. *Environment and Urbanization*, 4, 77-88.

Levine, R.V., Miyake, K. and Lee M. (1962). *Autobiography of a Mexican Family*. Penguin Books in association with Secker and Warburg (cited in Solvig Ekbald, 1993).

Mbizvo, M.T., Machekano, R. and McFarland, W. (1996). HIV seroincidence and correlates of seroconversion in a cohort of male factory workers in Harare, Zimbabwe. *AIDS, 10*, 895-901.

McNeill, W.H. (1979). Historical patterns of migration. *Current Anthropology, 20*, 95-102.

Merrick, T.W. (1983). *Access to Piped Water and Early Childhood Mortality in Urban Brazil, 1970-1976*. Working Paper No. 594. Washington D.C.: World Bank.

Moser, C.O.N. (1987). Women, human settlements and housing: A conceptual framework for analysis and policy-making. In C.O.N. Moser and Linda Peake (Eds.), *Women, Housing and Human Settlements*. London: Tavistock Publications.

Moser, C.O.N. (1993). *Gender Planning and Development: Theory, Practice and Training*. Routledge: London.

Mukhopadyyay, A. (1993). *State of India's Health*. New Delhi: Voluntary Health Association of India.

Needleman, H.L., Schell, A., Bellinger, D., Leviton, A. and Elizabeth, N.A. (1991). The long-term effects of exposure to low doses on lead in childhood: An eleven year follow-up report. *The England Journal of Medicine, 322*, 83-88.

Obrist, B., Tanner, M. and Harpham, T. (2003). Engaging anthropology in urban health research issues and prospects. *Anthropology and Medicine, 10*, 361-371.

Parson, T. (1951). *The Social System*. Glencoe: Free Press.

— (1957). The sick role and the role of physician reconsidered. *Health and Society, 53*, 257-78.

Peterson, C., Seligman, M.E.P. and Vaillant, G.E. (1988). Pessimistic explanatory style in a risk factor for physical illness: A thirty-five year longitudinal study. *Journal of Personality and Social Psychology, 55*, 23-27.

Pachuri, S. (1998). Unmet reproductive and sexual health needs in South Asia. *The Journal of Family Welfare, 1*, 29-39.

Pandey, M.R., Basnayat, B. and Neupane, R.P. (1989). Indoor air pollution in developing countries and acute respiratory infection. *The Lancet, 1*, 427-429.

Patel, S. (1990). Street children, hotel boys and children of pavement dwellers and construction workers in Bombay: How they meet their daily needs. *Environment and Urbanization*, 2, 9-26.

Planning Commission of India (2001). *Approach Paper to the Tenth Five-Year Plan (2002-2007).* New Delhi: Government of India. (www.planningcommission.nic.in).

Pennebaker, J.W. (1990). Opening up: Healing powers of confiding in others. New York: Morrow.

Price, T.G. (1984). Preliminary reports on maternal deaths in the southern highlands of Tanzania in 1984. *Journal of Obstetric Gynaecology of East and Central Africa, 3*, 103-110.

Qadeer, I. (2001). Debt payment and devaluating elements of public health. *Economic and Political Weekly, 37(1)*, 12-16.

Radley, A. (1994). *Making Sense of an Illness*. London: Sage.

Ray, O. (2004). How the mind hurts and heals the body. *American Psychologist, 59*, 29-40.

Ray, S. (2001). Living condition and health of two social groups inhabiting a squatter settlement in Calcutta, India. *Journal of Social Sciences*, *5*, 273-278.

Rice, A.L., Sacco, L., Hyder, A. and Black, R.E. (2000). Malnutrition as an underlying cause of childhood deaths associated with infectious diseases in developing countries. *Bulletin of World Health Organization, 78*, 1207-1221.

Rosenstock, I.M. (1966). Why people use health services. *Milbank Memorial Fund Quarterly, 44*, 94-124.

— (1974). The health belief model and preventive health behaviour. *Health Education Monographs, 2*, 354-386.

Rossi-Espagnet, A., Goldstein, G.B. and Tabibzadeh, I. (1991). Urbanization and health in developing countries: A challenge for health for all. *World Health Statistical Quarterly*, *44*, 186-244.

Rosenman, R.H. (1978). The role of the Type A behaviour pattern in ischamic heart disease: Modification of its effects by beta-blocking agents. *British Journal of Clinical Practice, 32* (suppl. 1), 58-65.

Sapir, D. (1990). *Infectious Disease Epidemics and Urbanization: A Critical Review of the Issues*. Paper prepared for the WHO Commission on Health and Environment, Division of Environmental Health, Geneva: World Health Organization.

Satterthwaite, D. (1993). The impact on health of urban environments. *Environment and Urbanization, 5*, 87-111.

Satterthwaite, D., Hart, R. Levy, C., Mitlin, D., Ross, D. Smit, J. and Stephen, C. (1995). *An Environment for Children: Understanding and Acting on the Environmental Hazards that Threaten Infants and Children and their Parents.* Draft Manuscript. London: International Institute of Environment and Development.

Scheier, M.F. and Carver, C.S. (1985). Optimism, coping and health: Assessment and implications of generalized outcome expectancies. *Health Psychology, 4*, 219-247.

Scheier, M.F., Weintraub, J.K. and Carver, C.S. (1986). Divergent strategies of optimists and pessimists. *Journal of Personality and Social Psychology, 51*, 1257-1264.

Scherg, H. (1987). Psychosocial factors and disease bias in breast cancer patients. *Psychosomatic Medicine, 49*, 302-312.

Shaper, A.G., Leonard, P.J., Jones, K.W. and Jones, M. (1969). Environmental effects on the body fluid, blood pressure and blood chemistry of nomadic warriors serving in the army in Kenya. *East African Medical Journal, 46*, 282-189.

Sharma, S. (1999). Social support, stress and psychological well-being. In G. Misra (E.), *Psychological Perspectives on Stress and Health*. New Delhi: Concept.

Songsore, J. and McGranahan, G. (1993). Environment, wealth and health; towards an analysis of intra-urban differentials within Greater Accra Metropolitan Area, Ghana. *Environment and Urbanization, 5*, 10-24.

Stephens, C. and Harpham, T. (1992). *The Measurement of Health in Household Environmental Studies in Urban Areas of Developing Countries: Factors to be Considered in the Design of Surveys*. London: Urban Health Programme, London School of Hygiene and Tropical Medicine.

Sundari, T.K. (1992). The untold story: How the health care systems in developing countries contribute to maternal mortality. *International Journal of Health Services, 22*, 513-528.

Surjadi, C. (1993). Respiratory diseases of mothers and children and environmental factors among households in Jakarta. *Environment and Urbanization, 5*, 78-86.

Swoboda, R.E. (1993). *Ayurveda: Life, Health and Longevity*. New Delhi Penguin Books.

Taylor, S.E. (1983). Adjustment to threatening events. *American Psychologist, 38*, 1161-1173.

Temoshok, L. (1987). Personality, coping style, emotions and cancer: Towards an integrative model. *Cancer Surveys, 6*, 545-567.

Thaddeus, S. and Amine, D. (1994). Too far to walk: Maternal mortality in context. *Social Science and Medicine, 38*, 1091-1110.

Uchino, B. N., Uno, D. and Holt-Lunstad, J.(1999). Social support, physiological processes, and health. *Current Directions in Psychological Science, 8*, 145-148.

UNEP and WHO (1990). *Children and the Environment*. Geneva: The United Nations Environment Programme and United Nations Children's Fund.

UNICEF (1986). *Children in Especially Difficult Circumstances.* Document based on the Executive Board Resolutions E/ICEF/1986/CRP 33 and 37. New York: UNICEF, Environment Section, Programme Division.

— (1991). *The State of World's Children*. Oxford: Oxford University Press.

— (1992). *Environment Development and Child.* New York: UNICEF, Environment Section, Programme Division.

Victoria, C.G., Smith P.G. and Vaughan, J.P. (1988). Water supply, sanitation and housing in relation to the risk of infant mortality from diarrhoea. *International Journal of Epidemiology, 17*, 651-654.

Ward, R.H. (1983). Genetic and sociocutural components of high blood pressure. *American Journal of Physical Anthropology, 62*, 91-105.

Weiss, K.M., Ferrell, R.E. and Hanis, C.L. (1984). A new world syndrome of metabolic diseases with a genetic and evolutionary basis. *Year Book of Physical Anthropology, 27*, 153-178.

WHO/UNICEF Joint Monitoring Programme for Water Supply and Sanitation (2000). *Global Water Supply and Sanitation Assessment, 2000 Report*. Geneva: World Health Organizations.

Wierzba, T., El-Yazeed, R., Savarino, S.J. and Mourad, A.S. *et al.* (2001). The interrelationship of malnutrition and diarrhoea in a peri-urban area outside Alexandria, Egypt. *Journal of Pediatrics, Gastroenterology and Nutrition, 32*, 189-196 (cited in Bartlett, 2003).

World Bank (2001). *India-Raising the Sights: Better Health Systems for India's Poor*. (Cited in www.icrier.res.in/pdf/RajivMishra.3.pdf).

World Health Organization (1992). *Our Planet, Our Health*. Geneva: Report of the Commission on Health and Environment.

— (1991). *Maternal Mortality: A Global Fact Book*. Division of Family Health. Geneva: World Health Organization.

— (2002). *Gender and Women's Health*. The Department Gender and Women's Health. Geneva: World Health Organization. (http://www.who.int/entity/gender/en).

World Health Report (1995). *Bridging the Gaps*. Geneva: World Health Organization.

— (1998). *Life in the 21st Century: A Vision for All*. Geneva: World Health Organization.

— (1999). *Making a Difference*. Geneva: World Health Organization. (Cited in Bartlett, S. 2003).

— (2000). *Health Systems: Improving Performance*. Geneva: World Health Organization.

— (2002). *Reducing Risk and Promoting Healthy Life*. Geneva: World Health Organization.

— (2003). *Shaping the Future*. Geneva: World Health Organization. (www.int/whr/2003/en/overview_en.pdf).

Zimmet, P., Taft, P. Guinea, A. Guthrie, W. and Thoma, K. (1977). The high prevalence of diabetes mellitus on a central Pacific island. *Diabetologia, 13*, 111-115.

Zinserr, H. (1935). *Rats, Lice and History: Being a Study in Biography, Which, After Twelve Preliminary Chapters Indispensable for the Preparation of the Lay Reader, Deals with the Life History of Typhus Fever*. Boston: Little Brown.

I

Health, Illness and Well-being

2

A Critical Review of Well-being Measures

A. SHARMA, N.R. SHARMA AND A. YADAVA

Nature of Well-being

Across time and cultures, people have been concerned with understanding 'happiness'. However, it is just a few decades ago that the behavioural scientists have started serious attempts in the direction of understanding and measuring happiness scientifically. And, any phenomenon can best be measured only when it is clearly and operationally defined. Currently, the behavioural scientists have re-labelled the concept of happiness under new rubrics such as subjective well-being, morale, positive affect, and life satisfaction. Literature suggests that various definitions of well-being can be clubbed into three major orientations as under:

First, well-being has been thought of as a virtue or holiness. In normative definitions happiness is described by possessing some desirable quality – a normative standard against which one's life can be judged. Here, no importance is given to the person's subjective judgement of his/her happiness. Rather, what is more important is the value framework of the observer who is looking for something desirable in the person concerned.

Secondly, researchers have been focusing on what leads one to evaluate his/her life in positive terms. This definition of well-being has simply been labelled as 'life satisfaction' and gives due importance to the subjective perceptions of the respondents about the standards that determine a good life. Interestingly, when a person's subjective assessment is the criterion of his state of happiness, then it clearly falls within the realm of subjective well-being.

Thirdly, happiness seems to be the closest to the present-day discourse: a preponderance of positive affect over negative affects (Bradburn, 1969) and mainly refers to the pleasant emotional experiences. It emphasizes that the person is experiencing mostly pleasant emotions and, if not currently, he/she is disposed to such emotions.

The above discussion clearly suggests that the field of well-being has three hallmarks (Diener, 1984). First, it is *subjective* because it heavily depends on one's personal experiences than on objective conditions/factors. For example, being healthy or wealthy is not a guarantee of happiness. Similarly, being poor is not an indication of unhappiness and misery. That is why, various objective conditions like health, wealth, virtue, etc., are not given much importance in the assessment of well-being. No doubt, they might influence subjective well-being but they are not an inherent and integral part of it. Secondly, well-being demands *positive measures*. It does not merely mean the absence of negative emotions but the presence of positive ones also. So, we cannot judge well-being by solely measuring anxiety, depression, stress, etc. We inevitably have to look for positive affect in the study of well-being. A final hallmark of well-being is that the field focuses on *long-term states*, not just momentary moods. Although each new event has its unique effect on one's mood, the well-being researcher is most interested in the person's moods over time. Well-being researchers generally focus on relatively enduring feelings of well-being, not just fleeting emotions (Diener, Suh and Oishi, 1997).

These hallmarks help explain the nature of the area of well-being. Well-being is not a unidimensional or unitary construct, and scholars in this area generally advocate examining different types of indicators. Well-being research gives due importance to the individuals' subjective experiences of their lives. The field is built on the presumption that to understand the individuals' experiential quality of well-being, it is appropriate to directly examine how a person feels about life in the context of his or her own standards. The underlying assumption is that well-being can be defined by people's conscious experiences – in terms of hedonic feelings or cognitive satisfactions. Some important definitions of well-being are as follows:

- Veenhoven (1984) defines subjective well-being as the degree to which an individual judges the overall quality of his or her life as a whole in a favourable way. In other words, subjective well-being is how well the person likes the life he or she leads.
- Verma and Verma (1989) have defined general well-being as "the subjective feeling of contentment, happiness, satisfaction with life's experiences and of one's role in the world of work, sense of achievement, utility, belongingness, and no distress, dissatisfaction or worry, etc."
- Myers and Diener (1995) define subjective well-being as "the relative presence of positive affect, absence of negative affect and satisfaction with life".
- Vandewater, Ostrove and Stewart (1997) used the term 'well-being' in an inclusive sense, intending to invoke all of the positive aspects of mental health and functioning appropriate to a particular life period.
- Shmotkin and Lomranz (1998) state: "Subjective well-being refers to the overall evaluation of one's quality of life on a positive-negative continuum and is more intuitively conceived as happiness or satisfaction. Reflecting the individual's essential outlook on life, it provides a positively termed, albeit crude, indicator of adjustment and mental health."
- And, in very simple words, Corsini (1999), in his dictionary of psychology, defines well-being as a subjective state of being well that includes happiness, self-esteem and life satisfaction.

On the basis of the above definitions, it can be safely concluded that well-being is clearly a multidimensional construct and proposes tripartite structure of well-being – positive affect, negative affect and life satisfaction. The first two components refer to the emotional aspects of this construct and the third is a cognitive-judgmental aspect. These can further be sub-divided into various components.

The following table presents the major divisions and sub-divisions of the field:

Table 1
Components of Well-being

Pleaseant Affect	*Unpleasant Affect*	*Life Satisfaction*	*Domain Satisfaction*
Joy	Guilt and shame	Desire to change life	Work
Elation	Sadness	Satisfaction with current life	Family
Contentment	Anxiety and worry		Leisure
Pride	Anger	Satisfaction with past	Health
Affection	Stress	Satisfaction with future	Finances
Happiness	Depression	Significant other's views of one's life	Self
Ecstasy	Envy		One's group

However, Sinha (1990) compared the concept of psychosocial well-being from the western and Indian perspectives. In the conceptualization of well-being, he gave due importance to the Indian scriptures that elaborate the role adjustment, health, adaptation, homeostasis, competence and quality of life play in the determination of well-being. Although western psychologists have been studying some of these variables in their cultural settings, yet a lot of empirical work is to be done by Indian psychologists giving due consideration to the basic cultural differences in the conceptualization of well-being (Kapur, 2001; Sinha, 1990)

Verma and Verma (1989) further stressed that these things (contentment, happiness, life satisfaction, etc.) are difficult to evaluate objectively, hence the emphasis is on the term 'subjective well-being'. Despite the impression that 'subjective' connotes lesser scientific credibility, well-being measures possess adequate validity (Diener and Suh, 1997). In fact, some theorists believe that well-being is determined largely by psychosocial states of individuals. For example, Markides and Martin (1979) have suggested that subjective assessments of various psychological states are more important determinants of well-being than objective assessments. For example, George and Landerman (1982) have argued that self-perceived health measures provide better estimates of global well-being than objective measures (e. g., physician's ratings). Larsen concluded that purely objective measures "are not necessarily the most accurate estimates of the extent to which a person's condition is painful and debilitating". So, the research concerns subjective well-being, for which the final judge is whoever lives inside a person's skin. For all these reasons, researchers take seriously people's reports of their subjective happiness, especially when supported by converging reports from informants and by observations of accompanying dysfunction (or social competence).

Measurement of Well-being

Use and Importance of Self-reports

Researchers have created a number of measures of well-being. The usual method of measuring one's well-being is through self-report surveys in which the respondent himself judges and reports his life satisfaction, and the frequency of his pleasant/unpleasant emotions. Self-reports of global well-being are popular because these have shown temporal stability in the 0.5 to 0.7 range over periods from six months to six years (Diener, 1994). Secondly, people's self-reported well-being converges with other measures (Sandvik, Diener and Seidlitz, 1993). Those who describe themselves as happy and satisfied with life seem happy to their friends and to their family members. Third, subjective well-being measures exhibit construct validity. They are responsive to recent good and bad events and to therapy and they correlate inversely with feeling ill (Sandvik *et al.*, 1993).

Single-item Measures

Usually, the researchers use simple one-time self-reports, which may consist of single-item or multiple-item scales. Several of the most frequently used measures during recent past are single-item survey questions. There is an exhaustive list of such measures but here is a brief description of some single-item scales:

(1) *The D-T Scale (Andrews and Whitney, 1976)*: This scale, also referred to as 'Life-as-a-whole Index', is a 7-point Delighted-Terrible (D-T) scale. This index is obtained by asking twice the subjects, "How do you feel about your life as a whole?" and averaging the responses. The response options are:
 (a) Terrible
 (b) Unhappy
 (c) Mostly dissatisfied
 (d) Mixed (about equally satisfied and dissatisfied)
 (e) Mostly satisfied
 (f) Pleased
 (g) Delighted

 Interesting to note here is that Headey, Holmstrom and Wearing (1984) write that unsurprisingly this index loads on the well-being factor and not on the ill-being factor despite having both 'positive' and 'negative' ends. This is because most people tend to reply towards the positive end. Although they might be having feelings of dissatisfaction also, yet they exhibit mainly feelings of satisfaction or what is thought of as desired as per current social norms.

(2) *Self-anchoring Ladder (Cantril, 1965)*: As the name suggests, this measure consists of a picture of nine-step ladder, the top of which is anchored with "the best possible life for you", and the bottom with "the worst possible life for you". The middle anchors are not provided. The subjects are asked to reply, "Where on the ladder do you stand at the present time?" Horley and Lavery (1991) report that when pointed towards 'present life quality' the self-anchoring ladder is a psychometrically sound instrument since it is stable and sensitive to changing circumstances.

(3) *Fordyce 1 (Fordyce, 1978)*: This measure of well-being asks, "In general, how happy or unhappy do you usually feel?" There are eleven-response alternatives – each anchored with different mood adjectives. For example, the top-most alternative taps whether the respondent usually feels "extremely happy, ecstatic, joyous and fantastic".

(4) *Fordyce 2 (Fordyce, 1978)*: This second measure deals with the 'percent happiness'. The respondents are asked to indicate, "What percent of the time do you feel happy, what percent of the time do you feel unhappy, and what percent of the time do you feel neutral?" The subjects have to report these percentages such that these add up to 100 percent.

(5) *Happiness Scale (Gurin, Veroff and Feld, 1960)*: This single-item scale asks, "Taking all things together, how would you say things are these days?" The respondents are provided with three-response alternatives: very happy, pretty happy, and not too happy.

Despite the obvious advantage of brevity, these and other single-item scales have been criticized on various grounds. For example, we are unable to average out the variance due to the specific wording of that single item. Also, we cannot obtain the estimates of internal consistency. The scores mostly are skewed towards positive side. But, the most serious drawback of these single-item scales is that they cannot tap separately various dimensions of this multi-dimensional construct.

Multi-item Measures

Recent measures of subjective well-being, however, contain multiple items. Some commonly used measures are:

(1) *Affect-Balance Scale (Bradburn and Caplovitz, 1965)*: This has been regarded as the first true well-being inventory. Bradburn (1969) postulated that well-being is a quality of experience (and not of the behaviours) which originates from the relative predominance of good and bad feelings or positive and negative affect (PA and NA). This strongly emphasized that well-being is a *subjective* experience. The ten items of the Affect-Balance Scale ask the respondents to indicate which of the five positive feelings and which of the five negative feelings took place during recent few weeks. Separate positive affect score (PAS) and negative affect score (NAS) are calculated. The directional difference (PAS minus NAS) serves as affect balance or the overall well-being score. The scores can range from –5 (through 0) to +5.

(2) *Satisfaction with Life Scale (Diener, Emmons, Larsen and Griffin, 1985)*: This scale contains five items requiring a general and cognitive evaluation of the respondent's life as a whole on a 7-point scale ranging from strongly disagree to strongly agree. So, the total score may range from 5 to 35. Scores on SWLS can be interpreted in terms of absolute as well as relative life satisfaction. A score of 20 represents the neutral point on the scale – the point at which the respondent is about equally satisfied and dissatisfied. Following is the scores' description:

Score	*Description*
5-9	Extremely dissatisfied with life
10-14	Dissatisfied
15-19	Slightly dissatisfied
20	Equally satisfied/Equally dissatisfied
21-25	Slightly satisfied
26-30	Satisfied
31-35	Extremely satisfied with life

Diener *et al.* (1985) reported that their scale had a test-retest correlation coefficient of .82 (over a two-month period) and a coefficient alpha of .87. Their factor analysis of the inter-item correlation matrix identified a single factor accounting for 66 percent of the variance. Since that time, other investigators have also shown satisfactory internal consistency and temporal reliability of the scale.

(3) *PGI General Well-being Scale (Verma and Verma, 1989)*: It is a 20-item scale to tap the general well-being of the subjects. Usually, five minutes are needed to administer and score this scale. While replying these items, they are instructed as, "How do you feel these days (past one month)? Kindly tick (T) the items applicable to you." For scoring purposes, the number of ticks are counted (scores ranging from 0 to 20) that indicate the well-being of that particular respondent at that particular time. Higher the score, the better is the well-being. Verma, Nehra, Malhotra and Sharma (2000) report that this scale is not affected

by various socio-demographic variables like age, sex, income, occupation, marital status, locality, family type, smoking habits, duration of illness, etc. Hence, they believe, this scale can be reliably utilized with different types of populations.

This scale is available both in English and Hindi languages and provides a single score on the well-being of the subjects. Although, it makes it easy to explain this single score of the respondents' general well-being but does not provide separate information about various dimensions of well-being. However, this is a good scale if the researcher is running short of time (i.e., he/she has to study a big sample in a little time) and requires a 'quick' and 'integrated' idea of one's general well-being.

(4) *Subjective Well-being Inventory (SUBI, Sell and Nagpal, 1992)*: This is a very comprehensive and robust instrument for assessing positive indicators of health. Developed by 'stepwise ethnographic exploration' process, this inventory initially consisted of 130 items that were supposed to be measuring various areas of concern possibly related to or parts of well-being and ill-being. This item pool was subjected to statistical treatment and factor analysis. The result was a 40-item version that assesses the subjective well-being of the subjects on 11 factorial dimensions. These dimensions are general well-being-positive affect, Expectation-achievement congruence, confidence in coping, transcendence, family group support, social support, primary group concern, inadequate mental mastery, perceived ill-health, deficiency in social contacts, and general well-being-negative affect. It is the strength of SUBI that this inventory has been adopted by WHO, has been standardized on adult Indian population, and covers a lot of significant dimensions of well-being. However, as the face value indicates, this inventory seems to miss the most important label, viz., 'life satisfaction' and adds a lot of new dimensions.

(5) *Psychological Well-being Questionnaire (Bhogle and Prakash, 1995)*: Finding other well-being instruments lengthy, Bhogle and Prakash (1995) attempted to develop not only a short and easy-to-administer questionnaire, but also a reliable and valid index of well-being. By following typical questionnaire

development procedures, they constructed a 28-item psychological well-being questionnaire. It measures 12 factors of well-being, viz., meaninglessness, somatic symptoms, self-esteem, positive affect, daily activities, life satisfaction, suicidal ideas, personal control, social support, tension, wellness and general efficiency. They reported that this was a very comprehensive, factorially adequate, reliable and valid tool. However, just like Sell and Nagpal's inventory, this questionnaire seems to miss 'negative effect' and added many more to the existing list. Whether the authors intend to measure negative effect by "meaninglessness, suicidal ideas and tension" is not clear. Also, they seem to be concentrating on increasing the number of factors to be covered by their questionnaire while decreasing the number of questions. It is to be ascertained whether only a few (say, two to four) items actually tap the 'well-being' which is *not* a simple and narrow construct.

On the basis of the popular conceptualization of well-being, we have covered here the most frequently used measures at national and international levels. In India, people generally do not use single-item measures because of their doubtful reliability, validity and applicability. Among the Indian, popularly used, multi-item measures, we find that they also suffer from flaws. What then is the solution? One safe approach could be using a 'battery of well-being'.

Battery of Well-being

As it is clear now, well-being is a multi-dimensional construct and different scale developers advocate examining well-being from their perspectives and dimensions. For example, Sell and Nagpal (1992) found 11 prominent dimensions of well-being, whereas Bhogle and Prakash (1995) reported 12 components measuring psychological well-being – having only a few dimensions in common. It leaves the researchers in a state of confusion over which scale is most appropriate and represents all or most of the well-being dimensions. Hence, to incorporate most of the dimensions of well-being, it becomes essential for any researcher to constitute a battery of well-being measures. Working on these guidelines, recently, in a study, Sharma (2002) constituted a battery of well-being measures by selecting SUBI (Sell and Nagpal, 1992), Satisfaction with Life Scale (Diener, Emmons, Larson and Griffin, 1985), and General Health Questionnaire-12 (Goldberg and Hillier, 1979), in an attempt to incorporate the most important dimensions of well-being as per the purpose of his study. So, the future researchers, in order to tap well-being, could use multi-item, multi-dimensional and multi-method battery. Here are a few suggestions that could be followed in the measurement of well-being (keeping in mind the research question, plan and resources).

Suggestions

(1) *Using measures other than self-reports:* The psychometric properties of various well-being scales tend to be strong. However, they provide only one approach to assess subjective well-being. Although single-occasion self-reports of subjective well-being have exhibited sufficient degree of validity, respondents' mood at the moment of responding to the scale, ordering of items and other situational factors and artifacts could influence reports of subjective well-being. Also people may respond to subjective well-being scales in socially desirable ways. If they believe that happiness is normatively appropriate, they may report that they are happier than other types of assessments may indicate. For this reason, in the future, researchers should more frequently combine other types of measures with one-time scales. Although based on self-reports, the naturalistic *experience-sampling method* (ESM) can avoid some memory and other biases that are bound to appear otherwise. In this method, respondents' subjective well-being is assessed at random moments in their everyday lives. Although it entirely depends on the purpose of the study, they are randomly signalled at many times over a period of one to four weeks. This way, studying their moods in their natural life settings gives a more refined and accurate record of their well-being.

Additional methods, such as recording of *non-verbal behaviours,* can supplement the self-reports. For this purpose, the subjects could be videotaped while they were being asked questions about their life experiences. Minute analysis of their particular gestures, postures, facial expressions and vocal tones can provide additional information about their emotional reactions.

Informant reports and *expert ratings* can be another powerful source of additional information about the subjects. Although their reports could be incomplete/biased, informant reports are valuable because these overcome the limitations of self-reports. And, these are not completely unreliable because these have been found to converge well converge with other measures of well-being. *In-depth interviews* about the respondents' lives can also provide some important information and supplement the self-reports.

Various *physiological indices* can provide important information about the mental and emotional states of the subject. So, electrophysiological measures such as electroencephalograms and electromyographic facial recordings should also be included in complete assessments of well-being.

Furthermore, Shedler, Karliner and Katz (2003) developed the *Early Memory Index* (EMI) believing that the self-report scales suffer from an inevitable problem, "they cannot distinguish genuine mental health from the facade or illusion of mental health created by psychological defenses". They labelled respondents who reported mental health but were judged distressed by clinicians as having *illusory mental health*. They also identified subjects who reported mental health and were judged healthy, and the subjects who reported distress and were also judged distressed. They classified the former as *genuinely healthy* and the latter as *manifestly distressed*. Shedler *et al.* (1993, 2003) claim that their technique can duplicate the mental health/distress judgements of expert clinicians and can discriminate between psychiatric patients and healthy controls.

(2) *Studying well-being from different dimensions:* Since well-being is a multi-dimensional construct, *multiple (separate) scores* could lead to clear understanding and explanation of various dimensions. A single-score explanation of this construct (as is provided by PGI General Well-Being Scale), therefore, should be avoided because this would hide much of the valuable information about the subject. Various dimensions of well-being can be highlighted on the following grounds: (a) *The affect-based versus cognitive-based*

well-being: As has been discussed above, major dimensions of well-being are positive affect, negative affect (affect-based well-being) and life satisfaction (cognitive-based well-being). (b) *The positive-negative distinction:* Whether positive affect and negative affect are independent dimensions or opposite poles is a continuous debate. (c) *The frequency-intensity dimension:* Research suggests that frequency of pleasant affect is crucial for well-being than the intensity of affect. (d) *Momentary versus long-term mood:* Although life events bring upward or downward changes in a person's momentary or daily affect, the individual soon returns to the person's mean level of emotional experiences which is known as long-term mood and forms the core of well-being. (e) *Discrete emotions versus global pleasantness:* Although studying long-term average levels of discrete emotions (such as joy, anger or anxiety) is certainly worthwhile, researchers should focus on studying well-being as the global or average level of pleasant and unpleasant emotions. Well-being can be assessed at either level, depending upon the requirements of the research. However, it is recommended that, since different components of well-being have been shown to have their own, different correlates, it can be more appropriate to obtain sub-global assessments wherever possible. In this way, a better understanding of underlying processes which influence well-being is likely to be attained. Researchers should be aware that there exist several measures that tap '*global*' well-being as well as several measures that tap the more '*specific*' components of well-being.

(3) *Studying positive emotions:* Furthermore, and most important, the world has given overemphasis on the negative emotions (anger, frustration, stress, and so on) but the *positive emotions* are of equal importance. So, the researchers should focus more on the positive affect and life satisfaction in the study of mental health and well-being.

Last but not the least, the researchers should be aware that they should select geriatric well-being scales (e.g., Philadelphia Geriatric Centre Morale Scale of Lawton, 1975) if they are to study older subjects. This is a 17-item scale measuring lonely dissatisfaction and attitudes towards one's aging. Since many of the items of these scales are age specific these become irrelevant and unsuitable for young and middle-aged subjects.

Conclusions

This is generally observed that we not only follow the conceptualizations of foreign researchers but also measures developed by them which can never do justice to the Indian culture, conceptualization, and population. Hence, we should develop understanding of a concept from the Indian perspective and develop measures that fulfill the psycho-socio-cultural needs of the Indian respondents, instead of blind-folded use or adoption of foreign tools to tap a phenomenon. However, the basic psychometric properties should be ascertained there in the new tools: they should exhibit high internal consistency; should show stability over time; and should be valid against other measures of the construct.

Whenever and wherever possible, the researchers should use multiple measures of well-being not only to study the well-being more accurately but also to assess most of the dimensions/components of well-being. No doubt, self-reports of well-being have adequate reliability and validity, use of additional measurements could strengthen the understanding of well-being and theory-building. Although each of the non-self-report methods has also its own shortcomings, psychologists can gain an especially strong assessment of well-being by using several methods in tandem because in this way a number of response artifacts can be eliminated. Because different methods of measuring well-being can produce different scores, a battery of diverse measures will produce the most informative composite. Although each of the alternative measures has its own limitations, the strengths of the different types of measures are often complementary to each other. Ultimately, the choice of which measures to use will depend on the format/purpose of the study and on the questions the researcher wants to answer.

References

Andrews, F.M. and Whitney, S.B. (1976). *Social Indicators of Well-being: American's Perception of Life Quality.* New York: Plenum.

Bhogle, S. and Prakash, I.J. (1995). Development of the psychological well-being (PWB) questionnaire. *Journal of Personality and Clinical Studies, 11,* 5-9.

Bradburn, N. (1969). *The Structure of Psychological Well-being.* Chicago: Aldine.

Bradburn, N. and Caplovitz, D. (1965). *Reports on Happiness.* Chicago: Aldine.

Cantril, H. (1965). *The Pattern of Human Concern.* New Brunswick, N.J.: Rutgers University Press.

Corsini, R.J. (1999). *The Dictionary of Psychology.* USA: Brunner and Mazel.

Diener, E. (1984). Subjective well-being. *Psychological Bulletin, 95,* 542-575.

— (1994). Assessing subjective well-being: Progress and opportunities. *Social Indicators Research, 31,* 103-157.

Diener, E., Emmons, R.A., Larson, R.J. and Griffin, S. (1985). The satisfaction with life scale. *Journal of Personality Assessment, 49,* 71-75.

Diener, E. and Suh, E.M. (1997). Measuring quality of life: Economic, social and subjective indicators. *Social Indicators Research, 40,* 189-216.

Diener, E., Suh, E.M., Lucas, R.E. and Smith, H.L. (1999). Subjective well-being: Three decades of progress. *Psychological Bulletin, 125,* 276-302.

Diener, E., Suh, E.M. and Oishi, S. (1997). Recent findings of subjective well-bcing. *Indian Journal of Clinical Psychology, 24,* 25-41.

Fordyce, M.W. (1978). *Prospectus: The Self-Description Inventory.* Unpublished manuscript. Edison Community College, Fort Myers, Florida.

George, L.K. and Landerman, R. (1982). *Health and Life Satisfaction: A Replicated Secondary Data Analysis, Research Synthesis of the Health-Life Satisfaction Relationship.* Symposium conducted at the annual meeting of the Gerontological Society of America, Boston.

Goldberg, D.P. and Hillier, V.F. (1979). A scaled version of the general health questionnaire. *Psychological Medicine, 9,* 139-145.

Gurin, G., Veroff, J. and Feld, S. (1960). *Americans View Their Mental Health.* New York: Basic Books.

Headey, B., Holmstrom, E. and Wearing, A. (1984). Well-being and ill-being: different dimension? *Social Indicators Research, 14,* 115-139.

Horley, J. and Lavery, J.J. (1991). The stability and sensitivity of subjective well-being measures. *Social Indicators Research, 24,* 113-122.

Kapur, M. (2001). Mental health, illness and therapy. In Janak Pandey (Ed.), *Psychology in India Revisited-Developments in the Discipline,* Vol. 2 (pp. 356-411). New Delhi: Sage Publications.

Lawton, M.P. (1975). The Philadelphia geriatric centre morale scale: A revision. *Journal of Gerontology, 30,* 85-89.

Markides, K.S. and Martin, H.W. (1979). A causal model of life satisfaction among the elderly. *Journal of Gerontology, 34,* 86-93.

Myers, D.G. and Diener, E. (1995). Who is happy? *Psychological Science, 6,* 10-19.

Sandvik, E., Diener, E. and Seidlitz, L. (1993). Subjective well-being: The convergence and stability of self-report and non-self-report measures. *Journal of Personality, 61,* 317-342.

Sell, H. and Nagpal, R. (1992). *Assessment of Subjective Well-Being: The Subjective Well-Being Inventory (SUBI),* Regional Health Paper, SEARO, No. 24. New Delhi: WHO Regional Office for South-East Asia.

Sharma, A. (2002). *Personality Correlates of Well-Being.* Unpublished Doctoral Thesis. M.D. University, Rohtak.

Shedler, J., Mayman, M. and Manis, M. (1993). The illusion of mental health. *American Psychologist, 48,* 1117-1131.

Shedler, J., Karliner, R. and Katz, E. (2003). Cloning the clinician: A method for assessing illusory mental health. *Journal of Clinical Psychology, 59,* 635-650.

Shmotkin, D. and Lomranz, J. (1998). Subjective well-being among Holocaust survivors: An examination of overlooked differences. *Journal of Personality and Social Psychology, 75,* 141-155.

Sinha, D. (1990). Concept of psycho-social well-being: Western and Indian perspective. *NIMHANS Journal, 8,* 1-11.

Vandewater, E.A., Ostrove, J.M. and Stewart, A.J. (1997). Predicting women's well-being in midlife: The importance of personality development and social role involvements. *Journal of Personality and Social Psychology, 72,* 1147-1160.

Veenhoven, R. (1984). *Data-book of Happiness.* Boston MA: Reidel.

Verma, S.K. and Verma, A. (1989). *Manual for PGI General Well-Being Measure.* Lucknow: Ankur Psychological Agency.

3

The Common Conceptualization of Mental Health: A Qualitative Investigation of Categories of Meaning

SHIKHA DIXIT

The present paper assumes that everyday meaning of mental health may significantly depart from the realist epistemological meaning that is prevalent in clinical psychology and psychiatry. This assumption follows from the trend of research that views knowledge about something as socially constructed. Studies within this trend have demonstrated that much of what we know about health and illness may not be learned through experience but may be an artifact of constructive social psychological processes (Herzlich, 1973). From this perspective, the objective clinical understanding of mental health may not provide a complete understanding of how people actually define and explain mental health in everyday life.

The fields of clinical psychology, psychiatry and psychopathology have described and defined mental health and illness in diverse manner. Historically speaking, the meaning of mental health and illness has changed from time to time. Various frameworks of meaning have been used to understand mental health (Korchin, 1986). Before the French and American revolutions, the concept of mental illness was inextricably associated with the 'madman', who was thought to be possessed of evil spirits and was treated as an outcast. The early 19th century saw the reforms instituted by Pinel and the insanes were now treated as sick people. Humane hospital treatment was advocated and asylums were established. However, the lay public still viewed the insane as sub-human and possessed. From mid-20th century onwards, the biomedical approach to mental health has been the most dominant view. This approach conceptualizes mental illness as a disease with biological causes that can be understood and treated scientifically. Later, in scientific medical history, the psychological approach emerged and psychopathology concerned itself not only with the diseases of psychological functioning but also the disorders of psychological origin. With the growth of scientific knowledge over the centuries, the medical concern in the realm of mental health has also grown.

Currently, the field of mental health and illness is understood in relation to three major orientations: (a) the biomedical, (b) the psychological, and (c) the psychosocial. These three orientations not only determine the conceptualization of mental health and psychological disorder but also the ways of understanding the meaning of mental health, the role of mental health professionals and the importance of institutional environment. The range of these three contemporary professional and scientific orientations suggests that mental health problems may be generated from diverse causal factors, ranging from the biochemical to the social.

The general scientific perspective views mental health problems as having objective mental symptoms and definite causal factors. However, in recent years, social constructionism has been adopted as an organizing framework for the fields of mental health and counselling (Daniels and White, 1994). The objective scientific orientation towards mental health may not serve the purpose when the meaning is viewed from a constructionist perspective. The meaning of mental health or mental illness may be formed in conversations among people and should be understood as being instrumental in organizing the everyday experiences of individuals and social groups. Within this perspective clinical problems are understood as inter-subjective linguistic creations formed during interactions between clients and clinicians (Guterman, 1994). The mental health practitioner, working within constructionist perspective, conceptualizes the locus of mental dysfunction in terms of socially constructed language determined systems, rather than objectively defined social systems. Social constructionists question the basis of knowledge. They view scientific facts as the product of social forces rather than an explanation of external reality. They do not believe in absolute truth. This line of thinking can be linked to Wilhelm Dilthey's work. Dilthey, in Palmer (1969), systematically studied the idea that social reality was a product of social conditions and not a mere description of the 'real' world.

In the light of the above view, the everyday conceptualization of mental health and illness may be different from an objective scientific view. These lay explanations may also shed some light on the social construction and transformation of objective knowledge into everyday knowledge. Jodelet (1991) has demonstrated that everyday assumptions about mental illness are influenced by traditions and practical knowledge and not exclusively based on ordinary scientific knowledge. According to Flick (1998), everyday knowledge is less explicit and less defined compared to scientific knowledge and is different from commonsense, as it takes into account the influence of scientific rationalization. Analyzing everyday knowledge can provide an understanding of social representations also.

In order to formulate effective ways to deal with mental distress and disorder, it is important to understand the local meanings and everyday articulations of that meaning. Socio-cultural factors, such as conceptualization of mental health and illness and community response, may be influenced by the local idiom. Research in cultural psychiatry and medical anthropology has paved the way for studies aiming to investigate the constructed meaning frameworks associated with mental health. A study by Carstairs and Kapur (1976) in south-west India is a pioneering work in the area of cultural epidemiological research, which outlines the importance of socio-cultural explanations of mental health problems and clinical patterns. Kakar (1982) has provided a brilliant insight into ancient Indian healing traditions, diverse cultural contexts in which the healers work and their unique approach to mental illness. The studies on the effect of socio-cultural context on aspects of mental health and illness provide the groundwork for the present study.

The major aim of this study is to investigate the constructed frameworks of meaning. This aim is in line with Radley's (1994) work on making sense of health and disease. Radley has investigated social psychological questions related to beliefs of people regarding health and illness, consequences of feeling ill, doctor's role, living with chronic disease, health promotion, healing relationship and a large number of other issues and questions regarding how people make sense of illness in everyday life. Levine and Moreland (1992) have also dealt with the relationship between social factors related to group processes and mental health.

According to Dalal (2001: 357), "staying healthy is contingent on lifestyle, cultural beliefs, health habits, family support, and other such factors. In this perspective, what is considered more salient is not the medical reality of a disease but the subjective experience of being ill (Klienman, 1974). From this perspective health psychology is concerned with the meaning and behaviour that structure the experience of an illness in a particular social-cultural context."

Sinha (1990, as noted by Dalal, 2001) examined the Indian conceptualization of health as depicted in ancient scriptures and found that health is described as a state of delight. Feelings of spiritual, physical and mental well-being were also found to be associated with the concept of health.

In view of the above discussion, it may be noted that the meaning and conceptualization of mental health in everyday lay understanding may be different from the current scientific orientation. The objective of the present study was to reveal the everyday conceptual frameworks associated with the meaning of mental health.

The Study

The study was descriptive and qualitative method was employed. Interpretative content analysis was used, without any reference to quantitative measures. The study was exploratory in nature and aimed at exploring the basic framework of the meaning of mental health, with an intent to analyze the content of the responses of all the participants. The basic assumption was that, the content would indicate the categories and themes employed by people to describe, explain and conceptualize the meaning of mental health. A more extensive inquiry based on the inputs of the present work may be undertaken, to validate and extend the findings of this study.

Participants

The participants were 60 under-graduate students studying in a premier institute of technology. They were first year, third year and fourth year students. The sample consisted only of engineering students. The implications of this fact for the purpose of generalization of results will be discussed in a latter section of this paper. However, a larger study based on the present conceptual framework is being planned, that will study more participants from various social groups and social contexts.

Data Collection

The method employed for data collection was in line with the descriptive orientation of the research. Such an orientation does not warrant the use of closely controlled methods of data collection. The participants were directly asked to write down their views regarding the meaning of mental health in the form of a short essay. This technique offers the participants with an opportunity to express their ideas and images regarding mental health. The assumption was that such a descriptive method would enable the participants to provide an account of the themes, categories, concepts, images, definitions and other possible elaborations of the core meaning of mental health.

Analysis

The aim of the analysis was to outline the general psychological content embedded in the essays. The analysis was purely qualitative in the tradition of the studies on health and illness, within the constructionist perspective (Herzlich, 1973). The first step was the preliminary summarizing of each essay. The first summary of each essay was used as a unit of analysis. Each summary was prepared by identifying the key concepts, ideas, images and descriptions. The summarizing was done to reduce the data and also to find themes of analysis. The first summary of the data was re-read and preliminary themes were identified. These themes were conceptualized as categories of meaning as used by the participants to understand mental health.

The summaries were further analyzed for recurrence of certain notions or themes and also for co-occurrence of two or more themes. This analysis resulted in the modified list of themes. The analysis of co-occurrence or perceived relationships provided a glimpse of the cognitive organization of themes.

In order to ensure the validity of identified themes, two judges independently conducted the same analysis of summaries. A considerable overlap was observed between the two sets of identified themes. On the basis of these two sets, a composite list of themes was prepared, which was finally used for further interpretation of results. These themes were treated as frameworks of meaning that are used by the participants to make sense of the notion of mental health in everyday life. Some of the responses reflecting the important themes and sub-themes will be quoted throughout the interpretation and discussion of results.

Results and Discussion

A summary of results is given in Table 1. This table provides a comprehensive list of themes or meaning frameworks used by the participants to conceptualize mental health.

Table 1

A Summary of Meaning Frameworks

1.	Mental health and social norms: 'Mental as Social' - Normative behaviour - Social desirability - Social responsibility
2.	Mental health and cognitive functioning - Attention, perception, memory and information processing - Intelligence - Constructive thinking
3.	Mental health and adaptation
4.	Mental health and goal attainment
5.	Philosophical notions regarding mental health
6.	Mental health and physical health
7.	Mental Illness and tension
8.	Mental illness and normative behaviour
9.	Personal characteristics of mentally ill

The results demonstrate that although the participants were instructed to write a short essay on the 'Meaning of Mental Health', they automatically involved an account of mental illness in their descriptions. This shows that the two are related in the minds of people. The core meaning of mental health is not complete without taking into account the notion of mental illness. However, the major themes of meaning were organized around the concept of mental health and not of mental illness.

The analysis clearly revealed that the major theme of mental health and social norms was closely related to social behaviour. Social behaviour was the term used for normative behaviour by some participants. The analysis of data demonstrated that the meaning of 'mental' was 'social'. As far as everyday understanding of mental health was concerned, these two notions were usually juxtaposed. An individual behaving in consonance with the norms of the social group, was perceived to be a mentally healthy individual. "Mental health of a particular individual can be defined on the basis of how that individual behaves in a social group." An individual who is engaged in "violation of social norms" was "unacceptable by the society".

Mental health, as commonly understood, is the tendency to conform to norms. The role of cultural and contextual factors was also emphasized with regard to normative behaviour. "The terms and standards used for evaluating mental health are defined by us, i.e., they may differ from one social group to another." Various social parameters, such as culture and social context, were seen as determinants of mental health. However, it was emphasized that different societies may have different meanings of mental health.

'Social desirability' was seen as one of the major indicators of mental health. A socially desirable individual was viewed as understanding social niceties and interactions, behaving according to accepted and customary rules of the society, responsible and benefiting the society. Social desirability was also understood in terms of social processes of communication and interaction. A scientist, obsessed with work and not engaging in 'social activity', was also seen as mentally unhealthy.

Another theme that was expressed as closely related to mental health was of 'social responsibility'. A socially responsible individual was seen as a mentally healthy individual. "A mentally healthy person is of course a very desirable person in the society. His thoughts and work definitely benefit the society. This is because, with pureness of thought, one will never indulge in antisocial or immoral activities, thereby becoming a desirable person. Such a person performs his duties with proper responsibility". Generally, 'social desirability', 'normative behaviour' and 'sense of individual and social responsibility' were closely interlinked.

Abnormal way of behaving was undesirable. It was the way in which "most people do not behave". Such behaviour was seen as different from general notion regarding appropriate social behaviour. The mentally healthy individual was perceived as optimistic, positive, rational, ethical, unbiased, confident, free of tension and being able to conduct everyday activities without any anxiety. Stability, calm and composed manner, mental strength, responding efficiently to the external world and a balanced state of mind were seen as indicators of mental health. Although some participants mentioned these personal characteristics of the mentally healthy, the overall emphasis was on the social characteristics and social efficiency. Behaviour in line with the social norms was the most important and consistently perceived indicator of mental health.

Cognitive functioning and mental health were seen as closely related. The ability to reason, recall, memorize, concentrate, associate, process information according to priority and think analytically were all seen as indicators of mental health. Cognitive overload, skewed perception, inefficient recall, excessive processing of a particular information and unnatural cognition were perceived as detrimental to mental health. Constructive thinking, that is beneficial to the society, was viewed as the most important cognitive function. Although normal cognitive functioning was considered as an indicator of mental health, a high intellectual ability was not seen as a necessary indicator of mental health. "Being a very intelligent person may not necessarily mean a mentally healthy person. This concept does not rely on intelligence or sharpness." An intelligent individual working against the social norms was considered as mentally unhealthy.

In addition, two major categories of meaning that emerged were related to the relationship between mental health and adaptation, and mental health and goal attainment. The ability to analyze the cases microscopically as well as macroscopically as per the requirement of the situation, and take decisions accordingly was seen as a sign of good mental health. The ability to keep pace with the ever-changing world and analyze the surroundings was described as one of the important characteristics of mentally healthy individuals. According to one subject, "one of the reasons why people tend to have a disbalanced state of mind is that in the fast moving life of today people cannot always keep pace with others. This leads to anxiety, worry, frustration, sleeplessness and other such troubles". The relationship between mental health and goal attainment was described as crucial to success. Success and attainment of goals were seen as enhancers of mental well-being. A successful person was seen as a mentally healthy individual. According to one subject, "the person who always has been successful and achieved in his life what he wanted can be a mentally healthy person because of his inner peace and contentment".

An interesting fact that emerged was that although the subjects were students of engineering, their descriptions did not include scientific notions regarding mental health. However, philosophical ideas regarding mental health were frequently expressed. Positive thinking, freedom of mind and a state of mental equilibrium were seen as important indicators of mental health. As described by one subject, "the meaning of mental health in my opinion is the harmony that a man establishes between his outer and inner worlds.... mental health is lost when someone either loses contact with his inner-self due to overburden of activities or misinterprets something".

A relationship was perceived between physical health and mental health. According to most participants, a healthy mind resides in a healthy body. Excessive physical activity, lack of sleep, headaches and bad physical health were seen as factors influencing mental health negatively. However, a healthy body was not perceived as a necessary indicator of mental health. A physically healthy individual indulging in activities not in consonance with social norms was seen as mentally unhealthy.

For most subjects a causal relationship existed between persistent tensions and mental ill-health. Mental tension was seen as the one of the most important causal factors in producing mental illness. It was also seen as one of the most common manifestations of mental illness.

In addition to the above themes of the meaning given to mental health, mental illness was seen as an opposite state of mental health. Non-normative behaviour and violations of societal rules were seen as indicators of mental illness. In this context, criminals and terrorists were thought of as mentally ill. To this extent the meaning given to mental illness was 'social'. In addition to this, a mentally ill individual was seen as lunatic, pervert, highly depressed, requiring counselling by some mentally healthy person, preoccupied with problems, worried about future, mentally not strong, more emotional than rational, negative, destructive, prone to addiction, restless, short-tempered, offensive, self-conscious, stupid, indecisive, having excessive sexual desires and fatalistic tendency. It thus appears that the locus shifted slightly from 'social' to 'individual' when people described mental illness as compared to mental health. However, the overall meaning of mental health was understood in predominantly social terms.

The most important fact that emerged was that everyday knowledge about mental health is socially constructed and that lay explanations do not include biomedical and psychological orientations. The everyday meaning of mental health was based on the premise that behaviour can only be judged in terms of the social context in which it occurs. This meaning is in line with the idea of normality as socially acceptable. According to this idea, behaviour that is in line with the normative expectations of the society is normal. Deviant behaviour is seen as abnormal. It has been argued that what clinicians understand as personality disorders should be seen as social deviance (Korchin, 1986).

The meaning of mental health as revealed in the present study is in line with the following view of Linton (1956: 637, as quoted in Korchin, 1986).

> The tests of absolute normalcy are the individual's ability to apprehend reality, as understood by his society during his developmental period. The test of relative normalcy is the extent to which the individual's experience has given him a personality conforming to the basic personality of his society.

It is thus evident that according to the results of this study the everyday meaning of mental health is not in line with the scientific orientation of the biomedical approach or the disease model that involves the understanding and sophisticated methods of medical science. The routine knowledge regarding mental health is also not in line with the scientific psychological approach which focuses on the individual personality and overlaps with the biomedical approach. As mentioned earlier, the current scientific orientation involves three major conflicting approaches, namely, the biomedical, the psychological and the psychosocial. The common meaning of mental health can be understood as overlapping with the psychosocial model which emphasizes the role of social systems in mental health and underlies community mental health approaches.

It, thus, appears that everyday knowledge regarding mental health is not in line with the orthodox view of madness and is also away from the medicalized version of mental health. It overlaps somewhat with a small part of the current scientific orientation but is not based on commonsense understanding of science. This study demonstrates that the 'social meaning' given to mental health mainly draws on social experiences and practical knowledge regarding conformity and deviance. This is quite in line with the view of Horwitz (in a review of Horwitz's book, *Creating Mental Illness* by O'Connor, 2002). According to him, any dysfunction of some internal psychological system results in a mental disorder when this dysfunction is considered as inappropriate in a particular social context.

The meaning of mental health is partly constructed because mental health is not commonly understood as a psycho-biological state but a social experience and social performance of conformity.

The 'social meaning' of mental health also points to the processes through which this construction takes place. The fact that 'mental' is understood as 'social' and that this is a pervasive socially shared meaning within the group of individuals studied, reflects the importance of active social processes such as communication, exchange and interaction. The constructed meaning of mental health also indicates the social reality of mental health. The commonly understood idea of mental health relates it to other social activities and it cannot be viewed as individualized biological or psychological phenomenon. This approach to mental health is in line with Gergen's (1985) assumptions of social constructionism and also with other examples of social constructionism (Berger and Luckman, 1966; Wright and Treacher, 1982).

Some Verbatim Samples and Excerpts of Participants' Responses

The results of the present study discussed in the previous section can be further interpreted and correlated with the verbatim samples quoted from the descriptions of the meaning of mental health provided by the subjects. Some excerpts have been quoted in the previous section. However, the verbatim responses selected and quoted in this section will serve to extend and further elaborate the discussion of results. The responses selected and quoted in this section represent some of the meaning categories used by the subjects in conceptualizing mental health. The responses quoted here have been edited for spelling and grammatical errors.

'Mental' as 'social'

- "Mental health of a particular individual can be defined on the basis of how the individual behaves in a social group....An individual can be called mentally ill, if he behaves in an 'abnormal way', i.e., in a way in which most of the people would not have reacted."
- "Any act, which is not in consonance with a social norm, can be attributed to mental illness."
- "Also to do something in society, which is not regarded correct or is not expected by society, is a case of mentally unhealthy

behaviour. There are certain norms, rules and regulations of the society. One should not harm society by breaking these rules. If someone does it and damages the society by his act, then that act can be regarded as a mentally unhealthy act."

- "The mental health of an individual is largely associated with the value framework of the society."
- "...for a good society, we need people to have good mental health. This will be good for the individuals and also for the entire society."

Mental health and adaptation

- "In modern era, life is changing at a fast pace. In this perspective, a person who balances well between the fast changing pace of modernization and value system of the society can be called a mentally healthy individual."

Mental health and goal attainment

- "If a man is mentally strong and is determined to do good work and achieve his defined goal, it goes to tell that his mental health is ok. Journey of life largely depends on how mentally strong you are, how bravely you face the problems and how good your thinking is."

Philosophical notions regarding mental health

- "Mental health is freedom of mind and is based on our thinking perspective, the way we think and the way we take things. A mentally healthy person is free from narrow-mindedness and vices. He takes things positively and sees the brighter side of things. Such a person has genuine reasons for all his actions...He enjoys every situation of life and would always love to struggle."
- "A person's mental state comprises of a long list of entities. But, on an average, we could say that a person is mentally healthy if he has a sort of equilibrium established. This equilibrium can't be attained easily. You have to free your mind. Free from all constraints."

Personal characteristics of mentally healthy and mentally ill individuals

- "The mentally healthy man is always active, energized, happy and frank. Mentally unhealthy are insisting, irritating and quarrelsome. They have a habit of criticizing everything, no matter how good it is."

Mental health and physical health

- "A person having good mental health could also influence his physical health positively even if he is not well physically. Mentally healthy provide an energetic environment to the surrounding society."

Mental illness and tension

- "The main reason of mental illness comes from tension and depression. The main reason is that something happens which you don't want and can't see, and also you can't stop it. When this happens repeatedly in day-to-day life.... it creates tension."

Implications for Generalizations of Findings

The present study was conducted on a group of engineering students of an institute of international repute. It was thus expected that their responses would be replete with scientific notions and explanations regarding mental health. However, two surprising facts emerged from the findings. First, the explanations and descriptions were not in line with scientific and biomedical aspects of mental health and illness. Secondly, in addition to the emphasis on social and cultural factors, philosophical and spiritual aspects were also cited frequently. It thus appears that being members of an elite scientific student community does not limit their explanations to the discipline of their formal education. The constructed meaning as revealed by the responses of the subjects depicts a much larger social context involved in meaning construction. It appears that the conceptual frameworks described by the subjects might have become the part of their conceptualization of mental health long before they took upon the study of engineering and technology. This meaning construction appears to be related to their membership in the middle class urban social community that values normative behaviour and social acceptance, lays emphasis on success and goal attainment, and takes pride in spiritual enhancement. The nature of the meaning of mental health revealed in the present study cannot be thus attributed to membership in a particular student community. The meaning categories reflect a social context that goes beyond the engineering institute. It might not be possible to generalize the findings of the present study to communities such as rural, tribal or some isolated groups, but the findings could be generalized to a large extent to middle class urban population to which most of the subjects belonged.

Conclusion

The main objective of the present work was to understand the terms in which people describe and explain the notion of mental health. The basic idea was to outline the commonsense conceptualization of mental health. An attempt was made to understand everyday knowledge regarding mental health that is generally less explicit and less defined than expert and scientific knowledge. Common knowledge and lay explanations of mental health have important attitudinal and behavioural implications both for individuals and groups.

In the present study, the meaning of mental health was seen as structured in terms of various content areas and themes, surfacing in the written descriptions of mental health provided by the respondents. The basic assumption of the study was that the meaning of mental health could be revealed by the content of everyday thinking about mental health. The content and structure of meaning as revealed by responses of the subjects was extended to understand the shared ideas regarding mental health and outline a framework of categories of meaning. Interestingly, this contemporary meaning of mental health was entirely different from the orthodox historical view of madness as well as from the medicalized scientific version.

Finally, the lay descriptions provided by the subjects revealed the constructed nature of the meaning of mental health. It appears that the complex world of mental health is understood in terms of relationship between the individual and the society where violation or adherence to social norms emerges as the core meaning around which other themes are organized in a relational network.

References

Berger, P. and Luckmann, T. (1966). *The Social Construction of Reality*. Garden City, NY: Doubleday.

Carstairs, G.M. and Kapur, K.L. (1976). *The Great Universe of Kota: Stress, Change and Mental Disorder in An Indian Village*. London: Hogarth Press.

Dalal, A.K. (2001). Health psychology. In J. Pandey (Ed.), *Psychology in India Revisited: Developments in the Discipline: Vol. 2, Personality and Health Psychology* (pp. 356-411). New Delhi: Sage Publications.

Daniels, M.H. and White, L.J. (1994). Human systems as problem-determined linguistic systems: Relevance for training. *Journal of Mental Health Counseling, 16*, 105-119.

Flick, U. (1998). Everyday knowledge in social psychology. In U. Flick (Ed.), *The Psychology of the Social* (pp. 41-59). Cambridge: Cambridge University Press.

Gergen, K.G. (1985). The social constructionist movement in modern psychology. *American Psychologist, 40*, 266-275.

Guterman, J.T. (1994). A social constructionist position for mental health counseling. *Journal of Mental Health Counseling, 16*, 226-244.

Herzlich, C. (1973). *Health and Illness: A Social Psychological Analysis*. London: Academic Press.

Jodelet, D. (1991). *Madness and Social Representations*. Hemel Hempstead: Harvester/Wheatsheaf.

Kakar, S. (1982). *Shamans, Mystics and Doctors: A Psychological Inquiry into India and its Healing Traditions*. Oxford: Oxford University Press.

Korchin, S. J. (1986). *Modern Clinical Psychology: Principles of Intervention in the Clinic and Community*. New Delhi: CBS Publishers.

Levine, J.M. and Moreland, R.L. (1992). Small groups and mental health. In D. Ruble, P. Costanzo and M. Oliveri (Eds.), *The Social Psychology of Mental Health: Basic Mechanisms and Applications* (pp. 126-165). New York: Guilford.

O'Connor, L.E. (2002). Review of creating mental illness by Allan V. Horwitz. *Human Nature Review*, 2, 4-6.

Palmer, R.E. (1969). *Hermeneutics: Interpretation Theory in Schleiermacher, Dilthey, Heidegger and Gadamer*. Evanston: Northwestern University Press.

Radley, A. (1994). *Making Sense of Illness: The Social Psychology of Health and Disease*. London: Sage Publications.

Wright, P. and Treacher, A. (1982). *Problem of Medical Knowledge*. Edinburgh: University Press.

4

Religiosity and Sense of Well-being: Spiritual Dimensions of Health

K. RAMAKRISHNA RAO

The topic of this paper by an Indian social scientist may be perceived as somewhat provocative and even audacious. Religion is not in the mainstream of Indian academia. We in the universities believe that we are wedded to reason and scientific outlook. Modelled after those in the west, our universities and what we teach in them consider religion as antithetical to science. With the 'holier than thou' attitude, we tend to outdo our western counterparts in upholding the sanctity of science in our shrines of higher learning, notwithstanding the fact that there is no such perception of opposition between science and religion in the native Indian tradition.

A couple of decades earlier the situation in the west was no different. When Jeff Levin (2001) began conducting epidemiological research and writing reviews in this area nearly two decades ago, his mentors and colleagues told him he was wasting his time. But, today, the situation is different in the US. There are many researchers actively engaged in this area. Koenig, McCullough and Larson (2001) review in their *Handbook of Religion and Health* 1,200 research reports and 400 reviews published in the 20th century. "Today, the epidemiology of religion and the larger field of clinical research on religion and spirituality are well established in the scientific world and in the public consciousness. The US National Institute of Health has convened invited conferences, established expert working groups, and funded considerable empirical research in this area. Prestigious scientific societies, including the American Academy for Advancement of Science, the American Public Health Association, the American Psychological Association, and the Gerontological Society of America have sponsored special symposia on religion and health" (Levin, 2001: viii). It is reported that more than two-thirds of all medical colleges in USA have course work or lectures on religion and spirituality.

Religion of one kind or another has existed in all societies; and it has had profound effects on the lives of those who practise it. Prayer is central to all religious practices. It is universal and ubiquitous, crossing cultural and geographical boundaries. It encompasses all religions, even those that do not specifically acknowledge an entity like God, as in Buddhism. Although the form and object of worship may vary, offering prayers is a pervasive phenomenon that is considered neither unusual nor abnormal. According to a survey published in 1996 by Princeton Religion Research Center, 96 percent of US population believed in God or a supernormal power. Despite the universally prevalent and largely shared religious behaviour and the belief that prayer is a means of propitiating gods or invoking supernatural forces/abilities to help improve human condition, it is a largely unexplored area until recently by contemporary social scientists. We psychologists in India paid little attention to this aspect of behaviour, which I presume is more pervasive and influential in our society than in the west.

In the absence of systematic studies of the effects of religious beliefs and practices on the health and well-being of people, health professionals in the past tended generally to either ignore or dismiss religious practices as no more than societal idiosyncrasies or dub them as sheer superstitious behaviour. Sigmund Freud (1927), for example, considered religion "a universal obsessional neurosis of humanity" and predicted its ultimate demise as people became more rational. Of course, this did not happen, even in the developed societies of the west that swear by science and reason. On the contrary, it is projected that the 21st century would be the most religious among the last five centuries (Novak, 1998).

Unlike his teacher and one-time colleague Freud, Carl Jung saw more to religion in the lives of his patients than neurosis. He wrote: "Among all my patients in the second half of life ... there has not been one whose problem in the last resort was not that of finding a religious outlook on life" (Jung, 1933: 229). In a review of relevant literature, David Moberg (1965) noted that "studies of happiness, morale, and personal adjustment have generally shown a direct relationship between good adjustment ... and religiosity ..." Psychologist Allen Bergin echoed a similar sentiment when he wrote, "religion is at the fringe when it should be at the center" of interest to social scientists. Jung, Moberg and Bergin were of course a small minority among health professionals who saw positive benefits of religion on human health and wellness. More vocal were those who advocated skepticism like Freud. A review published in the *American Journal of Psychiatry* concluded that "the contention that religion as an institution has been instrumental in fostering general well-being, creativity, honesty, liberalism, and other qualities is not supported by empirical data" (Sauna, 1969). Albert Ellis proclaimed nonchalantly that religiosity is inversely correlated with emotional health and that less religious people tend to be emotionally more stable. Here, then, we have a controversial area that needs some answers based on empirical data.

Beginning of Systematic Research

The above views, both pro and con, are no more than personal opinions. They are not based on a systematic collection of data, which began only in the late 1980s. Towards the end of the last century, there was in the US a perceptible shift and an increase of interest in scientifically studying the possible influence of religious beliefs and practices on human health and well-being. During the past ten years, there are literally hundreds of research reports published in refereed journals.

Harold Koenig and associates at Duke University carried out extensive studies on the role of religion in coping with the stress of ageing and disability. In one study, they (Koenig *et al.*, 1992) investigated the extent to which older patients tended to use religion to cope with stress and depression. The patient population was drawn from Duke University Medical Center and the neighbouring

Veterans Administration Hospital. The investigators evaluated the patients by means of Religious Coping Index (RCI), which they developed. The RCI consists of three items: "(1) an open-ended question about the most important factor that enabled the patient to cope, (2) a self-rating by the patient concerning the extent to which religion was used to cope, and (3) a rating by the examiner on the degree of religious coping, based on a discussion with the patient about how and when religion was used to cope."

The investigators found that, in answer to the first item, 20 percent of VA patients and 42 percent of Duke patients indicated that religion was the most important factor that enabled them to cope. When specifically asked to rate the extent to which religion was used in coping (item 2 in the index), about 70 percent of veterans and 90 percent of Duke patients responded that they used religion "at least to a moderate extent" and 55 percent of veterans and 75 percent of Duke patients indicated using it to a large or very large extent. In a series of studies, Koenig and colleagues looked into various aspects of the relationship between religious activity and health outcomes. They examined the effect of religious involvement on mortality, which showed a significant association between private religious activity such as prayer and longer survival in certain population groups (Helm *et al.*, 2000). They also found significantly less anxiety disorders among the people who attended religious services regularly (Koenig *et al.*, 1993) and an inverse relation between religious coping and scores on depression scales (Koenig *et al.*, 1992). Several studies with different groups ranging from terminally ill (Reed, 1986, 1987) to healthy adults (Mattlin *et al.*, 1990) suggest that a significant majority of people report that they use religion as a coping mechanism to deal with health problems and other stressful situations. As Koenig, McCllough and Larson (2001) observe, among the 16 studies that have examined possible relationship between religious involvement and blood pressure, 14 report lower blood pressure among the more religious. Steffen, Hinderliter, Blumenthal and Sherwood (2001) reported that among African Americans, religious coping is associated with reduced blood pressure.

Goldbourt *et al.* (1993) reported that in a 23-year follow-up study, the risk of death from coronary artery disease (CAD) was 20 percent lower among the most orthodox Jews than the less orthodox or non-believers. In their study of religious struggle as a predictor of mortality among medically ill elderly patients Pargament *et al.* (2001) found that the patients who experience religious struggle in comparison to those who religiously cope with their illness are at a greater risk of death. In a six-year follow-up study of 3,968 older adults, they observed that those who attended religious services at least once a week appeared to have a survival advantage over those who attended services less frequently. This effect of religious activity on survival, they contend, is equivalent to that of non-smoking vs. smoking on mortality (Koenig *et al.*, 1999).

There are several significant studies that explored the relationship between religiosity and a variety of health conditions. In about 150 studies on alcohol and drug abuse and religious involvement, most of the studies "suggest less substance abuse and drug abuse and more successful rehabilitation among the more religious" (Koenig, McCullough and Larson, 2001). Also, numerous studies investigated the effect of religion on mental health, delinquency, depression, heart disease, immune system dysfunction, cancer and physical disability (for a comprehensive review of research in these areas, see Koenig, McCullough and Larson, 2001).

Surveys of literature and meta-analysis of published research seem to confirm the claims of individual researchers linking religious practices with better health outcomes. For example, in a systematic and comprehensive review, Townsend *et al.* (2002) assessed the impact of religion on health outcomes. They reviewed all experiments involving randomized controlled trials published between 1996 and 1999 that assessed the relationship between religious practices and measurable health variables. The review revealed that "religious involvement and spirituality are associated with better health outcomes, including greater longevity, coping skills, and health-related quality of life and less anxiety." In a meta-analytic review of 29 independent samples McCullough *et al.* (2000) reported that religious involvement has a strong positive influence of increased survival ($p < .001$).

While the bulk of the studies are generally suggestive of the beneficial effects of religious practices on health, this area of research is not without its share of controversy. A few surveys do call into question the validity of the above claims on methodological grounds. For example, Sloan and Bagiella (2002) critically examined the claim made in many published articles that religious people tend to be healthier. They observed: "Of the 266 articles published in the year 2000 and identified by Medline search, only 17 percent were relevant to claims of health benefits associated with religious involvement. About half of the articles cited in the comprehensive reviews were irrelevant to these claims. Of those that actually were relevant, many either had significant methodological flaws or were misrepresented, leaving only a few articles that could truly be described as demonstrating beneficial effects of religious involvement. We conclude that there is little empirical basis for assertions that religious involvement or activity is associated with beneficial health outcomes."

Such criticisms notwithstanding, the evidence of the relationship between religious practices, especially prayer, and health is highly suggestive, even if inconclusive at this time. A good deal of skepticism is prompted by the western scientific mindset that looks with suspicion at anything that smacks of religion or spirituality, which is seen as antithetical to science. There is also a real fear of straying into the realm of the supernatural. The Indian mindset (of those who are not conditioned by the currently fashionable scientism) is somewhat different. In the native Indian tradition, there is no separation of science and spirituality, no dichotomy between natural and the so-called supernatural. For many in India, the putative positive effects of prayer on health and well-being is by no means surprising. It is not uncommon in India to offer prayers and engage in worship to overcome illness and misfortune. One wonders if these practices would have lasted as long as they did without reinforcement in real life. Of course, superstitions also survive for centuries; but then they too might have a useful role when not dysfunctional.

If religious involvement does have beneficial health outcomes, as many of the published reports in the west seem to suggest, then we may ask: How does this relationship work? What is its modus operandi, the process that underlies the presumed effect? What is the channel? Who is the source? These important, though often tricky, questions have no easy answers. The favoured explanation is a secular one. Religious beliefs and practices may have psychological effects, which in turn bring about somatic changes. If indeed religious beliefs and activities help to reduce anxiety, stress and depression, they could also help to shield their negative effects on general health and well-being.

As Koenig, Larson and Larson (2001) surmise, when people become physically ill, many rely heavily on religious beliefs and practices to relieve stress, retain a sense of control, and maintain hope and sense of meaning and purpose in life. It is suggested that religion (a) acts as a social support system, (b) reduces the sense of loss of control and helplessness, (c) provides a cognitive framework that reduces suffering and enhances self-esteem, (d) gives confidence that one, with the help of God, could influence the health condition, and (e) creates a mindset that enables the patient to relax and allow the body to heal itself. Again, the values engendered by religious involvement such as love, compassion, charity, benevolence and altruism may help to successfully cope with debilitating anxiety, stress and depression. All this may be true. Yet, there are issues that go beyond these explanations. For example, if the observed effects of distant intercessory prayer on the health of patients, who did not even know that some one was praying for them, are genuine, as they seem to be, the above secular explanations become clearly inadequate. We need more than a healthy mindset on the part of the patient to recover from illness because some one, unknown to him, had prayed for his recovery. There may be more to religion than being a social and psychological support system. Let us therefore consider briefly the case of remote intercessory prayer and its ramifications for future research in the area that explores the effects of religious activities on health and well-being.

The Case of Distant (Remote) Intercessory Prayer

As mentioned above, a number of studies gave positive evidence linking intercessory prayer with beneficial health outcomes. Intercessory prayer involves praying for others' benefit. In some of these studies, the patients did not know that someone was praying for them. Yet, their condition seemed to have improved compared to the controlled group of patients who did not have the benefit of someone praying for them. In a double blind study involving 393 coronary care patients, Randolph Byrd (1988) divided his subjects into two randomized groups: one group was the intercessory prayer group and the other was the control group. Neither the physicians attending on them nor the patients themselves knew which patients were being prayed for. Also, those who actually offered prayers did not know the patients for whose recovery they were praying. Results showed that the patients in the intercessory prayer group experienced significantly fewer episodes of congestive heart failures ($p < .05$), fewer cardiac arrests ($p < .05$), received fewer antibiotics ($p < .005$) and required less respirator support and medication ($p < .0001$). W.S. Harris *et al.* (1999) conducted a double blind study of distant intercessory prayer with 990 patients in the cardiac care unit. In this study with randomized controlled trials, it was observed that the experimental group (the prayed for patients) recovered better than the control group of patients. The results are statistically significant, even after correction for multiple analyses.

In a meta-analysis of published studies, Mueller, Plevak and Rummans (2001) found that randomized controlled trials had shown a significant positive effect between intercessory prayer and recovery from coronary disease. They observed that addressing the spiritual needs of the patient might enhance recovery from illness. However, all of these studies involved predominantly Christian population, with a smattering of Jewish and other religious people, raising the question whether these results are extendable to all of humankind.

In an interesting study, Cha, Wirth and Lobo (2001) investigated the effect of intercessory prayer on in-vitro fertilization. The study involved 219 women in Korea who were undergoing in-vitro fertilization and embryo transfer. The women in the experimental group were prayed for, unknown to them and their doctors, by individuals in other countries as far away as USA, Canada and Australia. It is reported that the women who were in the prayed for group showed 50 percent success rate compared to 26 percent success among the control group. The difference is statistically significant ($p = .0013$).

If these effects of distant intercessory prayer are genuine, as they seem to be, how do we explain them? The secular explanations of the sort we considered earlier are clearly inadequate. What is the mechanism involved? Who is the source? What is the channel? It was clearly understood by those who offered the prayers that it was God who was involved, responding to the prayer to influence the health outcome of the patients. Are we then experimenting with God? Can science go beyond itself and deal with spirituality and the divine. This could be scary and frightening to those who assume the essential incompatibility of science and spirituality.

Impressed with the extensive publications in the area, Chibnall, Jeral and Cerullo (2001) toiled for a couple of years to do a methodologically sophisticated and conceptually unambiguous study to test the influence of distant intercessory prayer on health. They found themselves unable to proceed beyond a critical review of the published reports. Their paper "Experiments on Distant Intercessory Prayer: God, Science, and the Lesson of Messiah" turned out to be more a debunking exercise rather than a constructive contribution. They conclude that this area of research is simply unproductive. They argue among other things that the notion of intervention by supernatural beings does not simply meet the basic testability and explanatory requirements of science. They write: "Science does not deny God, miracles, and the like, it merely neglects them ... Science cannot actualize spirituality, so why do we ask this of it?" This paper became quite influential among health professionals in the west for the reason that its rationale is quite consistent with their mindset that makes a clear separation between science and spirituality, between what is believed to be natural as distinguished from the supernatural, which is considered ex-hypothesis as beyond the scope of science. Such separation of the natural and the supernatural engenders among scientists the fear of trespassing into the sacred, which, it would seem, is one of the powerful reasons behind the efforts to fault researches in this and similar areas.

The argument that the researches in the religion-health area do not meet the testability requirements of science, is unconvincing. In addition, there is no intrinsic reason to bring in God or supernatural beings as the source of observed effects of distant intercessory prayer on health. Consider, for example, the wealth of studies that show similar effects of the influence of direct mental influence on remote biological systems. There is a large empirical database accumulated over the years by William Braud and associates that provides strong evidence suggestive of the possibility of influencing the physiology of a remotely situated person by sheer mental intention of another person. Braud and Schlitz (1991) review eight separate experiments in which the subjects attempted to influence remote biological systems by simply wishing such a change. The crucial difference between prayer and such wishing is that no supernatural being is invoked in the wish phenomenon, unlike in the prayer, which is generally directed at seeking the help of God to grant the wish. The results of the experiments by Braud and associates show that a subject by mental intention alone could influence in the desired direction (1) the autonomic nervous system activity of a remotely situated person, (2) the muscular tremor and ideo-motor reactions, (3) mental imagery of another person, and (4) the rate of hemolysis of human red blood cells in vitro. There is no reference in these studies to supernatural beings or non-testable entities. As Braud points out, based on the overall statistical results, the distant mental influence effects are relatively reliable and robust. The magnitude of the effects is not trivial and is comparable to self-regulation effects. The ability to mentally influence is apparently widely distributed. Thus, these experiments not only show the feasibility of scientifically studying such phenomena as healing through distant intercessory prayer, but they suggest also that the source of the effect may be a living person and not necessarily a supernatural entity like God.

Why then do we have the apprehension, such as the one expressed by Chibnall, Jeral and Cerullo, that in attempting to research in this area we ask of science to actualize spirituality? One possible answer is that the effects observed by Braud do not meet the explanatory criterion of science. Therefore, if the observed effects are genuine, they are anomalous. Either it will be shown later that these effects have natural explanations, such as an error somewhere, or they will remain forever outside the scope of science because they refer to supernatural phenomena. Such reasoning is a consequence of the assumption that there is an irreconcilable dichotomy between science and spirituality. It suffers from the tendency to secularize the sacred, which leads to what may be called the paradox of naturalizing the supernatural. William McDougall characterized the work of J.B. Rhine (1973) as such. Rhine's ESP work raised questions about the assumptive base of science itself. He used strict scientific methods and tools to investigate phenomena that do not obey the laws of science. For this reason, the successors of Rhine have to contend that the subject matter of parapsychology is the study of a certain set of anomalous phenomena. Telepathy is an anomaly. So are the abilities to foresee the future and perceive objects and events hidden from the senses.

The opposite of this attitude is the tendency to sanctify the secular and superimpose first-person categories on third-person phenomena. It is something with which we are quite familiar in India. Such an attitude leads to the paradox of spiritualizing science, again an unwholesome mix of categories. Science is science and it can hardly be fitted into spiritual categories. Similarly, spirituality is irreducible to scientific observations that have meaning and significance from the third-person perspective. It does not follow, however, that scientific observations are illusory or that spiritual experiences are delusional. Spiritual manifestations are first-person centred phenomena, whereas scientific observations of outer world are third-person focused. Science and spirituality may be considered as two distinctive perspectives. Their outcomes, the validity claims, need to be addressed and evaluated by different criteria. The paradoxes themselves have their origin in the postulated dichotomy between science and spirituality. Therefore, their resolution rests with a strategy that overcomes the dichotomy.

What is said above may not be construed as a criticism of western science. Its influence is too pervasive on our lives to ignore. Its validity in areas of its application is too obvious to deny. Yet, the assumption of the separateness of science and spirituality is neither intrinsic nor sacrosanct, as is often made. One could explore the possibility of an orderly and meaningful transition from one to the other without the reduction of one to the other. Observation is the key to scientific validation, because it allows for inter-subject agreement; but what constitutes an observation has changed significantly over time. It is no longer limited to naked sensing of the phenomena. Instrumental observation is too remote from the observer and requires several interpretative steps in between. Yet, we consider metre readings and other indirect measures as genuine observations. First-person experience, which is denied legitimacy in science as a reliable datum, without the agreement of similarly situated other persons, may be brought into science by valid manoeuvres as a kind of observation acceptable in science. When this happens, it might be possible to find a way of closing the explanatory gap between science and spirituality. For example, in the classical Indian tradition, there is no unbridgeable gulf between science and spirituality, no serious explanatory gap between first-person and third-person perspectives. Inquiry is considered possible in both the domains. In a sense, the scope of science would be significantly enhanced by allowing the possibility of transition from first person to third-person, possibly via second-person mediation. In this context, the traditional Indian practices such as yoga may have important lessons for learning about the process of transition from the first-person experience to third-person observation and for finding the common ground covered by science and the so-called spiritual phenomena (Rao, 2002). The case of meditation as a researchable area in science is worthy of consideration in this context.

Meditation and Prayer

Research in the area of meditation may be seen as a possible link between the secular and the sacred, between science and spirituality. Meditation has its origins in human spiritual quest. Like prayer, it is practiced in one form another in most communities. Devoid of its religious attributions, meditation is simply a mental process. As Naranjo points out, it is "the pursuit of a certain state of mind" (Naranjo and Ornstein, 1971). In meditation, there is a general focus of attention either in a diffused or concentrated form. Practice of meditation is believed to have beneficial outcomes in a variety of contexts, including health and well-being. As mentioned earlier, prayer generally involves propitiating gods to grant one's wishes. However, there are religious prayers that have no reference to God. For example, Buddha himself was agnostic. In non-theistic religions, the divide between prayer and meditation is almost invisible. Prayer itself, it seems to me, is a certain frame of mind, very much like the one that meditation helps to reach. God and the supernatural conjure up powerful archetypal images that command attention and help one to focus his mind. In fact, in the Indian tradition, *bhakti yoga* is one of the three important ways of reaching *moksha* or liberation – the ultimate goal of human condition. Since *bhakti* is prayerful devotion, we may not be far from truth if we assert that meditation is the secular equivalent of prayer.

There has been a great deal of scientific research on the effects of meditation on the states of mind and body. These effects seem to parallel those observed in studies that sought to link religious activities with health outcomes. A number of studies consider meditation as a self-regulation strategy that has relevance for managing stress, hypertension and drug addictions (Goleman and Schwartz, 1976; Patel, 1993). Davidson, Goleman and Schwartz (1984) report results that showed "reliable decrement in trait anxiety across groups as a function of length of meditating". A meta-analysis by Eppley, Abram and Shear (1989), involving about 130 studies, confirmed that meditation, especially TM, has the effect of reduced trait anxiety. John Astin (1997) among others reported the beneficial effects of meditation on stress reduction. A study by Alexander *et al.* (1994) investigated the effects of various types of meditation on the mortality rate of elderly persons. They reported that one hundred percent of the subjects in the study who practised TM survived during the follow-up period of three years, where the average survival rate was 62.6 percent. Alexander *et al.* (1994) also point out that epidemiological studies show that people practising TM had significantly lower inpatient and outpatient visits and expenditure than comparable control groups. In addition, there is credible evidence suggesting possible association between meditation and psychic abilities. The work of Braud and colleagues cited earlier and the positive relationship between meditation and psychic abilities provide a secular alternative to distant intercessory prayer. In fact, psychic healing practices are widely prevalent around the world. Therefore, study of prayer as a form of meditation has interesting possibilities for research.

Research Possibilities

As may be surmised from the above, religion-health relationship is a vastly important area. It opens up enormous opportunities for programmatic research that would have great relevance for social policy. The scope of the study of the beneficial effects of religion on human health and well-being is indeed very broad. It goes beyond medical settings, older population and health outcomes. Prayer is not limited to older people. People pray wishing a variety of beneficial outcomes such as health, wealth and happiness. However, at this stage, it is necessary that we limit the scope of research to areas of greater relevance and promise. I see three different stages in the progress of research in this area in India. As a major first step in Indian research in this field, we need first feasibility studies to gather ground information that could provoke greater interest in this topic among Indian social scientists. These would include preparing and testing the tools that would be required for further research in India.

At the same time, we would replicate in the non-western and non-Christian setting some of the western studies and extend them to non-clinical general population. There is already some evidence that practice of *yoga* and prayer has beneficial outcomes for health. In a survey of 3,148 rural adults in Rajasthan, Gupta and colleagues (1997) found persons engaged in *yoga* or prayer were more than 70 percent less likely to have coronary heart disease. This effect appears to be independent of other risk factors for cardiac artery disease.

During the first *exploratory* stage, we may address questions such as the following:

(1) How frequent is religious coping in medical and non-medical settings among the Indian population?
(2) Why do people engage themselves in religious activities?
(3) How do Indian people express their faith?
(4) What are the perceived consequences of faith to them?
(5) What kinds of people tend to be more religious? To put it differently, what are the effects of "being religious" on the personality of people with faith?

Of course, India is a pluralistic society. While the majority population is Hindu, we have in this country Muslims, Christians, Buddhists, Jains and others too in quite large numbers. Therefore, we need to gather data for different religious groups independently before attempting to generalize the results to Indian society as a whole. There is evidence to suggest significant differences in the prevalence of heart disease among different religious groups. For example, a survey conducted by Gopinath *et al.* (1995) showed wide variations in the prevalence of cardiac artery disease among Muslims, Sikhs, Hindus and Christians, with Sikhs showing highest rate of myocardial infarction and the Christians the lowest.

The second stage is the *confirmatory* stage. It would involve more focused and conclusive studies, which employ randomized controlled trials to study targeted groups such as patients admitted in hospitals for treatment of severe illness and prisoners serving long terms for serious crime. The goal is to learn if religious involvement, such as prayer, could bring about the transformation of the person that results in better health, well-being and adjustment and, if so, in what areas and contexts.

The third stage is the *explanatory* stage. It involves process-oriented research. It is not enough we know that religious activities have beneficial outcomes. We need to know how these effects come about. We need to know about the process, the source and the channel of these effects. Undoubtedly, other questions will arise and call for answers. The goal, however, is one of being able to put to use the knowledge we gain from these studies and draw out the implications for societal policies, medical education and intervention strategies for better health and all-round well-being of people.

At this point, it becomes necessary to note the distinction between religion and spirituality. Even though they two are often used interchangeably by researchers exploring the effects of religion on health and well-being, it is necessary to underscore the distinction. Religion is doctrinaire and denominational, having specific behavioural and social consequences. Therefore, being religious implies more than being spiritual. Spirituality is not circumscribed within the bounds of anyone religion. Rather, it is guided by a belief in what may be called the transcendental aspect of being. While all religions aim at promoting spirituality, there is the possibility that the manifest forms of religious worship and participation in religious activities may be dissociated from intrinsic spirituality. Therefore, a measure of religiosity need not be a measure of spirituality. Researchers are now becoming increasingly aware of this possibility. The Fetzer scale of 'Multidimensional Measurement of Religiousness/Spirituality' explicitly recognizes the distinction between religiosity and spirituality.

The Indian social scientists will have an advantage over their western colleagues in carrying out research at the explanatory level. At the outset, they would be less encumbered and constrained by what I consider a regressive notion that involves the dichotomy of spirituality and science. In the Indian tradition, we have appropriate concepts and viable research strategies to meaningfully deal with phenomena that appear anomalous on the surface. In my encounters with theoretical issues in psychology, I find Indian models very helpful. The concept of pure consciousness, the possibility of knowing by being, and the numerous mind-transforming techniques traditionally practised in India such as *yoga* would be useful in modelling process-oriented research in this area.

In the classical Indian tradition, consciousness is not conceived as an epiphenomenon or as a quality of experience. Rather consciousness is an autonomous principle, the ground condition of all knowing. However, in Indian tradition, not all knowing is the sensory kind, which gives us only representational knowledge. There is another kind of knowing, knowing by being, which arises when we access consciousness-as-such. In a state of pure consciousness, we are told, one has non-representational direct awareness. In such a state, there is no possibility of dissociation between knowing and being, cognition and conduct, and thought and action. As the Upanishadic statement proclaims, "to know Brahman is to be Brahman". If sensory awareness gives one understanding of the phenomena, knowing by being results in the realization of the phenomena in his being. The lives of true saints and those who have had genuine 'peak' experiences are instances of those who achieved realization in various degrees. Realization, on the one hand, removes any gap between belief and behaviour. On the other hand, it has important transformational consequences to the person and his well-being. It is important to recognize that the notion of pure consciousness is not an armchair metaphysical postulate. It is an empirical claim embedded in Indian tradition. We will do well to understand it and study its implications to psychological research.

The proposed phased and programmatic study would deal with one of the most profound and pervasive aspects of human conduct that received scant attention among the Indian academia in general and psychologists in particular. It would provide useful information on the extent and the role of religious coping in the lives of Indian people. It would also throw light on the inter-religious and inter-cultural validity of some of the findings of western researches in this area.

We would know more about the personality of religious persons as well as on the role of religious practices such as prayer on reducing anxiety and depression and for promoting a sense of well-being, especially among targeted groups, such as patients admitted to hospitals for treatment of severe illness and prisoners serving long terms for serious crime. The goal is to learn more about the beneficial outcome of religious involvement, the process of transformation of the person for better health and wellness. The exercise will involve applying and testing Indian models to study religious behaviour. The end result, I expect, would show the viability of Indian psychology for effectively studying those aspects of behaviour that western psychology has difficulty in adequately investigating.

References

Alexander, C.N., Robinson, P., Orme-Johnson, D.W., Schneider, R.H. and Walton, K.G. (1994). The effects of transcendental meditation compared to other methods of relaxation and meditation in reducing risk factors, morbidity, and mortality. *Homeostasis, 35*, 243-263.

Astin, J.A. (1997). Stress reduction through mindfulness meditation: Effects on psychological symptomology, sense of control, and spiritual experiences. *Psychotherapy and Psychosomatics, 66*, 97-106.

Braud, W. and Schiltz, M.J. (1991). Conscious interactions with remote biological systems. Anomalous intentionality effects. *Subtle Energies, 2,* 1-46.

Byrd, R.C. (1988). Positive therapeutic effects of intercessory prayer in a coronary care unit population. *Southern Medical Journal, 81,* 826-829.

Cha, K.Y., Wirth, D.P. and Lobo, R. (2001). Does prayer influence the success of in vitro fertilization embryo transfer? Report of a masked randomized trial. *Journal of Reproductive Medicine, 46,* 781-781.

Chibnall, J.T., Jeral, J.M. and Cerullo, M.A. (2001). Experiments in distant intercessor prayer: God, science, and the lesson of Messiah. *Archives of Internal Medicine, 161,* 2529-2536.

Eppley, K.R., Abram, A.I. and Shear, J. (1989). Differential effects of relaxation techniques on trait anxiety: A meta analysis. *Journal of Clinical Psychology, 45,* 957-974.

Freud, S. (1927/1962). Future of an illusion. In Strachey, J. (Ed.), *Standard Edition of the Complete Psychological Works of Sigmund Freud.* London: Hogarth Press.

Goldbourt, U., Yaari, S. and Medalie, J.H. (1993). Factors predictive of long-term coronary heart disease mortality among 10,059 male Israeli civil servants and municipal employees. *Cardiology, 82,* 100-121.

Goleman, D. and Schwartz, G. (1976). Meditation as an intervention in stress reactivity. *Journal of Consulting and Clinical Psychology, 44,* 456-466.

Gopinath, N., Chada, S.L., Jain, P., Shekhawat, S. and Tandon, R. (1995). An epidemiological study of coronary heart disease in different ethnic groups in Delhi urban population. *Journal of the Association of Physicians of India, 43,* 30-33.

Gupta, R., Prakash, H., Gupta, V.P. and Gupta, K.D. (1997). Prevalence and determinants of coronary heart disease in a rural population of India. *Journal of Clinical Epidemiology, 50,* 203-209.

Harris, W.S., Bowda, M., Kolb, J.W., Strychacz, C.P., Vacek, J.L. Jones, P.G., Forker, A., O'Keefe, J.H. and McCallister, B.D. (1999). A randomized, controlled trial of the effects of remote intercessory prayer on outcomes in patients admitted to the coronary care unit. *Archives of Internal Medicine, 159,* 2273-2278.

Helm, H., Hays, J.C., Flint, E., Koenig, H.G. and Blazer, D.G. (2000). Effects of private religious activity on mortality of elderly disabled and nondisabled adults. *Journal of Gerontology, 55,* 400-405.

Jung, C.G. (1933). *Modern Man in Search of Soul.* New York: Harcourt Brace Jovanovich.

Koenig, H.G., Larson D.B. and Larson S.S. (2001). Religion and coping with serious medical illness. *Ann Pharmacother, 35,* 352-359.

Koenig, H.G., McCullough, M. and Larson, D.B. (2001) *Handbook of Religion and Health: A Century of Research Reviewed.* New York: Oxford University Press.

Koenig, H.G., Cohen, H.J., Blazer, D.G., Pieper, C., Meador, K.G., Shelp, F., Goli, V. and DiPasquale, R. (1992). Religious coping and depression in elderly hospitalized medically ill men. *American Journal of Psychiatry, 149,* 1693-1700.

Koenig, H.G., Ford, S., George, L.K., Blazer, D.G. and Meador, K.G. (1993). Religion and anxiety disorder: An examination and comparison of associations in young, middle-aged, and elderly adults. *Journal of Anxiety Disorders, 7,* 321-342.

Koenig, H.G., Hays, J.C., Larson, D.B., George, L.K., Cohen H.J., McCullough, M.E., Meador, K.G. and Blazer, D.G. (1999). Does religious attendance prolong survival? A six-year follow-up study of 3,968 older adults. *Journal of Gerontology, 54,* 370-376.

Levin, J. (2001). Foreword in *Handbook of Religion and Health.* In H.G. Koenig, M.E. McCullough, and D.B. Larson (Eds.), New York: Oxford University Press.

Mattlin, J.A., Wethington, E. and Kessler, R.C. (1990). Situational determinants of coping and coping effectiveness. *Journal of Health and Social Behaviour, 31,* 103-122.

McCullough, M.E., Hoyt, W.T., Larson, D.B., Koenig, H.G. and Thoresen, C.E. (2000). Religious involvement and mortality: A meta-analytic review. *Health Psychology, 19,* 211-222.

Moberg, D.O. (1965). Religion in old age. *Geriatrics, 20,* 977-982.

Mueller, P.S., Plevak, D.J. and Rummans, T.A. (2001). Religious involvement, spirituality, and medicine: implications for clinical practice. *Mayo Clin. Proc., 76,* 1189-1191.

Naranjo, C. and Ornstein, R.E. (1971). *On the Psychology of Meditation.* New York: Viking Press.

Novak, M. (1998). The most religious century. *New York Times* (Open Editorial, Sunday, May 24).

Pargament, K.I., Koenig, H.G., Tarakeshwar, N. and Hahn, J. (2001). Religious struggle as a predictor of mortality among medically ill elderly patients: A two-year longitudinal study. *Archives of Internal Medicine, 161,* 1881-1885.

Patel, C.H. (1993). Yoga based therapy. In P.M. Lehrer and R.L. Woolfolk (Eds.), *Principles and Practice of Stress Management* (pp. 89-138). New York: Guilford Press.

Rao, K.R. (2002). *Consciousness Studies: Cross-Cultural Perspectives.* McFarland and Co.

Reed, P.G. (1986). Religiousness among terminally ill and healthy adults. *Research in Nursing and Health, 9*, 35-41.

— (1987). Spirituality ad well-being in terminally ill hospitalized adults. *Research in Nursing and Health, 10*, 335-344.

Rhine, J.B. (1973). *Extra Sensory Perception.* Brookline Village, Mass: Branden Press.

Sauna, V.D. (1969). Religion, mental health, and personality: A review of empirical studies. *American Journal of Psychiatry, 125*, 1203-1213.

Sloan, R.P. and Bagiella, E. (2002). Claims about religious involvement and health outcomes. *Annals of Behavioral Medicine, Winter, 24*, 14-21.

Steffen, P.R., Hinderliter, A.L., Blumenthal, J.A. and Sherwood, A. (2001). Religious coping, ethnicity, and ambulatory blood pressure. *Psychosomatic Medicine, 63*, 523-530.

Townsend, M., Kladder, V., Ayele, H. and Mulligan, T. (2002). Systematic review of clinical trials examining the effects of religion on health. *South Medical Journal, 95*, 1429-1434.

5

Perspectives on Health, Illness and Well-being: An Agenda for Future Research

A.K. SHARMA

Health, illness and well-being are words of everyday use. Health is seen as a basic service. The Government of India was a signatory to the Alma Ata Declaration, and the South East Asian Health Charter with the WHO for achieving the goal of "Health for All by 2000". Health is also seen as one of the major components of human development: improvement in life expectancy and reduction in infant mortality rate are viewed as indicators of progress in health. Yet, in the recent past, there has been a debate on constructions of health and illness. The issues are: What is health? Is health merely the absence of illness? Do many ill persons perceive themselves as healthy? How should one distinguish between reported illness, perceived illness and clinically established illness? What are the notions of well-being? Is health or absence of illness a necessary condition of well-being? This paper addresses some of these issues and suggests the agenda for future research.

Major Perspectives

For a long time biomedical model of health was the dominant perspective on health: sociologists who worked in the field of health used Durkheimian (or Parsonian) functional perspective. Attempts have been made by Marxists and others to examine class inequalities in health, both outside and in India, abandoning the biomedical model of health. The challenge to the functional perspective has come from those sociologists and others who stress that the concept of health is socially constructed. Thus, the subject of health is contextualized and made subjective. This leads to overlapping and multiple perspectives. Some of these are detailed below. There may still be some more perspectives, which can be developed further. Which perspectives are important is an issue that can be answered only in the structural context of the debate on sociology of health. For example, in the context of the less developed countries, the concept of 'health for all' may mean that primary facilities for treatment of malnutrition-infection syndrome are available to all. It does not mean eradication of all forms of illness. From subjective perspective health for all will never be possible.

Biomedical or Providers' Perspective

So far in India health has been studied from the perspective of planners for whom the goal of health intervention has been to raise and equalize life expectancy for all regions and classes of people. According to the Union Minister for Health (Thakur, 2002), India is committed to "a widely accessible and equitable system of health services addressing quality of care concerns. This is in line with the commitment made at the International Conference on Population and Development in Cairo, the conference at Beijing and subsequently at the United Nations General Assembly, which India has endorsed time and again".

Census and SRS data have shown that India has made a great leap in life expectancy from nearly 20 in the beginning of the last century (37 at the time of independence) to nearly 62. Now, women have a slightly higher life expectancy than men, which shows that overall sex discrimination in health practices is on decline. Regional differences are also declining as the low life expectancy states are progressing, although such differences still exist. A need is felt to bring the lagging states at par with the forward states. From this perspective, there is a need to examine morbidity and mortality rates among different classes and regions so that appropriate interventions can be made. Planners would also be worried about health problems among the older people and new risks such as HIV/AIDS for which treatment is either extremely costly or ineffective. Thoughts of ineffectiveness of modern medicines have given rise to thinking about alternative medicines. In this perspective, health is basically a function of absence of morbidity, and morbidity is itself a function of risk, availability of medicines and diet. Risk itself is a function of socio-economic status, family size and environmental factors.

Health = f (morbidity)

Morbidity = g (risk, medicines, diet)

Risk = h (socio-economic status, family size, environmental factors)

It may be noted that researchers, funded mostly by state or international organizations, share the above perspective. They have concentrated on life tables, age- and gender-specific mortality rates (sometimes morbidity rates), socio-economic and regional differences between them and trend analysis. Statisticians have applied mathematical hazard models to unearth laws of mortality. Biostatisticians and medical scientists have also adopted the same approach for the reason that it is easier to measure mortality and morbidity than health status (Verma, 2002).

The time has come to question the above paradigm. The limitations of this paradigm are as follows:

— It does not give importance to people's health beliefs, practices and social roles.
— It assumes that the planners' perspective (including social scientists' perspective) is scientific, and people's perspectives are unscientific (and therefore unreal).
— It equates well-being with absence of illness and forces the ill to accept 'sick roles' and social exclusion.
— It hides the gap between clinically established illness and reported illness. There are many persons who, if diagnosed, will be found to be ill but they do not feel so and consider themselves to be happy and healthy for long till the problem becomes severe.
— It often complicates problems by forcing the ill to accept scientific medicine without proper understanding of the risks of

modern medicine, and the unscientific component in the science.

— It provides supremacy to modern medicine and without proper scientific examination rejects the age-old wisdom of tradition.

— It does not provide understanding of how to live meaningfully in those situations in which it offers no hope.

It is amazing that although scientific perspective in medicine does not accept the finality of theories, it has been able to project itself real and create a myth that the traditional or age-old wisdom in communities is unscientific, i.e., false. It must be stressed that the modern scientific perspective needs support from business and political institutions. In corrupt societies, which most of the developing countries are, due to violation of anti-trust norms and inadequacy of public health facilities, modern scientific perspective has often played havoc with the health and life of people. In many areas, it has undermined faith in traditional management of health and made people dependent on *jhola chhap* doctors. Illegal abortions due to extreme shortages of MTP-trained doctors (Retherford and Roy, 2003), and eye operations by *jhola chhap* doctors taking away people's eyesight are not rare. In many cases, all effects of medicine are not known.

> ...in many cases the treatment causes more damage than the illness ever would, for example, the thalidomide drug where the effects on the unborn children greatly outweighed the advantages to the pregnant women. People suffering from depression are often given tranquillisers. This, in turn, can cause addiction. There is also much evidence to suggest that there are many unpleasant side effects to the contraceptive pill as it can cause cancer or thrombosis and intra uterine devices can cause all sorts of infections. However, they continue to be used by the majority of women, as there is little choice of other methods of birth control (http://www.essaybank.co.uk/free_course work/2611.html).

It has no doubt increased life expectancy by reducing infant and child mortality at the national level but it has increased misery among many. Moreover, with the epidemiologic transition caused by ageing, there is a shift towards degenerative diseases that demand more intervention in life style than medicine behaviour (Goldman, 2002; Pandey, 2002). The new situation demands appropriate legal, fiscal and other methods, which lead to changes in lifestyle, reduction in alcohol consumption and smoking, greater consciousness of consequences of sugary, salty and fatty diets, and improved physical activity, etc., to promote health in general population. Health issues are personal and familial issues. People have to adopt personal responsibility for health. This requires encouraging family cohesion and support (Ratzan *et al.*, 2000; WHO, 2002).

People's Perspectives

There is also a need to focus on health from people's perspective, necessitating studies of social representations of health and illness (Sharma *et al.*, 2002). This has become particularly important in the case of tribes.

The Tribal Perspective

NFHS-II (IIPS, 1995) has revealed that Scheduled Tribes (STs) are lagging behind in social development. All indicators of mortality and morbidity show that STs have not benefited from development as much as others. Among tribes death rates in general and maternal mortality rates in particular are very high.

Traditionally, tribes used herbal medicines for which the community depended on forest resources. *Hartis Malabarcia*, a book written by Henrick Van Rheed, the Dutch Governor of Malabar, during the 1670s, elaborates on tribal and other systems of medicine (Shankar, 1995). His biography shows that he formed a multidisciplinary research team and spent 12 years documenting information on cures for diseases afflicting human beings and animals. Even today, researchers from anthropology background are attempting to document the tribal medicines (Maiti, 2003). It would be interesting to examine whether different tribes living in different environments use the same herbs for the same purpose. It would also be interesting to separate the herbal part of the remedy from the associated rituals, and magical and religious practices.

Depleting forest resources and threatened common property resources raise serious questions about the availability and adequacy of herbs. Moreover, past studies carried out in various regions have shown that the tribal population suffers from poor nutrition, excessive alcohol consumption, and lack of safe drinking water and health facilities. Tribal villages have poor connectivity and in case they need to go to health centres, they have to walk for 8-10 km, carrying patients on cots. It has been observed that the tribes, especially the very poor, have a high incidence of infectious diseases. Communication between providers and clients is another serious problem in tribal areas. There is a need to have different PHC norms for remote tribes and particularly for the general health education among them.

Interestingly, the state governments support various forms of medicine: ayurvedic, unani, homeopathic, biochemic, acupressure and other local systems of medicines. The Directorate of Indian Systems of Medicines has a large infrastructure comprising a large number of dispensaries. In states like Chhattisgarh, another interesting initiative is taken by the State Forest Department, which has formed People's Protected Areas for conservation and utilization of medicinal herbs. The state government is making concerted efforts in maintaining the biodiversity of the state and reviving the traditional medicines.

A project for institutionalization of various horizontal and vertical linkages pertaining to traditional medicinal practices existing in the state of Chhattisgarh has been taken up by the Directorate of Indian Systems of Medicines and Health. Under this project, local healers are identified at village and district levels, and 'Traditional Healer Forums' are formed which in turn develops vertical linkage through ayurvedic doctors posted in state dispensaries. The forum selects the best and unique traditional medicinal practices along with the appropriate drug combination.

There is a need to involve people in the decision-making process in the health-related issues. There is also a need for demystification and deconstruction of medical knowledge. These efforts will require empowerment of people and community action for health: preparation of a workable health plan for each village.

In Chhattisgarh, the Panchayati Raj Institutions (PRIs) have been strengthened for better delivery of health service. Indira Swasthya Mitanin Yojana has been implemented whereby a community selects a health volunteer – the 'Mitanin' (i.e., a friend) – to help in developing a Village Health Plan. She also helps in 'Community Action in Health'. The concept of 'Mitanin' under the Indira Swasthya Mitanin Yojana is about empowerment of the PRIs in which the 'Mitanins' provide information to PRIs about the health status of people, help PRIs in developing a Village Health Plan, and bridging the gap between Gram Panchayat and the community. Similar efforts are needed in all parts of the country.

To quote Ray:

> Many health problems have their roots in various aspects of community life and cannot be influenced by health interventions alone. Non-medical interventions are also very vital, and for optimal results a reasonable coordination of both is essential.

In the past, the tribal communities of Chhattisgarh, as in other places, had lifestyles that were distinct from agrarian communities. The tribal practised shifting cultivation, survived on hunting and engaged in gathering of forest products (Naik and Sharma, 1985). All of the activities of the tribals closely related to and depended on the forests. The tribal society is now undergoing major transformation. The urbanized world has gradually engulfed their forest areas. Many of the tribes have now adopted permanent farming. Studies show that gradual depletion of common property resources and loss of forest rights have an adverse impact on the tribal economy, but more importantly on their health. Field visits by the author have also shown that the tribes have become more open to outside influences, but age-old beliefs regarding health are still quite prevalent among them. It is, therefore, necessary to understand their values and practices, how they look at health and illness, nature of health-seeking behaviour, and the relationship between gender and health (Lorber and Moore, 2000; Manning and Fabrega, Jr., 1973).

Women's Perspective

It is important to explore women's perspective on health because of the gendered nature of society and women occupying a subordinate place in social structure. Women also have some distinct problems and need distinct approach to health. Most often women share their problems with other women (in the family or neighbourhood) rather than with men, and thus develop a women's perspective.

> A woman's role is often looking after everyone in the family and because she tends to carry an added burden of stress with an attitude of having to shoulder her responsibilities she may be prone to physical and mental disorders. As victims of social and economic circumstances women tend to suffer from what is known as 'housewife syndrome'. The isolation and constant decision-making involved in housework are very stressful as is the responsibilities of looking after young children. In addition, there are certain illnesses that women suffer from because of their biology; because women live longer they tend to suffer from degenerative disorders (http://www.essaybank.co.uk/free_coursework/2611.html).

A few social scientists have looked at health and health delivery systems from the gender perspective. For example, Foucault (1973) looked at hospitals and their anatomy within the framework of power. To him, medical institutions are just another illustration of the nature of power distribution in society. Foucault averred that in modern societies, power is exercised through invisible observation of people's actions rather than visible demonstration of social force, leading to production of self-discipline. Looked at from this perspective, hospitals, like other institutions such as schools, asylums, army barracks, etc., are the places where *disciplinary power* is exercised. Arguing along similar lines, feminists have added that medicalization of modern societies has reinforced patriarchal control. The doctors are commonly the males. They are authorized to regulate and control women's bodies. They assert that medicine profession in the modern society does the same thing to control women that organized religion did to women in pre-modern societies.

Writing on gender and health, Lane and Cibula (2002) have analyzed the issues of sexual violence (including bride burning, dowry deaths, honour killing, rape and attempted rape), female genital mutilation, and the associated sexual and psychological problems. This change is reflected in India in increasing number of studies focusing on reproductive health and self-reported problems as against studies of patterns of morbidity.

Unnithan-Kumar (1999) has examined reproductive health care in the context of women's perceptions and experiences of illness in general and in terms of the material, ideological and political dynamics of household, kin and gender relations, in particular. She shows how perceptions of illness and health-seeking behaviour in a Rajasthan village are interlinked with outreach of health services, hospital experiences, age of marriage, beliefs about allopathic, unani and spiritual remedies, household composition, fertility, economic conditions, education and working conditions. Her fieldwork further shows that mere provision of health services is not enough. It has to be supported by proper attitudes and beliefs, and positive experiences. To quote:

> There is no doubt that the villagers in Sanganer want and need access to good health care services as is reflected in the high costs they incur as well as the distances they travel to seek out effective health cures. At the same time most of their experiences with the health services often have been negative, and given the exacting nature of their lives, women especially have a tendency towards inaction as far as seeking treatment for illness is concerned. At the same time, given reliable information about effective cures and doctors, women are quickly willing to explore the possibilities of seeking treatment from these sources, provided they have some support from their kinspersons to do so.

It has been observed that among women *the concept of health is functional*, while *the concept of illness is substantive* (Sharma *et al.*, 2002). Women talk about health as a condition in which they can do their work well (*sab kaam theek thak kar sakte hain*). Illness is a condition in which they have to meet a doctor. In illness, they also *look* depressed (*chehra latka hua ho*). Reportedly health also implies a state of happiness, lack of worries about money and children, and peace with oneself and others. In other words, health is social while illness is physical. However, a 'healthy' woman may be taking medicines and an 'ill woman' may be attending to duties.

Minority Perspective

There is no study of how members of cultural and religious minorities view health. In the absence of such studies, their reactions are often labelled and they are stigmatized. Newspapers have often reported that in Muslim areas people have prevented doctors' teams from delivering polio vaccines on religious grounds or due to the fear that the vaccine would lead to infertility (such statements are also made by the health providers at all levels). The same papers seldom report about near absence of health facilities in those areas. The absence of health facilities in the community is part of "the taken for granted".

Some systems of medicine are traditionally associated with some communities. For example, sections of Muslims may prefer yunani system of medicine (this is, however, to be tested empirically). How does it manifest: they believe that principles on which yunani system is based are better than the scientific principles; or that the poor and marginalized, outside the allopathic system, can benefit more from the traditional system; or that the traditional system is good but due to lack of support it has become non-functional; or that the traditional system is consistent with the religious beliefs of the community? Empirical researches only can help understand the issues of community, confounded with class and other social factors. Likewise, one can go deeper into Hindu perspectives on health. Hindus are not seen as a religious minority but only minority of Hindus believes in traditional Ayurvigyan. Does it have any link with the Vedic wisdom? Limited fieldwork done by the author shows that the minorities are more likely to hold traditional beliefs but the different fragments among them interpret traditions differently (Sharma, 1996). The interpretations depend on the following:

— Income and social class
— Urban-rural residence
— Educational and occupational background
— Ecological variations and neighbourhood
— Degree of isolation
— Degree of interaction with the clergy

It would be interesting to examine the effect of the above factors on the minority perspectives.

Perspective of the Sick

This question is never asked: how do the sick persons construct the ideas of health and illness? A problem that one would face here is that the sick persons are not a homogeneous group. One cannot put those suffering from common infectious diseases, cancer, HIV/AIDS, chronic disorders, diseases of old age, undiagnosed problems and accidents in one category. Some of them suffer from exclusion but others are normally active. There is also need to study social representations of health and illness from the perspective of the sick persons.

As such, there are no known studies on perspectives of the sick but the study of Addlakha and Grover (2000) touches upon this issue when they explore the health-seeking behaviour of the users of the Hepatitis B vaccine in East Delhi. Following Klienman (1980), they say that in the context of the plural medical culture people use a number of explanatory models. They are "notions about an episode of sickness and its treatment, and are employed by all those engaged in the clinical process". They seek to answer questions about *a particular episode of illness* (emphasis added) such as its aetiology, time and mode of onset of symptoms, pathophysiology, course and treatment, and prevention. "The user emerges as a strategist who selectively appropriates the biomedical and folk treatment spaces."

Alternative Medicines

The use of alternative medicines may be seen as an expression of post-modern society. It finds acceptance from the desire for self-determination and choice. It challenges the cultural dominance of traditional biomedicine and reflects a more general trend for maintaining the body through the purchase of consumer goods and services (Barry and Yuill, 2002).

Alternative medicines claim to treat the person rather than the specific disease. They are particularly suited in treatment of chronic ailments. They need experimental support. However, it has to be said that experimental support is not the same thing as scientific support which requires working of a drug in terms of principles of chemistry and quantum mechanics. Alternative medicines include Indian systems of medicine (ISM), folk medicines, *yoga* and related practices. Some of them even claim to cure degenerative ailments fully for which allopathic system has no solution except continuing medication that can often have adverse side-effects. Ayurveda recognizes social status of a person in prescribing treatment.

> A poor and friendless patient should live on alms, lead a life of perfect continence like an ascetic, forego use of shoes and umbrella and walk a hundred yojanas (A yojana is equal to eight miles) or more on foot without staying for more than one night at a single village. A rich man (suffering from Prameha.) should live on Shyamaka, Kapittha, Tinduka and Ashmantaka and live among the Deer. He should constantly follow the tracks of cows and take their urine (for food and drink). A Brahmana patient should live on the grain spontaneously fallen from plants, constantly study the Vedas and draw chariots occupied by Brahamanas. A patient belonging to the lower orders of society (shudras) should sink wells (under such circumstances). All these references highlight the importance of exercise (body activity) in case of Prameha (http://www.ayuherbal.com/diabetes.htm).

As mentioned above, all medicinal systems have their own philosophical basis. There is only need to have clarity on the philosophical basis of medicinal systems. This can be done at two levels: ontological and empirical. Ontology will show to what extent the beliefs lying behind alternative systems of medicine are consistent with scientific thinking, and the empirical tests will show whether the system works. For example, homoeopathy works although the underlying principles may not be acceptable to scientific system of medicine.

Corporate Perspective

Corporate organizations benefit from health. If the workers are healthy, they will be happy and motivated. Also, as part of practising corporate social responsibility, they provide health benefits to their workers. This takes the form of providing hospital services, full or partial reimbursement of medical bills, provision for medical leave, and safety measures.

So far government and many private business organizations have taken the responsibility of providing health care to their employees. While the employees were young, morbidity rates among employees were relatively low, and the organizations could bear the cost of providing health facilities. How will they react when increasing number of employees will be suffering from cancer, HIV/AIDS and other such problems which require very heavy expenditure and a sound management approach? How would the fellow workers react to such diseases? These are some questions which need answer. Some crucial issues are: how is corporate social responsibility defined? To what extent the corporate organizations feel responsible for employees and community? What can they do without losing the goal of profit? What will they gain by showing responsibility towards the various stakeholders?

Health Workers' Perspective

There are no known studies of workers in private hospitals. Studies of health workers in India are studies of public health officials, particularly those working at the grassroots level in the villages. Health workers are blamed for carelessness and inefficiency. It is disparagingly said that doctors posted at government health centres do not stay at the centre, do not update their knowledge, do not show sensitivity to community problems, engage in unethical and corrupt practices, are biased, go by caste and kinship considerations, and suffer from political interference. Similarly, grassroots workers do not stay at their place of work, do not work properly, have no power, lack support and look for political patronage. All this may be true. Yet, one has to understand the place of work in their life and conditions. What is their understanding of work and life? What is their understanding of organizational climate and organizational culture? What do the seniors tell about things and people when a new person joins? How do they define ethics and responsibility?

Health workers in the health profession are not necessarily by choice. They have the same goals and aspirations as others. In the globalizing society, ridden with various risks and anxieties, they are working in unacceptable situations. To make them effective organization can play a crucial role. Operations research only can tell how they can effectively combine their social and organizational roles.

The Issues

In the light of the above, further studies are required in the following fields:

(1) To explore the concepts of health and illness among the communities using fieldwork or ethnographic methods.
(2) To understand the existing beliefs, values and practices among people regarding the health-seeking behaviour.
(3) To explore the nature and availability of the traditional medicine system, especially to explore the availability of traditional herbal medicines.
(4) To analyze the background of the traditional health practitioners (including local healers), and modern health providers, and their ideas of work and life.
(5) To examine the effectiveness of community health system and ways of empowering people for health initiatives using participatory methodologies.
(6) To examine reach and effectiveness of health infrastructure in the tribal areas and among other disadvantaged groups.

The above discussion is an argument for study of what Caldwell calls the health transition. This includes the social, behavioural, cultural and ideational changes that accompany mortality decline and improved health (Caldwell and Santow, 2002). Health can no more be separated from cultural and ideational changes, whether at the micro level or the macro level, and one has to recognize that any theory of health is based on a perspective. There is a caveat here. In India, although the impact of health transition is obvious, the pre-transitional diseases and class inequalities in them have stayed. Therefore, the importance of social inequalities in various risks, utilization of health facilities and management of health institutions cannot be ignored.

Conclusion

The dominant perspective on health is the biomedical perspective. This needs to be changed. There is a need to look at health resources and health ideas from different perspectives. This would not only provide a fresh insight into the issues related to health but also make the health management in society more effective. Health studies would gain by incorporating the perspectives of tribes, women, minorities, the sick, alternative medicines, corporate world, and health workers who are actually working at the grassroots level in the public health programmes. Epidemiologic transition has already shifted attention from biomedical model to models incorporating lifestyles and life conditions. In any study of health at the social level these new factors cannot be overlooked.

Acknowledgement

The author wishes to thank Dr. Munmun Jha for going through the earlier draft of the paper and making useful suggestions.

References

Addlakha, Renu and Aruna, Grover (2000). User configuration and perspective: Hepatitis B introductory trial in east Delhi. *Economic and Political Weekly, 35*, 736-743.

Barry, Anne-Marie and Chris Yuill (2002). *Understanding Health: A Sociological Introduction.* Sage Publications.

Caldwell, J.C. and Santow, G. (2002). *Selected Readings in the Cultural, Social and Behavioural Determinants of Health.* Health Transition Series No. 1. Health Transition Centre. The Australian National University. Canberra: Highland Press.

Foucault, M. (1973). *The Birth of the Clinic.* Tavistock, London.

Goldman, N. (2002). Incorporating health into demographic training. *Genus, 58*, 3-4.

http://www.ayuherbal.com/diabetes.htm, 22 February 2003.

http://www.essaybank.co.uk/free_coursework/2611.html, 16 February 2003.

Kleinman, Arthur (1980). *Patients and Healers in the Context of Culture: An Exploration of the Borderland between Anthropology, Medicine and Psychiatry*. University of California Press, Berkeley.

Lane, Sandra D. and Donald, A. Cibula (2002). Gender and health. In Albrecht, Gary L, Ray Fitzpatrick and Susan C. Scrimshaw, *ibid.*, (pp. 36-153).

Lorber, Judith and Lisa, Jean, Moore (2000). *Gender and the Social Construction of Illness.* AltaMira Press.

Maiti, Sameera (2003 April). Study of ethnomedicine among the Bhotia of Chamoli (Uttaranchal). Paper presented at the National Seminar on Social Dimensions of Health, April 10-12, Centre for Behavioural and Cognitive Sciences, University of Allahabad, Allahabad.

Manning, Peter K. and Horacio, Fabrega, Jr. (1973). The experience of self and body: Health and illness in the Chiapas Highlands. In Psathas, George (Ed.), *Phenomenological Sociology: Issues and Applications* (pp. 251-301). New York: John Wiley and Sons.

Naik, S. and Sharma, A.K. (1985). Social structure and family planning: A case study of two tribal villages. *The Journal of Family Welfare*, December.

Pandey, Arvind (2002). Demographic transition and global health: An overview. In Kumar, Anil (Ed.), *Epidemiology, Health and Population.* Delhi: B.R. Publishing Corporation.

Ratzan, S.C., Garyn, L.F. and John, W.L. (2000). Attaining global health: Challenges and opportunities. *Population Bulletin*, 55.

Ray, Pratibha (2001). *The Primal Land*. Orient Longman.

Retherford, R.D. and Roy, T.K. (2003). *Factors Affecting Sex-Selective Abortion in India and 17 Major States.* IIPS Mumbai and East-West Centre Program on Population. Honolulu: Hawaii.

Shankar, Darshan (1995). Tribal medicine revisited. In Sunanda, K.S. (Ed.), *Grassroots Action*. Madras.

Sharma, A.K. (1996). Muslim fertility in urban U.P.: A qualitative study. *Demography India*, *23,* 41-49.

Sharma, A.K., Shikha, Dixit and Mamta, Misra (2002 December). Social construction of health and illness among women. Paper presented at the IRMS Silver Jubilee and XX Annual Conference of Indian Society of Medical Statistics, AIIMS, New Delhi, December, 19-22.

Thakur, C.P. (2002). Convocation address. *IIPS Newsletter,* IIPS, Mumbai.

Unnithan-Kumar, Maya (1999). Households, kinship and access to reproductive health care among rural Muslim women in Jaipur. *Economic and Political Weekly*, *34,* 621-630.

Verma, S.S. (2002). Statistical models for estimation of human performance. In Pandey, C.M., Pradeep Mishra and Uttam Singh (Eds.), *Biostatistical Aspects of Health and Epidemiology*. SGPGI, Lucknow.

WHO, *The World Health Report 2002*, http://www.who.int/whr/2002/Overview_E.pdf.

II

Indigenous Health Care Practices

6

Demographic Structure and Health Care Practices of Dhodia Tribal Population of District Valsad, Gujarat

GAUTAM K. KSHATRIYA AND A.K. KAPOOR

Over the past fifty years significant progress has been achieved in the context of economic, social and demographic attributes of India. Nevertheless, there still exists a strong inter-regional demographic disparity. Diverse social and cultural characteristics of Indian population are major contributory factors to such a varied demographic scenario besides many others. Moreover, inequalities continue to persist in the sphere of health care delivery system. The health problems need special attention in the context of tribal communities of India because of their settlements in difficult areas and circumstances. The health, nutrition and medico-genetic problems of diverse tribal groups inhabiting widely varying geo-climatic conditions present a formidable challenge for effective health care delivery. Similarly, the common beliefs, customs and practices connected with health and disease are intimately connected with the treatment of disease.

Few studies of this nature are available from the state of Gujarat. Basu (1995 and 1996) undertook social assessment studies of tribal health on Bhils and Rathwas of district Vadodara and on

Patelias of district Panchmahals. The study on Bhils and Rathwas was related with their perception, attitude and experience for the acceptability and the demand for the treatment of tuberculosis. The study on Patelias was undertaken to understand the utilization of the social services being offered by the government in tribal areas, to assess the perception and attitude related to health-seeking behaviour, and to conduct a need assessment of capacity building for better implementation of malaria control programme. Barring these two studies, which were oriented to specific national health programmes, little information is available on the health-seeking behaviour vis-à-vis the role of health providers in the tribes of Gujarat.

This paper, therefore, examines the demographic structure, health care practices and the role of health care providers among the Dhodias of district Valsad, Gujarat. The trends are discussed in the light of prevailing social, economic and cultural traditions. An attempt is also made to compare the fertility and mortality estimates with the population of Gujarat and Indian national population derived from Sample Registration System (1999) and *Census of India (2001)*.

Valsad District

The Valsad town of Gujarat does not find any reference before A.D. 1300. The opinion of some of the learned persons residing here is that the original name of this place was Nyagrodhpur. In Sanskrit, Nyagrodh means *Vad* (fig tree). Somebody might have thought about Nyagrodhpur keeping in mind the work *Val-Vad* occurring in Valsad. There might have been a cluster of fig trees here and so the name 'Valsad' might have been accepted. The name of the district has been kept Valsad from the name of Valsad town.

The district of Valsad is bounded on north by Navsari district of Gujarat, on the east by the state of Maharashtra, on the south by Dadra and Nagar Haveli and Maharashtra state and on the west by the Arabian Sea. It is situated between 20°07' and 21°5' north latitude and between 72°43' and 73°00' east longitude. The total area of the district is 5,244 sq. kms., comprising 2.68 percent of the total area of the state of Gujarat. The district headquarters is located at Valsad. Recently, the Government of Gujarat bifurcated Valsad district into two separate districts, namely, Valsad and Navarasi. At present, Valsad district has five *talukas*, namely, Valsad, Pardi, Dharmpur, Kaprada and Umergaon. As per the District Statistical Handbook (1997-98), there were 826 inhabited villages in Valsad district. Ever since the division of Valsad district into Valsad and Navsari, the former now has 452 inhabited villages. The total population of the district according to 1991 census was 21,73,672 comprising 11,10,632 males and 10,63,040 females. The ratio of females per thousand males was 957.

Dhodia is one of the major scheduled tribes mostly found in Surat and Valsad districts of south Gujarat. Regarding the origin of Dhodia, they do not have exact history but have different interpretations and beliefs. It is believed that the term 'Dhodia' has been derived form Dhulia – a place in Maharashtra from where two Rajput princes came to Gujarat and married Naika women. Another legend traces their origin to Dholka-Dhandhuka – a place near the south bank of the Narmada river. The term 'Dhodia' is also derived from the word 'Daudia'. According to the Dhodias, they were soldiers in the army of the local king. During the war, some soldiers fled from the battlefield. These soldiers had lost their courage to fight. The people who ran away from the battlefield are known as Dhodias. The literal meaning of the word 'Daud', both in Hindi and Gujarati, is "to run", hence the name 'Dhodia'. The term Dhodias might also have been derived from *'Dhur'* or 'soil' because the Dhodias are essentially agriculturalists and have to work on soil. Some also believe that the Dhodias were originally from Saurashtra, and belonged to the 'Yadav' *kul* (clan) of Lord Krishna of the Mahabharata. They believe themselves as the descendants of the prince of Dwarka, who later migrated to south Gujarat. Therefore, the Dhodia community domesticates 'cow' (symbolically associated with Lord Krishna) and worships it on a particular festival called *Bhagabarash*. Thus, it can be inferred that the Dhodias are not the original inhabitants of the district but have migrated from other districts of north and west Gujarat.

Material and Methods

In the present investigation, about 994 Dhodia households from 26 randomly selected villages belonging to three different *talukas*, namely, Valsad, Pardi and Umergaon, were studied. Fertility and mortality data as well as data on health care practices and the role of health providers were collected using a semi-structured interview schedule. Data on reproductive performance were collected by pregnancy enumeration. The collected information was further cross-checked from elderly members of the households and sometimes from village elders also. The average parity was calculated in each 5-year age interval for the women in the child-bearing ages. Thus, the mean parity of the women at the end of child-bearing age may be designated as the total fertility.

Since most of our information is based on oral reports, indirect estimation techniques were employed for calculating total fertility rate (TFR). The fertility levels as calculated by indirect estimation method suggests that the ratio of the average parity of women at the end of child-bearing age to the average parity of women in the younger age group (women in the age group of 25-29 years) is closely related to the relative mean parity of women early and late in their twenties, i.e., $T.F./P_3 = P_3/P_2$, where T.F. = total fertility, P_2 = parity of the women in the age group (20-24) years, and P_3 = parity of women in the age group (25-29) years (United Nations, 1967).

Similarly, in the absence of exact ages at death of offspring, indirect estimation (Brass and Coale, 1968; Brass, 1975) was used to assess mortality. This method translates proportions of surviving and dead among the children born to women in different age groups into conventional measures of mortality.

Assessment of the nutritional status of the Dhodia boys and girls was undertaken through a set of 12 measurements in the age group 0-6 years. These measurements include crown heel length/ standing height, body weight, skin fold at biceps, triceps, sub-scapular, calf and supra iliac, waist circumference, hip circumference, head circumference, chest circumference and mid-upper arm circumference. A total of 332 subjects (174 boys and 158 girls) were measured in different age groups for the above set of measurements. Measurements were undertaken following the procedure as described in Lohman *et al.* (1988). The anthropometric data from the present investigation were compared with the available anthropometric data on boys and girls as provided by ICMR (1984) and Ghosh (1992).

Further, 2 ml venous blood was collected in EDTA (anti-coagulant) bulb from each of the 131 adult males and 251 adult females through disposable syringes. Haemoglobin (Hb) estimation of the collected blood samples was undertaken for assessing the status of nutritional anaemia. These blood samples were also subjected to the test for sickling and thereafter those identified as sicklers were further confirmed through cellulose acetate electrophoresis for the status of heterozygous and homozygous. The analysis of blood samples was carried out following the procedure given by Verma *et al.* (1994).

Results and Discussion

Socio-economic Profile of Dhodias

An overwhelming majority of 99.90 percent (n=994) of Dhodia population follows Hinduism. The Dhodias are not very mobile as can be seen from a mean marital distance of 13.35 kms ±0.63 kms. Regarding family types, it can be seen from the Table 1 that nuclear families among the Dhodias preponderate with a frequency of 65.4 percent. As far as marriage is concerned, monogamy is the rule, which accounts for 99 percent of the total number of marriages (n=994). The mean age at marriage for males in the Dhodias was found to be 21.09 years ±3.36 years, with a range of 12 years through 39 years. Similarly, the mean age at marriage for females in the present study was recorded as 18.03 years ±2.86 years, with a range of 11 years through 35 years. Since the age at marriage of both males and females in the Dhodias conforms to the constitutional provisions, 99.6 percent of the newly married couples (n=994) start living together immediately after marriage. It is to be pointed out here that a relatively higher mean age at marriage also contributes to low crude death rate (CDR) among the Dhodias, which is surely a positive sign in the direction of health status. Age at menarche among Dhodia women was estimated to be 13.6 years ±1.08 years.

Table 1
Distribution of Family Types

Types of Family	*Number of Families*	
	No.	*%*
Nuclear	650	65.4
Joint	247	24.8
Extended	97	9.8
Total	994	100.0

Lifestyle

In the present investigation, it was found that for drinking purpose, majority (83%) of the households (Table 2) use water from bored well as the primary source and only a handful of households use other sources of drinking water. In 78 percent of cases, the source was located within the village and in rest within the house. Thus, quite a few number of Dhodia households have their own boring in the house. It can be seen from Table 3 that 50.8 percent of the houses of Dhodias are *kachha* (mud plastered, hay, wood, etc), 33.6 percent are *pucca* (cemented) and only 15.6 percent are semi-*pucca* (wood and cemented). About 99.4 percent of the respondents have their own houses. Table 4 shows that 98.6 percent of the houses are electrified. It is also significant to note that 50.5 percent of the houses use LPG as fuel for cooking and equally important is the fact that 48.7 percent of the houses still use cowdung and firewood for cooking

Table 2
Sources of Drinking Water

Source	*No. of Families/Users*	
	No.	*%*
River	1	.1
Boring	824	82.9
Tap (owned)	28	2.8
Well	141	14.2
Total	994	100.0

and other purposes. Likewise, 85.6 percent of the (n=992) houses do not have provision for own toilets and defecate outside and the rest possess own flush toilets. In the present study, it appears (Table 5) that 99 percent of the houses have no drainage, which is a perpetual source of poor environment and hygiene and is chiefly responsible for mosquito breeding and also a potential source for fungal and bacterial infections leading to communicable diseases.

Table 3
House Types

Types	*No. of Houses*	
	No.	*%*
Kachha	505	50.8
Pucca	334	33.6
Semi-*pucca*	155	15.6
Total	994	100.0

Table 4
Sources of Lighting

Source	*No. of Houses*	
	No.	*%*
Electricity	980	98.6
Kerosene	8	0.8
Others	6	0.6
Total	994	100.0

Table 5
Disposal of Waste Water

Disposal Categories	*No. of Houses*	
	No.	*%*
Closed drainage	3	0.3
Open drainage	8	0.8
No drainage	982	98.9
Total	993	100.0

Standard of Living Index

On the basis of the above description of various amenities that the Dhodias enjoy, a standard of living index was formulated. Each category of amenities that Dhodias own (9 in all) was ranked from 0 through 6, depending on its recency, technology and its probable relationship with the economic background of the household. The index was classified into three categories. The maximum score a household can get is 26 and the minimum is 0. An index less than 15 indicated a comparatively poor economic status, an index between 15 through 19 indicated a fairly good economic condition and an index above 20 indicated prosperity. The households thus classified are presented in Table 6, which makes it clear that 67 percent of the households thus ranked are relatively poor whereas only 10 percent are prosperous and the remaining 23 percent are between the two. Cows, buffaloes and bulls/oxen are the main domesticated animals among the Dhodias. About 76.4 percent of Dhodia households (n=980) have agricultural land, and only 52 percent of the occupied agricultural land (n=749) is irrigated.

Table 6

Standard of Living Index

Categories/Ranks	*No. of Households*	
	No.	%
<15 (relatively poor)	663	66.7
15-19 (fairly good)	230	23.2
>20 (prosperous)	101	10.1
Total	994	100.0

Occupation and Income

Table 7 presents the pattern of occupation among the Dhodias. It can be seen that there is a great degree of variability in the occupational pattern. Besides being primarily agriculturists, they have taken up private and government jobs and also have started their own business. The pattern of annual household income shows that 59 percent of the Dhodia households are relatively poor, 40 percent belong to middle-income group and only around 1 percent can be considered as prosperous (Table 8). This classification is almost similar to the one described above in the context of standard of living index.

Table 7

Types of Occupation

Types	*No.*	*%*
Labour	377	24.23
Private job	397	25.51
Agriculture	415	26.67
Government job	207	13.30
Business	160	10.29
Total	1556	100.0

Table 8

Annual Household Incomes During Last One Year (all sources pooled)

Categories	*No. of Households*	
	No.	*%*
<Rs. 25,000 (poor)	585	58.85
Rs.25,000-60,000 (lower middle)	286	28.77
Rs. 60,000-1,50,000 (moderate)	109	10.97
>Rs. 1,50,000 (Prosperous)	14	1.41
Total	994	100.0

Literacy

Literacy rate, as evident from Table 9, turns out to be 82.57 percent among the Dhodias, which is a very significant observation in the present study. Female literacy rate was found to be 73.6 percent. Out of those who are literate, 29 percent are primary educated, and similar percentage of subjects is middle school and high school educated. Literacy rate among the Dhodias is much higher than its corresponding figure of 26 percent in Indian tribal groups: 61.29 percent for Gujarat and 65.38 percent for Indian national population. Thus, literacy is a very good social indicator, which goes a long way in moulding the attitude of people towards modern medical practices and decision-making.

Table 9
Literacy Rate

Literacy	*No.*	*%*
Illiterate	770	17.45
Literate	3642	82.55
Total	4412	100.0
Literates		
Primary School	1072	29.43
Middle School	1017	27.92
High School	977	26.83
Higher Secondary	332	9.12
Graduate and others	244	6.70
Total	3642	100.00

Note: Children less than 6 years of age excluded.

In short, the Dhodias are in a transitional phase, i.e., a mixture of both prosperity and deprivation and traditional and modern syntheses. Traditions have bonded them to rigid cultural practices, but they are opening up to modern developmental and health schemes that are being introduced by both governmental and non-governmental agencies. The social and economic profile and the lifestyle of the Dhodias have a linear relationship with the health status of community. Many amenities of Dhodias have a direct bearing on various vector-borne diseases as well as communicable fungal and bacterial diseases. They are being educated and have now come a long way to combat many distressing morbid conditions with the help of various NGOs and governmental agencies.

Demographic Trends

In the present study, a population of 5,198 individuals of the Dhodia community was covered from three different *talukas*, viz., Valsad, Pardi and Umergaon, on the coastal belt, representing a total of 994 households from 26 villages.

Effective Population Size

It is impossible to estimate the effective population size from census population because they have overlapping generations. Nei (1965) obtained a simple equation for deriving effective population size in such a situation:

$$N_e = t\, N_m$$

where N_e = effective population size,
t = generation time, i.e., mean age at reproduction in years,
N_m = number of individuals who reach the mean reproductive age per year.

Alternatively, N_e can be estimated as N_e = tbpN
where

$$t = \frac{\sum[\text{no. of individuals of age x}][\text{no. of birth per year born of a parent of age x}]}{\sum(\text{no. of birth per year born of a parent of age x})}$$

b = crude birth rate,
p = probability of survival upto the age of reproduction,
N = total number of breeding individuals.

The effective population size refers to the breeding individuals who actually contribute to the gene pool of the next generation, which is small as compared to the size of the general population. This provides clue to the differential fertility and mortality and to the number of individuals really reaching the reproductive age.

The effective population size of the Dhodias is estimated to be 2,280.

Age and Sex Composition

The age structure of the Dhodias (Table 10) indicates that 32.77 percent of males and 30.83 percent of females are less than 15 years of age. If males and females are taken together, 31.82 percent of total population is below 15 years of age. Similarly, it can be seen that 60.51 percent of males and 62.14 percent of females are below 30 years of age. The age structure indicates that the Dhodias have a broad base and then from 15 to 40 years, the structure is fairly stable without any tapering. The structure starts tapering towards the apex only after 50 years, indicating that the period between 15 and 50 years does not experience any significant mortality in different age groups.

Table 10
Age and Sex Composition

Age Group (in years)	*Males*		*Females*		*Total*	
	No.	*%*	*No.*	*%*	*No.*	*%*
0-5	397	14.99	303	11.89	700	13.47
5-10	241	9.10	267	10.47	508	9.77
10-15	230	8.68	261	10.24	446	8.58
15-20	222	8.38	239	9.38	461	8.87
20-25	234	8.83	295	11.57	529	10.18
25-30	279	10.53	264	10.36	543	10.44
30-35	235	8.87	195	7.65	430	8.27
35-40	193	7.28	167	6.55	360	6.93
40-45	131	4.95	125	4.90	256	4.92
45-50	179	6.76	149	5.85	328	6.31
50-55	103	3.89	76	2.98	179	3.44
55-60	67	2.53	79	3.10	146	2.81
60-65	53	2.0	67	2.63	120	2.31
65-70	30	1.13	42	1.65	72	1.39
70+	57	2.15	65	2.55	120	2.31
Total	2649	100.00	2549	100.00	5198	100.00

The sex ratio of the Dhodias was found to be 962 per thousand males, which is higher than that of Gujarat (921) and Indian national population (933) at 2001. A comparative view of sex ratio thus reflects a very encouraging and positive trend in the overall demographic features of the Dhodias.

Fertility Indicators

Total fertility rate (TFR) among the Dhodia women in various childbearing age groups is 3.44 (Table 11), estimated from the average parity of women in the age group 45-49 years. Indirect estimation of the total fertility calculated from $(P_{(3)})^2/P_2$ has been found to be 3.97 which differs little from the observed fertility rate for the women in the age group 45-49 years.

The age specific fertility rates (ASFRs) of the Dhodias are comparable to India and Gujarat (Table 12). Moreover, TFR estimated on the basis of ASFRs comes out to be 3.86, which is comparable to direct and indirect estimates of TFR. TFR for

Gujarat has been estimated as 3.0 and for Indian national population as 3.2 (Table 13). The general fertility rate (GFR) for the Dhodias was estimated to be 123, which is comparable to Indian national population of 125.2 and Gujarat of 110.3 (Table 13). Crude birth rate (CBR) for the Dhodias has been estimated to be 24.5, which is below the Indian national population (26.1) and for the population of Gujarat (25.4) (Table 13).

Table 11

Estimation of Fertility and Mean Age at Child Bearing from Age Specific Average Parities

Age Group (in years)	*Number of Women*	*No. of Births*	*Mean Parity*
15-19	17	12	0.706
20-24	168	226	1.345
25-29	200	462	2.310
30-34	193	479	2.482
35-39	132	378	2.864
40-44	117	350	2.991
45-49	91	313	3.440
Total	918	2220	2.418

Estimated total fertility $= [P_{(3)}{}^2/P_{(2)}] = 3.97$

Mean age at child-bearing = m = 27.81

Table 12

ASFRs of the Dhodias, Gujarat and Indian National Population

Age Group (in years)	*ASFRs*		
	Dhodias	*Gujarat*	*India*
15-19	118	87	107
20-24	202	230	210
25-29	240	148	143
30-34	78	52	69
35-39	23	18	28
40-44	34	5	8
45-49	77	3	3

Table 13
Fertility and Mortality Indicators in Dhodias, Gujarat and Indian National Population

Statistic	*Dhodias*	*Gujarat*	*India*
GFR	123	110.3	125.2
TFR	3.86	3.0**	3.2**
CBR	24.5	25.4**	26.1**
CDR	7.8	7.9**	8.7**
IMR	73	63**	70**
Sex ratio	962	921*	933*
Growth rate		2.03*	1.93*
Rate of natural increase	16.7	17.5**	17.4**

Figures in parentheses represent natural increase.

Sources: * 2001, Census of India (Provisional)
** SRS, 1999

Mortality Indicators

Crude death rate (CDR) among the Dhodias has been estimated to be 7.8, which is lower than the Indian national population (8.7) and the population of Gujarat (7.9) (Table 13). Infant mortality rate (IMR) is a very sensitive indicator of mortality indicating a prenatal, natal and post-natal care of mother and infants. IMR among the Dhodias has been estimated to be 73/1,000 live births, which is comparable to the Indian national population (70/1,000 live births) and to the population of Gujarat (63/1,000 live births) (Table 13).

Rate of natural increase for the Dhodias was found to be 16.7, which is comparable to the Indian national population (17.4) and population of Gujarat (17.5) (Table 13). Once again, this variable, i.e., rate of natural increase, is very similar in all the three groups.

Life Expectancy at Birth

The distribution of age-specific mortality among the Dhodias together with multiplying factors K_a and the resulting q(a) values is presented in Table 14 along with life expectancy at birth. These estimates are based on q_5 values and interpolated from Brass one parameter model life table (Carrier and Hob Craft, 1971). Life expectancy at birth among the Dhodias is estimated as 61.9 years for total population, while this figure is comparable to the Indian national population (males=62.3; females=65.27) (Statistical Abstract of India, 1997); it is much higher than the reported figure of life expectancy at birth for various tribal groups in India (Kshatriya, 2000).

Table 14

Estimation of Age-Specific Mortality among the Dhodias

Age Group (in years)	*No. of children dead*	K_a*	*Age-specific child mortality*	
			*D***	*q (a)* ***
15-19	-	0.886	-	-
20-24	14	0.956	0.062	0.059
25-29	33	0.961	0.071	0.068
30-34	37	0.973	0.077	0.075
35-39	32	1.013	0.085	0.086
40-44	36	0.990		0.102
45-49	40	0.988		0.126

e_0 based on 61.9 years

$^{o}q_5$ values

*Multiplier for age (a), Brass (1975). Ages 1-5 based on P2/P3; ages 10-20 based on m=27.81

** Proportion of children dead

*** Probability of dying by age (a)

Thus, the demographic information on Dhodias clearly indicates that they are progressive and that their attitudes, beliefs and awareness are being canalized in a desired route under the influence of changing social and economic conditions and also the impact of various developmental and health programmes.

Morbidity Pattern and Common Diseases

Information gathered from the district hospital regarding morbidity profile is presented in Table 15. It can be seen that intestinal disorders, arthropod-born diseases (malaria, unspecified fevers), nutritional deficiencies (marasmus, protein calorie malnutrition), diseases of blood forming organs (anaemia), respiratory disorders, diseases of oral cavities, diseases of digestive system, skin disease and genetic disorders (sickle cell anaemia) are fairly common. This is understandable, because the morbidity pattern reflects the existing health care practices, environmental sanitation, food habits and lifestyle of the people of Valsad.

Table 15

Morbidity Profile of the Dhodias (2001-02)

S.No.	*Ailments*	*No. of individuals who had taken treatment*	
		No.	*%*
1.	Intestinal disorders	2790	11.48*
2.	Tuberculosis	636	2.62
3.	Other bacterial diseases	150	0.62
4.	Viral diseases	420	0.73
5.	Arthropod borne diseases (fever and malaria)	2145	8.84*
6.	Endocrine and metabolic diseases (diabetes)	130	0.54
7.	Nutritional deficiencies	1165	4.80
	(i) Marasmus	255	1.04
	(ii) Protein calorie malnutrition	910	3.75
8.	Disease of blood and blood forming organs (anaemias)	4225	17.39*
9.	Diseases of the nervous system (meningitis and epilepsy)	17	0.06
10.	Disorders of the eye	195	0.81
	(i) Glaucoma	28	0.11
	(ii) Cataract	142	0.59
	(iii) Conjunctivitis	25	0.10
11.	Diseases of the ear and mastoid process	550	2.26
	(i) Oritis and mastoiditis	540	2.22
	(ii) Deafness	10	0.04
12.	Rheumatic fever	74	0.30
13.	Hypertensive diseases	503	2.07
14.	Heart diseases	802	3.30
15.	Respiratory disorders (tonsillitis, bronchitis, pneumonia, influenza, pleurisy)	4107	16.90*
16.	Diseases of the oral cavity	1034	4.25*
17.	Diseases of the digestive system	1443	5.95*
18.	Disease of the urinary system	290	1.19
19.	Diseases of the male genital organs	186	0.77
20.	Diseases of the female genital organs	363	1.49
21.	Abortion	333	1.37
22.	Direct obstetric causes (haemorrhage of pregnancy childbirth, toxaemia of pregnancy, major puerperium, infections of genito urinary tract in pregnancy, obstructed labour and other complications)	140	0.58
23.	Diseases of skin	2258	9.29*
24.	Diseases of the musculoskeletal system (arthritis and ankylosing spondylitis	27	0.11
25.	Congenital malformation	10	0.04
26.	Fractures	299	1.23
	Total	24292	100

* Frequent morbid conditions

Common Health Problems among Dhodias

Responses of 994 Dhodia individuals were grouped (after consulting with government and private health providers and after interpreting the local name of the disease and symptoms of the illness into defined category) into 10 broad categories (Table 16). These categories are leptospirosis, intestinal/oral disorders, acute respiratory infection (ARI)/upper respiratory tract infection (URTI)/ear nose and throat (ENT), urinary tract infection (UTI)/sexually transmitted disease (STD)/reproductive tract infection (RTI), arthritis/body pain/fracture, jaundice, skin disease/leprosy, malaria/unspecified fever, tuberculosis (TB) and anaemia. Table 16 summarizes the responses of the 994 Dhodia individuals regarding their perception of common ailments. From the table it appears that the Dhodias feel that intestinal/oral disorders, respiratory infections, urinary and reproductive tract infections, arthritis, jaundice, skin diseases, anaemia, malaria and TB are the common problems. Out of these, gastroenteritis/oral disorders, respiratory infections, arthritis and jaundice are the commonest of common, which is in accordance with the data available from the civil hospital. Further, 16 percent of the 382 individuals tested for abnormal haemoglobin were found to be sicklers, and three of the 61 sicklers were homozygous for haemoglobin S (HbS). HbS gene is found to occur with a frequency of 8 percent and is a cause of great concern.

Table 16

Common Health Problems among the Dhodias (self-reported)

Categories	*f**	%
Leptospirosis	17	1.70
Intestinal/oral disorders	882	88.73
ARI/URTI/ENT	874	87.93
UTI/STD/RTI	328	32.99
Arthritis/body pain/fracture	550	55.72
Jaundice	524	52.72
Skin disease/leprosy	424	42.65
Malaria/unspecified fever	366	36.82
TB	278	27.97
Anaemia	442	42.45

*N=994

Table 17
Pattern of Traditional Treatment

Indigenous Plants	*Ailments*
1. *Garadia* Bark of Garadia tree/plants is crushed with vala root to paste and them paste is mixed with water and is taken in divided doses in the morning for two days, empty stomach.	Jaundice
2. *Ber* Bark of the Ber trees is crushed to a paste and the paste is mixed with water and the syrup is then taken according to the need in fever.	Fever
3. *Arjun Shadhoda* Bark of the Arjun Shadhoda tree is pounded to a paste and is then mixed with water for consumption in diarrhoea.	Diarrhoea
4. *Karan Javeli* Leaves, stem and root of the tree are boiled in water. Half a cup of the drink is taken in the morning, empty stomach, every day.	Acidity/gastric problems
5. *Tulsi* Tulsi leaves are boiled in water or taken in the form of tea.	Cough and cold
6. *Adusha* Leaves of the tree are boiled in water and the drink is taken for treatment in cold and cough.	Cough and cold
7. *Neem* Leaves of the tree are boiled with water and the drink is taken to cure fever.	Fever
8. *Shangh Jeera* Drink is prepared by mixing lemon juice with water and shangh jeera and is consumed in gastric problem.	Diarrhoea
9. *Chanothi Herb* Chanothi herb is pounded and is taken with juice.	Worm infection
10. *Shitafal* Root of the tree is pounded to a paste and the paste is applied on the wound.	Dog bite
11. Local healer use mantras to take out the poison.	Snake bite
12. Dough made out of following items is used for treating burn victim: (i) Tamarind (ii) Cowdung (iii) Haldi (turmeric) (iv) Oil (edible) or coconut oil (v) Banana plant juice (vi) Cold water	Burn cases
13. *Lili* Leaf of the tree is pounded to a paste and the paste is mixed with water and is consumed in divided doses.	Gall bladder

Mean Hb values for men (14.25 g/100 ml blood) and women (12.27 g/100 ml blood) are towards lower range of the normal values. Nutritional anaemia as reflected from haemoglobin determination, both in men and women, is of a mild nature.

Health-seeking Behaviour

Concept of Illness

Health-seeking behaviour of a person is determined by his social and economic background, knowledge, education, cultural practices, availability of providers together with accessibility and affordability. The Dhodias believe both in supernatural (i.e., evil eye and ancestral spirit) and physical (such as food, accident, weather and natural calamities) as causation of disease. A person is considered to be sick when poor health incapacitates a person from undertaking normal routine.

Traditional Way of Treatment

For the treatment of various diseases, the Dhodias seek help from the traditional healers (*Bhagat-Bhua*), allopathic and ayurvedic services providers, both private and government. If the treatment given by the local healer is not effective, then they go to consult a doctor or vice versa.

The traditional method of treatment includes use of charm, animal sacrifice, propitiation of disease-related spirits, worshipping of deities and belief in protective function of rituals. Thus, magico-religious practices, as a part of religion, are also effectively used in the treatment of various ailments.

Further, traditional treatment using various medicinal plants for various ailments is undertaken as remedial measure. Table 17 presents various traditional medicines used for the treatment of various diseases.

Allopathic Medicine/Treatment

Most of the Dhodias prefer allopathic system of medicine rather than any other system, although their preferences remain with traditional healing practices. The main reason might be the immediate effect of the medicines as most of them are wage earners in industries. Ayurvedic or homeopathic medicines do not give immediate relief. The other reason might be the increased awareness among people about competency of qualified doctors and potency of drugs.

Primary Health Centres (PHCs)/sub-centres are the nearest health institutions located near the users. All the respondents opined that services like immunization, ante-natal check-up (ANC), post-natal check-up (PNC)/family planning (FP), clinical check-up and laboratory facilities were available only at the district hospital and at the community health centre. About 36 percent of all respondents stated that PHC was within 5 kms from the place of residence. Over 99 percent of them responded that four of the five essential services were available with PHCs (immunization, ANC, PNC/FP, clinical check-up). However, only 50 percent said that diagnostic laboratory facilities were available at PHC. Similarly, at sub-centre, laboratory facilities are not available. About 42.5 percent of the respondents reported that the sub-centre is located nearest to their places of residence. Some 14.2 percent informed that private health institution was near their place of residence. One distinctive feature of private health providers was that in general they did not provide ANC services, immunization and FP services. It was taken for granted that such services were the responsibility of the government. Respondents unanimously opined that private health providers provided clinical and laboratory services.

Around 88.7 percent of respondents felt that intestinal and oral disorders were common in the community. More than 40 percent were of the opinion that respiratory disorders, TB, anaemia, veneral diseases, jaundice, sickle cell, skin diseases, malaria, unspecified fever, diarrhoea, dysentery, arthritis, body pain, fractures were common among the tribal population of the Dhodias. Of all the medical facilities available to them, 58.1 percent of the Dhodia respondents preferred private health providers. The second in order of preference is PHC.

In fact, a total of 30.27 percent of the Dhodias preferred going to PHC as their first choice. In spite of the differences of the responses given by Dhodias, it was observed that their responses had an element of bias, as it was found that utilizing private health services was also linked with economic status and infrastructural set-up at PHC.

However, their preference was based on the proximity of the health institution and the availability of health services. The two main reasons for preferring the services of private providers were: (a) private health providers were always available (91.8% of users of private health services opined that way), and (b) they did not have to wait for a long time for check-up and that medicines were given on credit as well (84.5% of the Dhodia users had such opinion).

At least 651 individuals reported to have fallen sick during the last three months. Respiratory infections, gastric and oral cavity problems, arthritis, jaundice, TB, skin diseases are the common health problems among the Dhodias. They consult private health providers (54.2% of all cases) and government health providers (28.7% of all cases) in order of preference. About 85.2 percent of the respondents (844/991) have visited PHC and 81.16 percent of those who visited PHC (685/844) were satisfied with the services; 79.5 percent (671/844) of respondents felt that medical services were available with PHC.

In all, 65.29 percent of the respondents (649/994) told that they used the services of *Bhagat-Bhua* for treatment. However, 91.14 percent of the Dhodia respondents believed that traditional methods were not very useful. Most of them preferred allopathic medicines. In fact, they did not have much choice because allopathic providers were abundant.

It is interesting to note that Dhodias have compartmentalized their preference for seeking health services in different situations. For example, in the case of the younger children falling sick, the Dhodias would consult local healer first and government and private doctors later. In the case of an adult (male/female) individual falling sick they would either visit private or government health providers. But anything related with reproductive and child health (RCH), they would largely utilize the services of government health providers (this includes pregnancy, gynecological and obstetric problems and inoculation).

Maternal and Child Health Care

Utilization of ANC Services

In the present investigation, 261 women were found to have given at least one birth during the last two years and 91 women were found to be currently pregnant. It was observed that 99.6 percent of CMW (currently married women) with a birth in last two years had been registered for ante-natal services. It was further observed that 50 percent of the women were registered in the third month of pregnancy and 29 percent in the fourth month. Thus, an overwhelming majority of the pregnant women were registered in the third or the fourth month of pregnancy. Majority of CMW (96.16%) reported that one or the other health functionary had visited them during the ante-natal period.

In the present study, 59 percent of the women had at least three ante-natal check-ups, and government health providers examined 80 percent of these women. As for as Tetanus Toxoid (TT) injections are concerned, 95 percent CMW had received two doses of TT and only 5 percent CMW had received a single dose; and again, 81 percent of these women had received TT injections from government sources. As far as iron and folic acid ((IFA) consumption is concerned, the Dhodia women are not aware about the quantity to be consumed during pregnancy. About 89 percent of the CMW had consumed 10 to 120 IFA tablets during the pregnancy period, and that 88 percent of women had received IFA tablets from government sources.

Place of Delivery

In the present study, an inquiry was made about the place of delivery of those women who had given birth to a child during the last two years, and the persons who assisted at the time of delivery (Table 18). The analysis indicated that a high proportion of deliveries (66.41%) were institutional. More than two-third of these deliveries were conducted at private institutions and 32 percent in government health institutions (mainly at PHCs). A significant proportion (34%) of all deliveries was conducted at home. It can be seen that trained persons conducted 70 percent of the deliveries while traditional birth attendants (TBAs) conducted 28 percent of the deliveries.

Table 18

Distribution of the Dhodia Women by Place of Delivery and Assistance during Delivery

Place of delivery and assistance received	*Percentage (n=261)*
Women who had institutional deliveries	66.41
Types of institutions	
Government	32.2
Private	67.8
Types of assistance during delivery	
Doctor	56.3
TBA	28.0
ANM	13.8
Others	1.9

Cord Cutting

The mother and other household members were asked about the instrument used in cutting the placental cord. One of the important observations of the study is that a typical leaf of *Boru* grass is used for cutting the placental cord, which has very sharp edges like a blade on both the sides. This grass is fairly abundant and is used traditionally for cutting. In the present study, in 19 percent of the cases, *Boru* grass was used for cutting placental cord. However, the most common instrument (65%) used for cutting placental cord was a pair of scissors.

It was observed that 41 percent of the expectant mothers do not consume any specific diet during pregnancy and take same diet as they were taking before pregnancy, and 80 percent of the women were found to perform hard work (cutting and bringing woods, fetching water, lifting heavy articles etc.) even during last trimester.

Childcare Practices

Table 19 presents childcare practices among the Dhodias. It can be seen that 85 percent of the infants get their first feed as mother's milk with colostrum. Thus, infants get essential nutrition in the form of colostrum. Further, 86 percent of the infants also receive their feed within two hours of their birth. As far as initiation of supplementary diet is concerned, 78 percent of infants get their first supplementary diet between 6 and 12 months of age. Similarly, 74 percent of the Dhodia new-borns are breast-fed up to two years. Only 7 percent of Dhodia new-borns leave their mother's milk by the end of the first year of life. In the present context, two years of breast-feeding is a long duration and can be reasoned out from the fact that most of the Dhodia women are involved in household activities and in those income-generating activities that do not require them to leave their kids at home.

Table 19

Childcare Practices among the Dhodias

Childcare Practices	*Percentage*
First feed given to infant (n=259)	
Mother's milk with colostrums	84.9
Mother's milk without colostrums	12.0
Jaggery water	1.9
Any other	1.2
Age at first supplementary diet (n=229)	
6 months	48.0
6-12 months	30.2
After one year	21.8
Duration of breast-feed (n=615)	
1 year	6.7
2 years	74.5
3 years	16.5
More than 3 years	2.1

Immunization Status and Nutritional Assessment of Children

Table 20 presents the status of child immunization among the Dhodias. It is clear that Dhodias are highly motivated for immunization. In this regard, efforts of the government have been appreciable.

More than 95 percent of the children have been vaccinated for DPT, Polio and BCG. The performance in the administration of vaccination for measles and Vitamin A prophylaxis needs further strengthening of the efforts in this direction. Incidentally, government institution is the primary source of vaccination in more than 95 percent of the cases. By and large, immunization coverage is very high in the Dhodias of Valsad district. Lack of awareness and slackness among the Dhodias were the main reasons for not immunizing their children.

Table 20

Status of Child Immunization among the Dhodias

Vaccination	*Percentage*
DPT (n=259)	
Yes	95.0
No	5.0
Polio (n=257)	
Yes	96.1
No	3.9
BCG (n=259)	
Yes	96.1
No	3.9
Measles (n=256)	
Yes	69.9
No	30.1
Vit A (n=254)	
Yes	70.1
No	29.9

Anthropometric Measurements

Anthropometric measurements were made on the Dhodia children of six years of age to assess their nutritional status. Anthropometric data were collected from 332 children belonging to the Anganwadi centres of different villages, households and primary schools. Out of these 332 subjects, 174 were males and 158 females. In all, 12 body measurements were taken, viz., crown-heel length (up to two years)/standing height, body weight, skin folds (skin fold at biceps, triceps, sub-scapular, supra iliac and calf sites), waist circumference, hip circumference, head circumference, chest circumference and mid-upper arm circumference.

The results of each of the 12 measurements indicated that differences between the two sexes were not statistically significant for most of the measurements, revealing similar pattern of growth among boys and girls. A comparison of these measurements on Dhodia boys and girls with data on rural Indian boys and girls

(ICMR, 1984) and girls and boys from better socio-economic class (Ghosh, 1992) did not reveal any great differences with them. A least 58 percent of the boys and girls suffer from mild to moderate form of malnutrition with respect to weight for height and height for age. Mean mid-upper arm circumference among the Dhodia boys and girls in the age group and above (> 13.5 cm.) does not suggest any unusual nutritional status.

Family Planning

It was found in the present investigation that 44.3 percent of the total eligible couples were not practising any methods of family planning (FP). Among those who adopted any form of FP practices, 90 percent underwent tubectomy. In other words, the terminal method for family planning is the most accepted method among the Dhodias. Only 6 percent of the current users have adopted spacing methods. The inference which one draws from such data is that in spite of the emancipation of women among Dhodias, there is a considerable gender bias regarding the usage of FP methods. Male participation in FP is lacking in the Dhodias, which constitute only 5 percent of all current users. It was also found in the present study that 43 percent of couple starts using contraceptive after two children and another 38 percent after three children. It is thus amply clear that a majority of the Dhodias are restricting their choice to two or at the most three children, and the decline is in favour of two children.

Role of Health Care Providers

Many researchers have often been very critical about the various aspects of health care delivery system. There is a general degradation of value system over the time and health care system is no exception to it. However, if the demographic profile of Indian national population and subsequently decline in mortality during the past few decades are of any significance, such reactions undermine the efforts of the government health providers and the constraints under which they are functioning. Appreciating the efforts and hard work put in by the health providers along with highlighting the difficult areas would have given considerable impetus to their morale. It is important to realize that the government health providers are catering to a very large section of the Indian national population whereas other non-government health providers are catering to a very small section of the society.

Our experiences in tribal areas - be they primitive or non-primitive - indicate that providing health care at grassroots level is a complex issue. By and large, the programme officers of the district, medical officers at CHCs and PHCs and paramedical staff at grassroots level are providing reasonably good services against the backdrop of their problems and constraints. While talking about the health services by the government providers, we often neglect the linking issues that have vital relationship with the quality of services. And, in such circumstances, medical officers at PHCs and paramedical staff unfortunately become the scapegoat. Similarly, communication and all-weather roads linking the villages with the primary care centre are necessary for improving the health status of the population in question.

The Valsad district of Gujarat, where the present investigation was undertaken, meets many of the criteria stated above. Firstly, the district is situated on the Delhi-Mumbai rail highway and most of the villages are well connected with all-weather roads. The people are sufficiently aware about the health care, primarily because the district has been quite sensitive in participating in various movements before independence. Moreover, Mumbai being closeby and having Vapi as an important industrial town, Valsad is a centre of happening.

In Valsad, the district hospital, CHCs and PHCs are functioning reasonably well. Paramedical staff in general, and female health workers in particular, are doing exceptionally good job. These workers are providing services at the doorsteps. Their main focus is on RCH, minor ailments and primary care. They compile important baseline information regarding births and deaths and also maintain the record of the children below five years of age, pregnant and lactating mothers. They impart vital health education to the people and are instrumental in bringing down the IMR, to some extent birth rate and morbidity as well. They play a key role in informing the health officers when any epidemic breaks or any health problem arises in the community. They are in direct touch with the community and are very well accepted. This is not to understate the role of medical officers at primary and tertiary levels.

There are other non-governmental health providers who are also playing their roles reasonably well. Qualified private health providers are few in the district and they have few diagnostic facilities and those are expensive. Difficult cases are referred to hospitals. FP and immunization services are not popular with private health providers. Treatment is by and large symptomatic and private medical practitioners have few surgical options. People opt for private health providers because of good personal relationship, credit options, use of instruments, prompt treatment without waiting, availability of medicine and affordable services. Private health providers, to some extent, have been able to take over the services of government health providers, who cater to a larger segment of the society.

Thus, it can be inferred that the Dhodias are increasingly getting their presence felt in the mainstream. Except for HbS, there is no tribal-specific disease among Dhodias. Health status of the Dhodias is slowly but steadily improving. They have made big strides in various developmental activities. Various social and economic indicators among the Dhodias are shaping them for better future and health. Demographic changes are apparent and must be sustained. They are highly aware about availability of health services and their attitude towards utilizing modern medicine is encouraging and positive. Private health providers are also contributing their share towards the health status of the community.

Governmental efforts are often undermined and criticized. The government is catering to a large section of society with small infrastructure. There are a large number of ambitious health schemes and programmes. Nevertheless, the efforts of the government health providers are stupendous. They are trying a daunting task and have a long way to go. Participation of NGOs is not only essential but necessary. Community health is a joint venture and must be viewed that way.

References

Basu, S.K. (1995). Social assessment study: Perception, attitude, experience of tribal communities vis-à-vis the role of health providers for the acceptability and demand for tuberculosis treatment in tribal areas. Unpublished World Bank Study.

— (1996). *Malaria Control Project: Beneficiary Social Assessment*. Unpublished World Bank Study.

Brass, W. and Coale, A. (1968). Methods of analysis and estimation. In W. Brass *et al.* (Eds.), *The Demography of Tropical Africa*. Princeton: Princeton University Press.

Brass, W. (1975). *Methods for Estimating Fertility and Mortality from Limited and Defective Data. Laboratory for Population Statistics.* Occasional Publication. Chapel Hill: Carolina Population Center.

Carrier, N. and Hob Craft, J. (1971). *Demographic Estimation for Developing Societies*. London: Population Investigation Committee.

Census of India (2001). Registrar General and Census Commission of India, New Delhi.

District Statistical Handbook (1997-98). Valsad District Panchayat (in Gujarati). Valsad: Statistical Department.

Ghosh, S. (1992). *The Feeding and Care of Infants and Young Children*. VHAI: New Delhi.

Indian Council for Medical Research (ICMR) (1984). *ICMR Technical Report Series No. 78*. New Delhi: ICMR.

Kshatriya, G.K. (2000). Ecology and health with special reference to Indian tribes. In M.K. Bhasin and V. Bhasin (Eds.), *Man-Environment Relationship.* Delhi: Kamla-Raj Enterprise.

Lohman, J.G., Roche, A.F. and Martorell, R. (1988). *Anthropometric Standardization Reference Manual.* Chicago: Human Kinetics Books.

Nei, M. (1965). Effective population size with overlapping generations. *Annual Report of National Institute of Radiological Science*, 5, 49-52.

Office of the Civil Hospital (2001-2002). *Annual Report of Valsad District*. Valsad: Office of the Civil Hospital.

Sample Registration System (1999). *Fertility and Mortality Indicators*. New Delhi: Registrar General of India.

Statistical Abstract of India (1997). New Delhi: Ministry of Home Affairs.

United Nations Manual IV (1967). *Methods of Estimating Basic Demographic Measures from Incomplete Data* (Population Studies, 42). New York: Department of Economic and Social Affairs.

Verma, I.C., Kaur, M. and Das, G.P. (1994). *Laboratory Manual for Health Professionals in Tribal/Rural Areas.* New Delhi: Genetics Unit, All India Institute of Medical Sciences.

7

A Study of Ethnomedicine among the Bhotias of Chamoli (Uttaranchal)

SAMEERA MAITI

In recent years there has been an increasing interest shown in ethnomedicines, especially those that are derived from plants, mainly because of the widespread belief that 'green medicines' are healthier and safer than the synthetic ones. Thus, herbals are staging a come back with a sort of 'herbal renaissance' taking place across the world today.

The World Health Organization (WHO) has estimated that 80 percent of the people in the world rely on traditional medicine for primary health care needs. And, of the 119 plant-based drugs used today by modern medicine, about 74 percent are from plants traditionally used as herbal cures (Farnsworth, 1990). Keeping these facts in mind, WHO in its 29th and 30th Assembly (1976 and 1977) gave formal recognition to traditional medicines and recommended the association of traditional healers with the national health care programmes.

A systematic review of the literature suggests that the area of ethnomedicine is not a new one in anthropology. Over the years, several important works have been carried out in this direction dealing with various aspects of medical anthropology. Mention may be made here of a few important ones such as those of Ackernecht (1942), Clements (1982), Lieban (1977) and Park and Park (1991).

Several researches have also been carried out on various aspects of health among tribals including those of Uttaranchal, viz., Joshi (1978, 1981 and 1993), Rizvi (1986 and 1991), Singh and Maheshwari (1992), Solanki (1995) and Tiwari (1995). However, none of these deal with the Bhotias in particular. Hence, the present paper makes an attempt to study ethnomedicine, especially indigenous herbal medicines, among the Bhotias. It also attempts to take note of the present condition of this system of treatment and ultimately makes suggestions for the conservation of this valuable indigenous knowledge.

Ancient Indian and world literature on medicine suggests that indigenous and tribal people use several kinds of medicinal plants for combatting diseases. Knowledge of these medicinal herbs has been handed down through generations and some of these knowledge have survived through time among the various tribal communities of India. It has been estimated that there are around three lakh village-based herbal healers in India, who with their knowledge, cure various ailments and diseases (Darshan, 1998). These medicine men possess a comprehensive knowledge of medicinal plants, herbs, tubers, roots, barks, leaves, etc., found in their surroundings from which they extract medicines. Over the years, from generation to generation, through personal experience, they have established correlation between the properties of various ethnomedicinal elements and amelioration of particular diseases. Such knowledge is ecological and culture-specific and, therefore, varies from tribe to tribe. According to Government of India (GoI, 1994) report, out of 7,500 wild plant species used by the tribes in India for medicinal purposes, about 950 are found to be new claims and worthy of scientific investigations. However, today, when on one hand the world is taking to researches in this field and to the use of natural drugs, on the other hand, the inheritors of this indigenous knowledge are withdrawing from it. Similar is the case of the Bhotias.

The Himalayan and sub-Himalayan regions in India are abounding with unique medicinal plants that have potential to be used in modern medical therapy. The healing properties of some of these plants are also mentioned in Vedic literature. Since time immemorial, ethnic communities and local populations residing in this area have been using these herbal medicines for curing various ailments. One such ethnic group, who is known for their knowledge of various medicinal herbs available in their habitat, is the Bhotias, inhabiting the district Chamoli, Uttaranchal.

Material and Methods

Etymologically, the word 'Bhotia' is popularly believed to have originated from the term *Bhot* or more correctly *Bod*, which means Tibet, and which has given rise to the name used for tribes living in the areas between the two countries (Atkinson, 1882). According to Singh (1994), the Bhotia tribe is divided into eight sub-groups, namely, the Jad, Tolchha, Marchha, Johari, Jethora, Darmi, Chaudansi and Byansi. But, despite sharing a common ecology and a common name, these groups exhibit socio-cultural and religious variation (Das, 1994). The Bhotias claim to be Rajputs although they have not yet been able to put forward any proof for the same. Turner (1931) made the earliest record of this while working for the census. According to him, the Bhotias were one of the several tribal and lower caste groups who found this opportunity most appropriate for putting forward their claims to a 'higher caste'.

A special feature of the Bhotias is transhumance, which involves their upward/northward migration along with animals during summer and downward/southward migration during winters. Consequently, they have two dwellings with all basic amenities in both summer and winter villages.

The Bhotias are a landowning community, although their traditional occupation had been trade, with their trade zone extending from Tibet in the north to the plains in the south. Agriculture, animal husbandry and cottage industry formed their subsidiary occupations. However, the Chinese occupation of Tibet and their subsequent invasion in 1962 led to the sealing of the border with India. This adversely affected Indo-Tibetan trade and the main sufferers were the Bhotias who were thrown out of their traditional and prosperous trading economy. Thus, today, they have taken to various occupations ranging from agriculture to cottage industry and from government jobs to government contracts.

In Uttaranchal, the Bhotias reside in the districts of Pithoragarh, Chamoli, Almora, Uttarkashi and Nainital. The region inhabited by them falls in the north-eastern part of the state and is locally known as *Bhot* or *Bhot Pradesh*, consisting of several valleys bordering Tibet. These valleys from west to east are Vishnuganga (Niti), Dhauliganga (Mana), Johar, Darma, Chandans and Byans. The Bhotias living in Vishnuganga (Niti) valley of district Chamoli belong to the Tolcha sub-group and as such the present paper deals with the practice of ethnomedicine, specifically herbal medicines, among them.

The district of Chamoli is located in the northern part of Uttaranchal covering 7691 sq. kms. in the central part of western Himalayas. The district lies between 300 and 310 North latitude and 790 and 800 East longitude (Bhatt, 2003). The high altitude regions of Uttaranchal can be divided into three main climatic zones: the alpine zone, the temperate zone and the sub-tropical or sub-temperate zone. The alpine zone nearing the Tibet border is rich in wild medicinal and aromatic plants and happens to be the main habitat of the Bhotias, whose summer/traditional villages are situated here. During winters, the Bhotias migrate downwards to their lower habitat in the temperate and sub-temperate zones, which also have an abundance of various medicinal plant species and orchids of medicinal importance.

The data presented in the paper have been collected primarily by in-depth interviews consisting of open-ended questions administered on 40 individuals apart from non-participatory observations and group discussions. Interviews were taken both from tribals as well as non-tribals, viz., doctors (3) and nurses (4) at Public Health Centres (PHCs), private practitioners (5), tribal medicine men (8) and tribal-folk (20). Data collection was carried out in October 2001 during fieldwork in the lower valley of block Dasholi and Karnaprayag where the Tolcha settle during winters.

Ethnomedicine among the Bhotias

Diseases and ailments are common problems in every community, be they simple or complex, and every culture evolves its own method of treatment for health problems faced by its members. On the basis of observations made during the study and information gathered from the above mentioned sources, it was deduced that the Bhotias do not suffer from any particularly serious diseases, although they cannot be called healthy in any way since minor ailments are a regular feature. Table 1 shows that cold and cough seem to be the most common ailments affecting the members of all the age groups. Apart from this, children between 0-14 years of age are regularly found suffering from dysentery, diarrhoea and worm infestations, while young and adults (in the age group of 15-60 years) commonly suffer from headache, weakness and giddiness. Men belonging to this age group were also found suffering from bronchitis, while women commonly suffered from leucorrhoea, anaemia and backache. In the age group of 51+ years, both men and women suffer from arthritis/joint pain, bronchitis, asthma and blood pressure. A glance at the ailments indicates the major causative factors too, viz., difficult terrain, extreme cold, fluctuating climatic conditions and non-availability of potable water. Like every other community, the Bhotias too have their indigenous or popular healing practices for curing various ailments as well as specific emotions, attitudes and strategies related to health and diseases. The Bhotias, in general, do not have a very clear concept related to the cause of diseases and ailments. However, they believe that there may be two causes for the same – natural or climatic and supernatural. At the first instance, all illnesses and ailments are attributed to natural or climatic causes, but persistence of even minor ailments and all major diseases and illnesses are attributed to supernatural causes such as the wrath of gods/goddesses, the evil eye, evil effects of malicious spirits and black magic done by an enemy. The major source of illness being supernatural, treatment too lies in propitiation of the responsible force through adequate ritualistic performances or sacrifices if necessary. Thus, when struck by some illness, a Bhotia can either contact a non-Bhotia Brahmin, a Bhotia sorcerer/exorcist, or a herbalist. Usually, the herbalists, apart from giving treatment, also function as sorcerers. A combination of these two knowledge makes them effective healers. For minor health problems such as cold, cough, fever and backache, home remedies are administered first of all attributing it to climatic effect. Generally, every elder member of a Bhotia household has some knowledge pertaining to common herbal medicines available in the area and uses them frequently. However, for serious problems or when home remedies do not work, the help of a herbalist is sought. According to a Bhotia belief, some of the herbs found in and around their habitat have supernatural powers and are *shubh* (auspicious) and therefore cure the patients miraculously. When home remedies seem to have no effect, the help of either a Brahmin (non-Bhotia) is sought to propitiate the gods and goddesses and calm down the responsible planets *grah nakshatra* (planets), or a sorcerer is contacted to propitiate and drive away evil spirits.

Table 1

Common Ailments Affecting Various Groups

Children (0-14 years)	*Young-adults (15-50 years)*		*Old (51+ years)*
Male and Female	*Male*	*Female*	*Male and Female*
Cold and cough Diarrhoea Dysentery Worm infection	Cold and cough Headache, weakness and giddiness	Bronchitis Lucorrhoea Anaemia Backache	Cold and cough Arthritis/joint pain Bronchitis and asthma Blood pressure

Earlier, it was only when all the indigenous methods of treatment failed and the patient's condition became serious, the Bhotias turned to allopathic doctors in PHCs or hospitals. However, presently, a gradual shift in health-seeking behaviour can be noticed among the Bhotias, and more so among the younger generations who are turning away from herbal medicines. Thus, now-a-days, when home remedies prove ineffective, nearly 20 percent of the Bhotias adopt allopathic treatment. To get an idea about the treatment preferences of the Bhotias, the eldest male or female members of 50 households were asked to rank (according to their own and their family's choice) the three methods of treatment, viz., allopathic, herbal and home remedies. Treatment preferences indicated by them can be seen in Table 2(a). Eighty-five individuals indicated home remedies, nine allopathic and six herbal medicines to be the first preference for treating an illness or ailment. Seventy-two individuals stated herbal treatment while five home remedies and three individuals allopathic treatment to be the second preference. As a third preference, 68 individuals went for allopathic treatment, 32 for herbal, while none took up to home remedies.

Table 2(a)

Treatment Preference

First Preference		*Second Preference*		*Third Preference*	
Method	*No.*	*Method*	*No.*	*Method*	*No.*
Home remedies	85	Home remedies	05	Home remedies	-
Herbal	06	Herbal	72	Herbal	32
Allopathic	09	Allopathic	23	Allopathic	68
Total	100		100		100

Note: Data for this table were collected from the eldest male and female members of 50 households.

Table 2(b)

Treatment Preference

1st preference (85%)	Home remedies
2nd preference (72%)	Herbalist and appeasement of supernatural forces
3rd preference (68%)	Allopaths/hospitals and appeasement of supernatural forces

Analysis of Tables 2(a) and 2(b) depicts an overall preference for treatment adopted by the Bhotia tribe. During this survey, it was also mentioned by the respondents that at the initial stage of any ailment only medical treatment is given as it is attributed to natural or climatic causes. However, if the medication does not prove effective and the ailment persists, it is assumed that the cause is supernatural and so apart from trying out other methods of treatment, the Bhotias contact a non-Bhotia Brahmin or Bhotia exorcist/sorcerers to appease the supernatural forces. It is for this reason that Table 2(b) includes the list of preferences 'appeasement of supernatural forces' along with the second and third preferences. On the basis of data thus gathered, it is derived that majority (85%) of the population go for home remedies as their first preference, 72 percent go for herbal treatment as their second preference if the first fails while 68 percent go for the allopathic treatment as their third preference if the earlier two methods do not work. Apart from this, to be on the safer side and make treatment more effective, almost all the people also go for rituals and sacrifices to appease the supernatural forces if the initial medical treatment fails.

Although till date a majority of the Bhotias prefer herbal treatment to allopathic treatment, as is evident from Table 2, the profession of herbalist and use of herbal medicines is on a decline here. The Bhotias put forward following three main reasons for this changed attitude:

- According to many of the Bhotias, herbal medicines take long time to cure and at times have several restrictions and taboos that are to be adhered to while taking these medicines. On the other hand, allopathic medicines cure nearly instantaneously, putting one back to work in a few hours or days and rarely have any accompanying taboo.
- Collection of medicinal plants needs long hours of wandering in the wild and precise knowledge of each variety takes years to master. Further, payment made to herbalists by the locals being very nominal, it is not considered a lucrative job and therefore no young Bhotia is ready to take it up as a full-time profession. Again, the knowledge is passed on only from father to son and if the son is not interested (as in most of the cases), passes away with the father, who is generally not ready to share it easily with others.
- The ban imposed by the forest department on collection of 'green medicines' from the wild resulted in private/personal illegal trade (PIT). PIT by wandering communities and unsustainable exploitation of rare medicinal herbs from the wild for ethno-pharmacological practice and various socio-religious functions by the locals including the Bhotias have led to the near extinction of some of these precious plants, in the absence of which herbal treatment becomes difficult and sometimes impossible.

All the three reasons mentioned above indicate towards the precarious condition of herbal medicines in the community. It also makes it quite clear that, in a decade or so, the indigenous knowledge pertaining to the uses of various herbs that the Bhotias have acquired over the generation through trial and error will be lost forever with the passing away of the elders of the community.

Table 3
Medicinal Plants Used by the Bhotias

Sl. No.	Bhotia Name	Botanical Name	Used for Curing
1.	Atees	*Acontium heterophyllum*	Diarrhoea, dysentery, stomach ache, high fever and jaundice; mixed with *katuki* and ginger juice can cure typhoid, cold, cough and bodyache
2.	Aadu/Kirov Chuhi	*Prunus ponsica*	Backache, stiffness of muscles and joint pains
3.	Arand	*Ricinus communislum*	Arthritis
4.	Balchhar/Laljari	*Macrotomia benthamii/ Arnebia benthamii*	Hair fall, dandruff, wounds and arthritis
5.	Baanj	*Onerans laucotrichophosen*	Constipation and scorpio bites
6.	Bichhu ghas/ Kanali/Kandali	*Urtica dioica*	Constipation, early stage of paralysis, Chhora (blisters around joints) and dog bite
7.	Biskanara	*Morduna longifolia*	Wounds and blisters
8.	Brahma-Brahmi	*Centella asiatica/ Hydrocotyle asiatica*	Increases memory, dysentery
9.	Choru	*Angelica glauca*	Gastric and constipation; also provides energy and vigour
10.	Chalmodi	*Oxalis corniculata*	Ear pain and skin problems
11.	Chirauto/Chireta	*Swertia Chirayita*	Malaria and fever; is also a blood purifier
12.	Datura	*Datura stremonium*	Arthritis and teeth pain
13.	Dolu	*Rheum emodi*	Cuts, boils, wounds, ulcer and joint pain
14.	Ekalbeer	*N.A.*	Cataract and eye problems
15.	Feren	*Allium consanguineum*	Jaundice, cold and cough; absorbs extra fat when added in curry
16.	Fankaml/Faina	*Saussurea gossypiphora*	Severe burns; believed to keep away evil spirits
17.	Gainthi	*Dioscoreaceae*	Ear pain
18.	Gahat	*N.A.*	Stones
19.	Gizar	*N.A.*	Diabetes
20.	Haran	*N.A.*	Whooping cough
21.	Hatajari	*Dactylorhiza hatagirea*	Deep wounds and check bleeding; is a rejuvenating tonic

Contd...

Contd...

22.	Jatamasi/Mansi	*Nardostachya grandiflorum*	Asthma, blood pressure, joint pain and burns
23.	Katuki/Kaduwi	*Picrorrhiza kurroa*	Acute fever, acidity, stomach ache, constipation, gastritis; is also a blood purifier and liver tonic
24.	Kuth	*Sanssurea costus*	Asthma and cough
25.	Kalihari	*Gloriosa superba*	Fractures and joint dislocation
26.	Kaagazi Neebu	*Rutaceae (Citrus medica)*	Stress, cold and cough
27.	Kumkum	*N.A.*	Dog bite
28.	Meetha	*Aconitum falconeri/ Aconitum violaceum*	Back pain, sores and tuberculosis
29.	Meen	*N.A.*	Snake bite (prevents spread of poison)
30.	Nagphani	*Sansevieria roxburghina sehult*	Ear pain
31.	Pashan Bhed	*Bergenia storychii*	Stones
32.	Salam Misri	*N.A.*	Leprosy
33.	Shaimaru	*N.A.*	Skin diseases, pimples and itching
34.	Sheesham	*Dalbergia sissoo/Roxb. Fabaceae*	Sprain and fracture
35.	Thunyor	*Taxus wallichian/Taxus baccata*	Breast cancer, throat cancer, stress, asthma, cold and blood pressure; provides vigour
36.	Titora	*Rtmicya bhalgirs*	Leprosy
37.	Temar	*Xenthozylum oxifilum*	Teeth problems
38.	Tantri	*Rheum moorcroftianum*	Constipation

Note: N.A. Botanical name not available.

Hence, it is of great importance for researchers to salvage as much as possible of the valuable knowledge on medicinal plants known to these tribals before they disappear forever. In keeping with this view, a humble attempt has been made to take note of some of the 'miracle herbs' found in the Bhotia habitat and the ailments that they can cure. For convenience the various medicinal herbs used by the Bhotias and the ailments these cure are given in a tabular form in Table 3. As stated earlier, use of some of these herbs, such as *atees dohi* and *katuki* are known to all elders of the tribe, and therefore every house with members of the old generation keeps some of these herbs at home to be used as home medicines. It can be noticed from Table 3 that a single herb can be used for curing various ailments. The examples of *atees* and *bicchu ghas* can be given here. One-fourth teaspoon of dried and powdered *atees* root is taken with warm water to cure diarrhoea, dysentery and stomach ache. One-fourth teaspoon of this powder is given every hour to cure high fever and jaundice. A mixture of one-fourth teaspoon each of *atees* and *katuki* powder is given with a teaspoon of ginger juice to cure typhoid, cold, cough and bodyache. *Bichhu ghas/kanali* is used to cure constipation, paralysis, cholera and dog bites. Boiled tender leaves of the plant are chewed for curing constipation. Stem and leaves of the plant are beaten on the affected area to cure paralysis during its initial stage. Ground seed of *kanali* is applied on the affected area to cure *chhora* while a paste of *kanali* leaves and green chilly is applied on the area bitten by a dog to stop spread of infection or poison.

It can also be seen from the table that a single ailment is curable with the use of more than one herb. Thus, to treat cold and cough (the most common ailment found among all the members of the Bhotia, irrespective of age and sex) *atees, feren, kuth, kaagazi neebu* or *thunijor* may be used according to availability of the plant and severity of the problem. At the initial stages, *kaagazi neebu, atees* or *feren* may be used, but on persistence, *kuth* or *thunijor* is used. Similarly, for curing constipation, *baanj, bichhu ghas, choru, katuki* or *tantri* may be used according to its availability.

Suggestions for Conservation

Although, in general, a decline in carrying forward the profession of herbalist and use of herbal medicines has taken place among the Bhotias, a group of educated youngsters, realizing its value, among them, has taken up the task of saving these plants from extinction and the knowledge from dying out. In fact, a society named Dronagiri Biorenish Society was registered in 2001 by a group of Bhotias with the following aims: to preserve and protect herbs and herbal medicines; educate people (specially the local community) about their environment, forest and its importance; cultivate rare and useful herbs around Niti valley; and to work for the Nanda Devi Biosphere Reserve (NDBR). Realizing the importance of the rich biodiversity of the area, NDBR was established under the auspices of UNESCO's Man and Biosphere (MAB) project in the early 1980s with the aim to conserve some Himalayan floral and faunal species in their natural habitat. However, setting up of this 'national park' or 'protected area', compounded with the ban imposed by the forest department on collection in the wild, led to an agitation by the Bhotia community living in and around the area against violation of their communal rights by the government. For generations, the Bhotias have been employing old and experienced sustainable environmental practices, such as collection of plant species after the seed dehiscence is over, and after the rainy season, when maximum germination and multiplication of almost all species has taken place naturally. According to Cunningham (1993), pressures on medicinal plants in such areas are low and in general one can say that use of medicinal plants is not a cause of concern. Under such circumstances, the anger of the local tribal community is quite justified since they are not in a position to cash on their own natural resources and indigenous knowledge.

Researchers the world over are suggesting that the most important way to protect natural habitat and maintain survival of rare plant species is *in situ* conservation, which may be defined as the continuing maintenance of a plant population with its ecosystem in the environment to which it is best adapted. Guidelines provided by the World Health Organization (WHO), the World Conservation Union (IUCN) and the World Wide Fund for Nature (WWF) (1993) state that such conservation can be achieved both by setting aside areas as nature reserves and national parks and by ensuring that as many wild species as possible can continue to survive in managed habitats, such as farms and plantation forest. However, it also rightly states that such schemes cannot succeed in a poverty-struck region like the Himalayas unless the fullest support and involvement of the local people are ensured. Even the park managers should ensure that some of the benefits of conserving threatened species within the park area accrue to local people and that the dependence of these people living nearby on the forest resources should not be ignored. If this is not ensured, agitations by locals will continue as also the illegal procurement and trade of these plants. Cunningham (1993) rightly observes that regulations have been largely ineffective in controlling medicinal plant exploitation. In fact, sometimes, such regulations increase manifold pressures on species growing in the wild, especially endemic ones, which cannot be supplied to the concerning agencies from any other region. Given these facts, it is suggested that the Bhotias and other local communities be involved in any scheme adopted by the government and non-government organizations henceforth to protect the rich floral and faunal wealth of the area. Emphasis should also be laid on the traditional way of collection through sustainable harvest. Further, locals should be educated to protect their habitat from illegal and unscientific exploitation by wandering traders and collectors who do not care in the least about the environment and are out to cash on the species as long as they exist. The government should also provide the locals with some kind of incentives for their efforts to conserve and cultivate the rare and rich medicinal herbs of the area, because only when the tribals find their efforts being paid for, will they be ready to put in their might. If this is not done soon, the growing disinterest in the use of herbal medicines and knowledge related to medicinal plants that has come about in the Bhotia community will take its toll and the indigenous knowledge of these 'magical plants' and their significance will disappear forever.

References

Ackernecht, E.H. (1942). Problems of primitive medicine. *Bulletin of the History of Medicine*, 2, 503-521.

Atkinson, E.T. (1882). *The Himalayan Gazetteer*. New Delhi: Cosmo Publications (Reprint 1973).

Bhatt, S.C (2003). *The District Gazetteer of Uttaranchal*. New Delhi: Gyan Publishing House.

Clements, F.E. (1982). Primitive concept of diseases. *American Archaeology and Ethnology*, 32, 185-252.

Cunningham, A.B. (1993). African medicinal plants, setting priorities at the interface between conservation and primary health care. *People and Plants: Working Paper I*, France: UNESCO.

Darshan, S. (1998). Conserving a community resource: Medicinal plants. In A. Kotari *et al.* (Eds.), *Communities and Conservation*: *UNESCO*. New Delhi: Sage Publications.

Das, J.C. (1994). From trade to agriculture: The case of Bhotia of Pithoragarh. In K.S. Singh (Ed.), *Economics of the Tribes and Their Transformation*. New Delhi: Concept Publishing Company.

Farnsworth (1990). The role of ethnopharmocology in drug development. In D.J. Chandwick, and J. Marsh (Eds.), *Bioactive Compounds from Plants*. New York: John Wiley and Sons.

Government of India (1994). *Ethnobiology in India: A Status Report*. New Delhi: Ministry of Environment and Forest, Government of India.

Joshi, P.C. (1978). *Perception of illness among the Khasa tribals of Jaunsar Bawar*. Paper presented at the Tenth International Congress of Anthropological and Ethnographical Studies, New Delhi.

— (1981). Perception and classification of illness among the Khasa tribal of Jaunsar Bawa, *Tribe*, 13: 16-20.

— (1993). Culture, health and illness: Aspects of ethno medicine. In S.K. Biswas (Ed.), *Central Himalayan Panorama*. Calcutta: Institute of Social Research and Applied Anthropology.

Lieban, R.W. (1977). The field of medical anthropology. In D. Landy (Ed.), *Culture, Diseases and Healing*. New York: Macmillan Publication.

Park, J.E. and Park, P. (1991). *Preventive and Social Medicine*. Jabalpur: Banarasidas Banot.

Rizvi, S.N.H. (1986). Health practices of Jaunsaris: A socio-cultural analysis. In B. Chaudhury (Ed.), *Tribal Health: Socio-cultural Dimensions*. New Delhi: Inter-India Publications.

— (1991). *Medical Anthropology of the Jaunsaris*. Delhi: Northern Book Centre.

Singh, K.K. and Maheshwari, J.K. (1992). Folk medicinal use of some plants among the Tharus of Gorakhpur district, Uttar Pradesh, *Ethnobotany 4*, 39-43.

Singh, K.S. (1994). *The Scheduled Tribes: People of India National Series*, Vol III. New Delhi: Oxford University Press.

Solanki, B. (1995). Mechanical strategies in folk medicine in Rawai Garhwal Himalaya. In Joshi and Joshi (Eds.), *Uttaranchal Himalaya*. Almora: Shree Almora Book Depot.

Tiwari, S.C. (1995). Health and disease in the tribes of Uttarakhand. In Joshi and Joshi (Eds.), *Uttaranchal Himalaya*. Almora: Shree Almora Book Depot.

Turner, A.C. (1931). *Census of India 1931*, Vol. XVIII. United Provinces of Agra and Oudh. Allahabad: Government Press.

WHO, IUCN and WWF (1993). *Guidelines on the Conservation of Medicinal Plants*. Geneva: WHO.

8

Koya Perception of Health and Illness: An Ethnomedical Analysis

NANDA KISHORE KANNURI

Anthropologists believe that culture has a far-bearing influence on all human activities, whether social or biological. After the role of culture on health was widely recognized, some anthropologists in 1960s continued their quest in the direction that led to the development of medical anthropology as a new sub-field of socio-cultural anthropology. Ethnomedicine later emerged as an important branch of medical anthropology when anthropologists started studying the indigenous medical features of a particular community. Usually, the communities of interest for most anthropologists were so-called 'primitive' and 'non-literate' societies. Hughes (1968) defines ethnomedicine as a term that has been used to refer to those beliefs and practices relating to diseases that are products of indigenous cultural conceptions and are not explicitly derived from the conceptual framework of modern medicine. Ethnomedical approach is to study how a particular group of people perceives and deals with its health and illness. This approach thus includes the study of medical beliefs, healing techniques, and medical practitioners and the association of these with culture and society in which they are found. The emic perspective in ethnomedical approach helps the anthropologists to look at the natives' point of view.

Culture determines to a large extent not only the type and frequency of disease/illness but also the way people perceive, explain and treat diseases as well as the manner in which they respond to the delivery of modern medicine. Thus, culture is an invariable determining factor of a community's understanding of health and illness. Every culture, regardless of its simplicity or complexity, has its own conception of health, illness and health-seeking behaviour, which is referred to as 'health culture' – a component of the overall culture of the community (Kar and Gogoi, 1993). The socio-religious medical responses to illness in various forms – including the belief forms established, conducts approved – make the health culture. As a part of this health culture, members of each community tend to develop a specific belief frame relating to several illnesses/diseases recognized by them. The symptom recognition, evaluation and health decisions related to regaining of health recovery are influenced by belief frames relating to disease causation, spread, diagnosis, and cure of each of the many categories of diseases recognized.

Health and illness are two antagonistic concepts, one defined as the absence of the other. It can be said that these two concepts lie on two opposite poles of the continuum. Health in general is understood as absence of illness.

Illness is a socio-culturally defined departure from health and it can be differentiated from disease, which is a biomedical category. Anthropologists' concern would be more towards illness rather than disease since illness is a subjective phenomenon related to social and cultural factors, whereas disease is an objective phenomenon defined purely in bio-medical terms by medical professionals. The response to illness – illness behaviour – is the way in which symptoms are perceived, evaluated and acted upon. This may vary from one individual to another. However, this behaviour is also greatly influenced by the culture, of which the sick person is a member.

Since the beginning of evolution, humankind has always been able to find some medicines in the nature that surrounds them. Early therapeutic treatments were derived from the surrounding environment of human beings, who were forest dwellers. They made use of plants, animals and other substances naturally available to them to treat illness. The knowledge of many medicinal herbs is derived from the direct observation of animals that consume herbs when ill. Complex health care systems of simple societies evolved, based on deep observation of the nature and environment. This is more prominent among tribals who can be differentiated from the mainstream society by their ways of life. Tribals have a distinct health culture, different from the majority non-tribal population. The medical system in these simple societies is structured on the lines of herbal and psychosomatic treatment. Their practices of healing, apart from herbal remedies, incorporate a touch of mysticism, supernatural and magic, resulting in specific magico-religious rites.

Several anthropologists have undertaken studies among tribals to understand their indigenous perceptions of health and medical practices. In ethnographic studies of tribal communities by pioneering Indian anthropologists such as S.C. Roy and D.N. Majumdar, some data on indigenous health practices are available. Studies on Balahis of Central India described the types of medicine men among them and on Hill Saoras of Orissa gave an inventory of the gods associated with various diseases in Saora pantheon (cf. Ali, 1994). Moreover, studies on tribes like Mundas, Idu Mishimi of Arunachal Pradesh, Pandu, Waynad of north Kerala, Santhals (cf. Ali, 1994) and on Gonds, Kolams and Chenchus (Hussain, 1992) have documented the ethnomedical practices and allied aspects of the tribals. These studies help us to understand the importance of indigenous practices of medicine, which are interwoven with their culture and the tribal perceptions of health and diseases.

There are 427 tribal communities in India and each community is not only geographical area-specific but also culture-specific. Hence, what is true in the case of one tribe may not hold good in the case of another (Swain, 1994). This signifies the need for further studies on the other tribal communities of India.

The Study

The present study deals with the health behaviour of the Koyas – a tribe of Khammam district of Andhra Pradesh. They are the largest group among the tribal population of Andhra Pradesh. According to the 1991 census, Koyas form about 12 percent of the total ST population of Andhra Pradesh. Majority of their population in the state inhabit along the riverbanks of Godavari and Sabri, stretching over the three districts of Khammam, East Godavari and West Godavari. The emphasis of the study is on looking at how they perceive the notions of health and illness and various socio-cultural aspects interrelated with health and illness.

The main objectives of the study are:

(1) to study the Koya perception of health, illness and cure; and
(2) to study their illness behaviour and health-seeking behaviour.

This is more of an ethnographic study with an ethnomedical approach in order to try and understand the perception of health and illness and the socio-cultural behaviour of the Koyas associated with it.

Methodology

The present study is based on the fieldwork carried out for a period of two months (April and May) in the year 1998 in a village called Repaka, inhabited by the Koyas. This particular village is in Kunavaram *mandal* of Khammam district of Andhra Pradesh.

Participatory observation, household schedule, interviews, case studies and group discussions were the primary methods used for data collection. These were supplemented by secondary sources.

Koya Perception of Health and Illness

The Koya concept of health is functional and is associated with the fulfilment of roles ascribed to an individual. In other words, a person, who is performing her/his regular duties well, is considered healthy. On the other hand, a person who is unable to perform her/his duties due to bodily discomforts is considered ill. This system of categorization as healthy and ill according to Bauman (1961) can be called as 'performance orientation'. The Koyas, following this concept of performance orientation, do not consider some skin ailments, dental problems, gynaecological problems (in case of women), etc., as illness because they do not hinder them from performing their regular duties.

The etiological understanding of this tribal group can be said to fall under Foster's dualistic classification of personalistic and naturalistic medical systems. In the personalistic system, illness is believed to be affected by the action of supernatural beings like deity or god, or a non-human agent like a witch or sorcerer, whereas in the naturalistic system, illness is said to be caused by the disturbance in equilibrium of the impersonal and insensate elements of the human body (Foster and Anderson, 1979).

Koyas classify the illness caused by natural/physical reasons into three categories as under: (1) illness caused by humoral imbalance, (2) injuries, and (3) animal bites.

They believe that human body is constituted of five natural elements, viz., sky (*Akasam*), fire (*Nippu*), water (*Neeru*), earth (*Bhumi*) and air (*Gali*) in a balance. This balance may be disturbed leading to ill-health due to consumption of certain foods, which they categorize as hot and cold (*vedi* and *chaluva*). They consider over-consumption of vegetables like tomatoes, pumpkin, okra, bottle gourd, ridge gourd, snake gourd, onions, cabbage, potatoes and beans, citrus fruits like lemon and toddy, gruel prepared out of *jowar* and left-over cooked rice, as cold causing factors that disturb the humoral balance. Similarly, the Koyas believe that excessive consumption of fruit of eggplant, meat of wild boar and deer and sweet pumpkin would lead to inflammation of joints, which they call *vatham*. Excessive intake of guava, meat of hare, spiny fruit of eggplant, sorghum, toddy in the early morning would lead to accumulation of phlegm which they call *nanju pattadam*. Other illnesses caused by the intake of cold foods are cold (*rompa*), cough (*daggu*), headache (*edekku*), migraine (*varagoba*), abdominal aches (*kanchuka*), swollen stomach (*dokka ubbu*), vomiting (*vantulu*) and malaria (*chalijwaramu*). Over-consumption of foods, like fish, chilly, chicken, beef, pork, mutton and jaggery, some leafy vegetables like spinach, grains like maize, consumption of liquor brewed of *mohuva* flowers and jaggery, will cause heat in the body disturbing the humoral balance. The illness/diseases associated with the humoral imbalance caused due to excess heat are fever (*jwaramu)*, conjunctivitis (*kandlakalaka*), sores and boils, backaches, pains of pregnant women (*chula nopulu*), sunstroke (*vadadebba*), giddiness (*tetakallu)*, epileptic fits (*murchalu*), lack of milk in a lactating mother (*rommu enduka*), etc.

Other categories of illness include those caused due to injuries while working, hunting and playing, and burns and bites like those of dogs, wild boars, snakes, scorpions and insects.

The supernatural causes of illness are spirits, gods and goddesses. Like most tribal groups, this group too considers spirits as both benevolent and malevolent. The diseases and illnesses are caused owing to the effect of malevolent spirits and souls. These spirits are of people who died of unnatural deaths. As these spirits are dissatisfied, they enter a human being and cause various illnesses like epilepsy (*moorcha*), atrophy (*sompidi*), diarrhoea, mental imbalance, tuberculosis (*mudurudaggu*) and whooping cough among children. This they call as *deyyam pattadam* or *gali sokudu*. Most of the psychological illnesses and behavioural anomalies are associated with these spirits. Diseases like chicken pox (*ammatalli*), dysentery (*thimmi* or *sandhi*) among children and jaundice (*kameralu)* are such diseases caused because of the rage of goddesses, gods or ancestral spirits. Chicken pox is thought to be caused due to the wrath of their village goddess *Muthyalamma*. Similarly, many skin diseases like itching (*duradalu*), scabies (*gajji*), leucoderma (*sobem*) and ringworm (*tamara*) and some venereal diseases (*korukudujabbulu*) are believed to be caused due to the violation of some taboos, especially sexual taboos like copulating with menstruating women. Among women, some generic problems are supposed to be caused because of the breach of taboos like defiling gods and ancestral spirits. The evil eye (*dishti*) is believed to cause sickness among children, young women and men.

Sorcery is an important factor to which the Koyas attribute disease and illness. Diseases like atrophy, paralysis (*devarasattu*), carbuncle (*nari kurupu)* and some sudden illness with unknown symptoms are attributed to sorcery, which they call *chetabadi*, performed by some magicians (*manthragadu*). *Chetabadi* is performed upon a person by acquiring his/her body parts like hair and nails or by introducing some objects like bones of birds, fish or some herbs (believed to have magical powers) into the body of a person through food.

The Koyas also believe that any individual's act of committing and omitting certain activities can cause illness to that person or to the family members or to the entire village.

Labelling

The knowledge of the Koya tribe regarding various 'new' diseases is limited. Illness or a disease for them is identified through visible symptoms or acute bodily discomforts. Common ailments like cold, headache, cough, joint pains, fever and epidemics like cholera and chicken pox are diagnosed through visible symptoms. Persistent symptoms for a long duration are considered severe. They are also unaware of diseases like cancer, diabetes, typhoid and tuberculosis. Diseases unknown to them and which persist for a long time are classified as 'severe fever' as in the case of malaria or typhoid, or as severe cough in the case of tuberculosis. A disease with severe symptom is called *muduru rogam*.

Illness Behaviour of the Koyas

Mechanic (1962) defined illness behaviour as the way in which symptoms are perceived, evaluated and acted upon by a person who recognizes some pain, discomfort and other signs of organic malfunction.

As noted, the first step in the illness behaviour is to perceive symptoms. The Koyas identify a disease through its symptoms, and prolongation of symptoms. Various factors like age, gender, religion and education effect their perception.

Age

It is observed that youngsters are more attentive to observing the deviations in their normal health condition. In contrast, the elderly do not give much attention towards such deviations, as they believe old age brings illness and disease. Though children perceive symptoms of illness like fever and dysentery, they ignore skin diseases and do not report them.

Gender

Women seldom report their gynaecological problems unless they are severe and problematic.

Religion

Religion among the Koyas has had a major influence upon their perceptions of health and illness. This is evident among the Christian converts who are more aware of different diseases and their symptoms than their counterparts practising animism.

Education

Though most of the members of the tribe are non-literate, some youth who are formally educated have knowledge about diseases like tuberculosis, malaria and dysentery.

As noted earlier, illness behaviour is characterized when a sick patient recognizes her/his symptoms. According to Kochar (n.d.), the illness behaviour can be categorized into four stages:

(1) normal performance of one's ascribed roles,
(2) reduced capacity of performance and getting into sick role,
(3) involving in sick role, and
(4) leaving the sick role.

These four stages can also be attributed to the Koyas.

Parson (1964) developed the concept of sick role and describes its essential aspects as follows:

(1) Depending upon the nature and severity of illness, the sick person is exempted from some or all of her/his normal social responsibilities.
(2) Sick persons cannot help being ill, and cannot get well by an act of decision or will.
(3) The sick person is expected to want to get well as soon as possible.
(4) She/he is expected to seek medical care and co-operate towards getting well.

This ideal conceptual sequence of sick role, which is associated with illness behaviour, hardly occurs and it is also the same in this particular tribe. Though a sick individual is exempted from working, those who are not severely ill or who are suffering from chronic illness like tuberculosis deny the sick role and perform their roles and responsibilities at least on a reduced scale. Denying sick role is equally found among men and women. Men deny sickness when they are involved in agricultural works and women when helping their family members in agricultural labour and also while performing household chores. It is interesting that most children aged between 10 and 14 years also deny the sick role and go for cattle grazing or playing.

Similarly, the second postulate of Parsons' sick role can be contradicted among the Koyas since in their medical worldview, breach of taboos plays an important role. Persons cannot help being sick if an illness is caused because of sorcery or natural cause, but they can avoid sickness by non-violation of taboos.

Health-seeking Behaviour

The Koyas administer self-medication of herbs for minor ailments like cold, cough and fever and visit the herbalist or a shaman, if the illness does not subside. Treatment for the illness, which the herbalist classifies as natural, is carried out by administering herbal medicines. For diseases caused owing to supernatural forces, a shaman gives treatment by propitiating gods, goddesses and ancestral spirits. For the illness caused owing to sorcery and spirit intrusion, treatment is given by performing magical rites and counter-sorcery.

Herbalists, shamans and priests are the traditional medical practitioners among the Koyas. Herbalists, who administer herbal medicines to cure illness, are called '*Vaidyudu*'. Shamans are classified into two categories, viz., *Vejju* and *Mantragadu*. A *Vejju*, according to them, carries out propitiating rituals, identifies the causes of sorcery and treats the disease. On the other hand, the *Mantragadu* performs counter-sorcery by magic after identifying the cause of sorcery. The services of the village priest (*Pujari*) are taken at the time of ceremonies like marriage, death, festivals and propitiation of gods and goddesses to cure illness caused by breach of taboo or else.

A herbalist diagnoses illness by going through the symptoms and visible bodily changes. Often, patients themselves reveal the probable causes like consumption of foods causing over heat or cold. The herbalist administers a particular medicine or a combination of herbs depending on the availability of herbs in that season, body constitution of the patient, patient's willingness to follow certain diet restrictions, etc. Normally, the cause for an illness, which is not guessed by the patient and one that persists for more than a 'reasonable' period, in spite of home remedies and treatment by herbalists, is attributed to supernatural reasons, and a specialist is consulted. In the case of illness afflicted by wrath of gods, or spirit intrusion, the shaman gets into a trance and then finds the cause for sickness. If it is a case of wrath of gods, some propitiating rituals are suggested to please gods. In the case of sorcery, the shaman identifies the source of sorcery and counters it to cure the illness by performing certain rituals, offering sacrifices and invoking the spirits.

The Koyas also practise some preventive measures to avoid diseases/illness. They wear amulets on the upper arm or on the neck as preventive and protective measure from the evil eye or sorcery; children wear amulets to ward off evil spirits. The priest or a shaman ties the amulets on the waist or upper arm of the children on the day of naming ceremony, generally performed on the eleventh day or the twenty-first day after the childbirth. Sometimes, when a child is sick, the shaman treats it and then ties an amulet as a preventive measure.

Conclusion

Though each tribal community of India is distinct and unique in culture, it can be observed that there are certain features common among them. Some important features of tribal culture, which also influence their health, are isolated inhabitation, presence of traditional health care practices, and their belief patterns. Natural and supernatural causation is the basic premise on which the tribal worldview on health and illness is based.

Akin to health cultures of many other tribal groups of India, the Koyas also have a distinct health culture, which is based on personalistic and naturalistic systems of health. They have developed their traditional medical system through observation of nature since ages. This traditional medical system is embedded in their concept of magic and religion and is a part of their culture. They depend largely on their traditional medical practitioners for their health needs. Owing to increasing contact with the non-tribals, they have also started approaching the modern medical facilities, but usually they did it as a last resort.

To conclude, in order to achieve the much aspired health for all, ethnomedical understanding of various health cultures is needed.

It is essential to research into the beliefs and response patterns, treatment patterns, indigenous *materia medica*, utilization of modern medical care and associated problems among the tribals as their perceptions of health and illness are quite distinct from those of the majority of non-tribal population. Therefore, there is a resistance to the mainstream health programmes since some therapeutic practices are in direct conflict with their traditional beliefs and culture. A scientific understanding of such factors will be of great help in framing specific health policies so as to encourage tribal participation in various communities based national health programmes, in implementation of certain modern medical programmes and in disseminating health care to the poorest and marginalized sections of the society.

References

Ali, Almas (1994). Indigenous health practices among tribals: Relationship with prevalent diseases. In S. Basu (Ed.), *Tribal Health in India*. New Delhi: Manak Publications.

Bauman, B. (1961). Diversities in conception of health and physical illness. *Journal of Health and Social Behaviour, 2*, 39-46.

Foster, G.M. and Anderson, B.G. (1979). *Medical Anthropology*. New York: John Wiley and Sons.

Hughes, C.C. (1968). Ethnomedicine. *International Encyclopedia of the Social Sciences, 10*, 87-93.

Hussain, Khan, C.G. (1992). Relevance of ethnomedicine. *Man and Life, 18*, 1-2.

Kar, R.K. and Gogoi, J. (1993). Health culture and tribal life: A case study among the Noetes of Arunachal Pradesh. *Man and Life, 19.*

Kochar, V. (n.d.) *Readings in Medical Sociology and Medical Anthropology*, Part II. Unpublished Manuscript, Department of Sociology and Anthropology, University of Hyderabad.

Mechanic, D. (1962). Concept of illness behaviour. *Journal of Chronic Diseases, 15*, 189-194.

Parson, T. (1964). *Social Structure and Personality*. New York: The Free Press.

Swain, S. (1994). Health disease and health seeking behaviour of tribal people in India. In S. Basu (Ed.), *Tribal Health in India.* New Delhi: Manak Publications.

9

Anthropological Perspective on Health

RAJAT KANTI DAS

I

It goes without saying that in the animal kingdom humans occupy a place of utmost importance for many considerations. In one sense, they may be regarded as animals who have made the best possible use of the evolutionary development. Admittedly, both biology and socio-cultural attributes shape human development. This realization has an important place in the current anthropological thinking and in the field of health this has assumed considerable importance. Broadly speaking, humans as social beings are all subject to a process of socialization around the bio-medical model. Consequently, health and illness, the latter having a strong mental component, are structured by social forces acting upon biology. It is true that disease with a strong somatic component has only a bio-medical application, but it becomes a part of the social phenomenon when looked from the people's point of view, particularly the meaning it holds for them in a specific social setting. The implication is that ultimately the mental level controls the somatic. The relation between somatic and mental health and between health and illness is a complicated one, but one has reasons to believe that these are not totally separable. In modern times, at the human level, behaviour and functioning are important determinants, but here more and more abstract attributes of the person (physio-chemical, anatomical, physiological, bio-chemical) are increasingly given prominence.

When these attributes become salient, the idea or concept of disease is essentially bio-medical. In such a situation, the attention shifts from the person to the process. On the other hand, our understanding of illness is one which focuses attention on the person. The contributions of medical anthropologists so far are mainly with regard to illness, though sickness involving disease and/or illness is their actual domain. In the ultimate analysis, there is considerable interdependence and interpenetration between the domain of individuals or persons and that of people and their culture. When sickness is defined as the process through which worrisome behavioural and biological signs, particularly ones originating in disease, are given socially recognizable meanings, the emphasis shifts more to culture and society. After all, it is the specific culture which provides a specific group of socially bound people with ways of thinking and creates a meaningful existence for them. Cultural manifestations reflect the human ability to develop behaviour patterns in the context of each and every ecological niche.

Health today is one particular area, which has engaged the attention not only of medical professionals, which is but natural for them, but also of social scientists, including anthropologists and sociologists, policy makers and administrators, development specialists and human welfare activists. The reasons for this are two-fold: (i) change in concept, and (ii) change in emphasis. At the conceptual level, sickness behaviour, representing health behaviour, is used as a concept to distinguish between disease as a biological category and illness as a social category. At another level, human populations like any forms of life undergo a continual process of adaptation to disease and illness. This calls for examining more closely and evaluating effects of disease and illness on human populations in producing sickness behaviour. Sickness behaviour, and for that matter, the whole gamut of health behaviour, requires close observation and here anthropologists, with a long history of field work behind them, may prove quite handy. Previously, in anthropology, behaviour in the field of health used to be considered along with other forms of social behaviour in a total setting. Now, health in itself represents a separate area marked by diversity of health beliefs and practices. While it may be hard to make valid generalizations about health behaviour because of the existence of a variety of health traditions, it is probably fair to say that the need is for an eclectic health model which may be able to combine scientific concepts and the ways of culture. After all, culture shapes the mode of life and it is culture which could maintain and sustain the fundamental rights, value system, traditions, worldviews and belief system of a people. Concepts of health and disease are a part of every culture. In one sense, understanding of disease means understanding of its causes, which concentrates more on biology of health. But, there is the question of relationship between biological and social phenomena. Illness representing social forces acts upon biology of health. For example, cholera is regarded as a disease of poverty, but malnutrition, which is also a condition of poverty, is taken to be an important factor in determining the state of health. Even the occurrence of depressive illnesses and all forms of psychological disorders may be attributed to socio-economic and cultural changes. The problems of adjustment in family affecting the children, working women and the aged have never been so strongly felt as they are today. Some psychosocial problems and disorders have assumed the forms of social pathological problems and social disorders. In case of specific diseases, terminal or chronic, we are now harping on social rehabilitation. Social behavioural development of children has come first among health priorities, but side by side it has to be remembered that the behavioural inconsistencies shown by the children are the results of growing expectations of the parents for their children. Here, the society undoubtedly has a role to play. Of late, the nature and intensity of the supports that a mentally retarded person needs to function in society have been highlighted. People with considerable degrees of intellectual disability, or those who are commonly identified as mentally retarded, need support from their families and from social service agencies. According to the American Association on Mental Retardation (AAMR), "mental retardation refers to substantial deficits in certain aspects of personal competence. It is manifested as significantly sub-average abilities in cognitive functioning, accompanied by deficits in adaptive skills."

Both cognitive functions and ability to function in society are impaired in the case of an individual with intellectual disability.

II

Though psychosocial problems and disorders are highly prevalent, these are not always properly recognized or taken note of making their treatment rather difficult. Moreover, traditional societies sometimes follow their own modes of social and cultural expression of health beliefs. It is not always easy to modify feelings, particularly when they are deeply rooted in cultural myths and beliefs. Following Pelzer (1996), psychological problems and disorders can be classified in the following way:

(1) social disorders (economic and occupational problems, family problems, sorcery, witchcraft, theft, ostracization, security and legal problems);
(2) psychoneurotic disorders (hysteria, depressive neurosis, anxiety neurosis);
(3) functional psychotic disorders;
(4) psychosomatic disorders (menstrual problems, impotence, asthma);
(5) disorders related to the use of alcohol, cannabis and other substances;
(6) psychosocial problems in patients with infertility, epilepsy, sterility, organic psychosis, mental handicap and development disabilities; and
(7) terminal or chronic diseases requiring psychosocial rehabilitation.

The scientific concepts regarding the above-mentioned psychosocial problems and disorders could not, on all occasions, be blended with the beliefs of popular culture because the emotional needs of the people mainly originate in a particular cultural context. Public health authorities have now recognized the positive influences of culture on health, which could be used to promote better health. And, the positive influences of culture involve body's natural abilities. In case of psychic suffering culture has a role to play because culture can affect the evolution and communication of depressive symptoms. It has been recognized that disillusionment on the part of individual and feelings of being lost may lead to destructive behaviour, criminality, gang-building, violence and abuse. Losing one's cultural identity or cultural uprootedness may lead to destructive behaviours in the form of alcoholism, criminality, domestic violence, anomie, and the like. At Barua, barely 3 km away from the heart of Midnapore town, the Santals, who are the original settlers, lead a more marginal existence than their neighbours, who were predominantly refugees from the erstwhile East

Bengal. Enterprising as they are, the Bengali migrants are now in a much better economic condition. Of course, in this case, the patronage of the dominant political party has to be taken into account. They enjoy a greater share of economic benefits; the number of service holders and entrepreneurs are more among them and they could derive better educational benefits. Not only that, they have more representation in the political bodies. Right from the beginning, the Santals were more at the receiving end. Their lands were taken away and they were increasingly drawn into a situation of deprivation. With lesser opportunities and means of their disposal, they have fallen well behind their Bengali neighbours in the field of education and employment. More and more of their people have become alcoholic. Relation with their neighbours is anything but cordial. There were even open outbursts against them, which, if anything, were evidences of psychological distress. They used to suffer from a cultural uprootness. Obviously, there are social and political origin of psychological distress. It is now common knowledge that suicide deaths, cases of poisoning and inflicting violence are on the increase. Insecurity has become the order of the day as has been demonstrated by frequent accidents causing serious injuries and deaths. The non-specific characteristics in relation to functional disorders of individual mind, which seem to be almost universal, are a fundamental change of mood, a diminution of interest and initiative, a lack of enjoyment of life, sleeping troubles, and loss of appetite or libido. In a WHO study conducted in 1983, it was revealed that 76-100 percent of the patients in all four countries involved, namely, Canada, Iran, Japan and Switzerland, showed a core of symptoms comprising "sadness, lack of joy, anxiety, tension, lack of energy, lack of interest, loss of concentration and feelings of inadequacy, incapacity or loss of esteem".

In the early nineties of the last century, the World Bank and WHO drew up tables of the burden associated with different diseases in terms of disability adjusted life years. Depressive disorders account for almost 30 percent of the disability from neuro-psychiatric disorders among women, but for only 12.6 percent among men. On the other hand, alcohol and drug dependence accounts for 31 percent of neuropsychiatric disability among men, but for 7 percent among women. It appears that symptoms of depression and anxiety as well as unspecified psychiatric disorders and psychological distress are more prevalent among women, whereas substance disorders are more prevalent among men. This difference in the pattern of the mental disorders between sexes varies in different phases of life. Most studies show a higher prevalence of mental health problems in young boys than in girls, the former experiencing more conduct disorders, with aggressive and anti-social behaviour. During adolescence, the difference becomes smaller because girls experience more emotional problems, with fearful, anxious or over-controlled behaviour. In adulthood, men have more problems related to alcohol, drug abuse and anti-social behaviour, while women suffer more from anxiety, depression and eating disorders. If alcohol and drug abuse are problems equally affecting the women, the instigation comes more from the men. Men are used to see women as their companions and supporters of their cause. After all, gender violence makes women suffer most. It may very will be the cause of psychiatric morbidity in women. In a displacement-oriented study of a village in the Sagar Island of the Sundarbans of West Bengal conducted by Salil Kumar Dutta, a Ph.D. scholar to the Department of Anthropology, Vidyasagar University, it has been revealed that in family matters women's participation and involvement are substantially higher than the menfolk. Day in and day out, they perform their household duties without any break, looking into the requirements of dependent family members – the old and the children. It is they who literally run the families and in the process also earn taking part in tiger prawn seed (*Penacus modon*) collection, which happens to be the major source of earning for the villagers. Their husbands, on the other hand, spend a lot of time outside remaining away from the family. They are also not so consistent in contributing their share to the family. Of late, they have developed a tendency to spend more time in playful activities – gossiping with friends, taking to alcohol and popular opium products and even gambling. Some of them have become addict. When they run short of money, they demand from their wives and, if refused, resort to physical torture. Pressure on the women is considerable, placed as they are in a difficult situation of managing the family matters effectively with the uncertain support of their husbands. At the top of it, they have to yield to the sexual demands of their husbands. No wonder, the women show more mental stress, which has been confirmed from the results of the scale employed in the study. Needless to say, gender violence is closely tied to a women's sexuality, fidelity, pregnancy and childbearing. In this way, it becomes a reproductive health problem. Domestic violence takes a terrible toll on women's self-esteem. More than physical pain, it creates emotional anguish of being forced into sex life. Attempts are now being made in some limited quarters comprising the most enlightened section of the womenfolk to stall the onslaught. There are even instances of retaliatory measures being adopted by the women. But this also generates more stress.

The social origins of psychological distress for women has been acknowledged by classical research works. It was found that depression was more prevalent among working class rather than middle class women. Poor women are more likely to deal with chronic sources of social stress in the form of low-quality housing, dangerous neighbourhoods, higher risk of becoming victims of violence and of encountering problems in parenting and childcare. Even when severe harm is inflicted on them or they become serious victims of male-dominating behaviour, they cannot automatically count on the support of the different organizations and representative bodies managed by the educated and enlightened people. More and more women are now drawn into the field of politics. Naturally, political compulsions, strong commitments to political ideal leave them with little opportunity to provide unqualified support to women's cause in each and every social context. The problem lies more with their poverty than with their status as women. After all, poverty represents a state of suppression and a part of the population is always suppressed. One may suggest that psychiatric morbidity in women has a direct relation with socio-economic factors. Robert Desjarlais *et al.* (1995) observed:

> Poverty, domestic isolation, powerlessness resulting from economic dependence or low levels of education and patriarchal oppression are all associated with a higher prevalence of psychiatric morbidity in women. This morbidity is, however, exclusive of substance abuse.

It is the cumulative effect of various socio-economic deprivations that matters most. In the context of removing social ills and countering socio-economic deprivations, community consideration is receiving much attention not only from the government, but also from a host of development specialists and social scientists. It has now dawned on us that promoting healthy, non-violent communities contribute to good health and a relatively tension-free atmosphere. Michele Tonsella, Professor of Psychiatry, Institute of Psychiatry, University of Verona, and formerly Director of the WHO collaborating centre for Research and Training in Mental Health and Service Evaluation, in one article in *World Health* (1998), has made a valid point regarding the relative weight of the biological and psychological behaviours causing mental disorders. He writes:

> It is more helpful to think of two main groups of causes of mental disorders: physical and biological on one side (such as genetic component, birth trauma, maternal infections at a particular point in a pregnancy); and social, situational and interactional on the other side (such as stressful factors but buffers that serve to diminish the impact of unfavourable external events). Again, the relative contribution to mental disorder made by the biological/physical or by the social/cultural sets of factors is not unclear.

There is, of course, an urgent need to improve psychological and social well-being of the people and for this purpose apart from identifying clear-cut biological factors, special attention needs to be given to factors related to roles, stereotypes and social circumstances of people's lives.

III

It may be said that human lifestyles and human behaviours hold the key to the future of health of humankind. Lifestyle again is intricately connected with social habits and cultural values. These, of course, keep on changing. Recent studies have shown evidence of a definite change in the clinical profile of depressive states in developing countries. A wide range of ailments such as headache, stomach upsets or back pain, as well as the fear of illness and death, are increasingly associated with the lifestyle. These express not only a feeling of being unwell but also a desire to die, which are indicative a depressive states. An epidemiological study made among the general public in Tunisia in 1995 revealed, in a sample of 5,000 persons, prevalence rates of depression that were entirely comparable with those of the industrialized countries. It does seem as if 'western style' depression is common in parallel with socio-economic development, urbanization and the consequent dislocation of traditional community structures. A recent WHO survey in general health care setting in 14 countries confirmed that depressive disorders were as common in developing countries as they were in developed countries.

Charles Hughes and John Hunter (1972: 93) coined the term 'diseases of development' to refer to "those pathological conditions which are based on the usually unanticipated consequences of the implementation of development schemes". Such diseases may be divided into three general categories. First, there are those diseases that result from integrating people into large-scale industrial societies: diabetes, obesity, hypertension and so on. For example, the people of Nauru found themselves with a dramatic increase in disposable wealth in the 1960 as a result of renegotiations of the royalties paid to them for mining phosphate on their isolated South Pacific island. In fact, they soon had one of the highest per capita incomes in the world. Along with this sudden increase in wealth came a rise in consumption of food containing more sugar and salt but low in nutrition's value. Their food consumption reached a daily average of around 6,000 calories per person. The impact of this on their health was equally dramatic. In 1983, out of a total population of some 5,000 Nauruans, about 400 were known or believed to be suffering from diabetes. The second category includes instances where development programmes have upset existing environmental conditions and introduced or increased bacterial and parasitic diseases. African river blindness, which was once rampant in the Volta river basin in West Africa, is a clear example of that. The slowly debilitating disease *bilharziasis*, caused by a parasitic blood fluke found in certain water snails, is another instance of the impact of development projects. Many more such instances could be cited. The third category comprises diseases resulting from the failure of development programme that seek to overcome the conditions that result from the unsatisfactory integration of people into large-scale societies. These include the innumerable diseases associated with poverty, undernourishment and unsanitary living conditions. Even arctic hysteria, which was detected among the arctic people, falls into this category. This is a condition marked by periods of silence followed by seizure characterized by certain behaviours like tearing of one's clothings, flight and wandering about in the snow.

It is now an established fact that cultural representations of the human body, time, life, death and disease vary from society to society. Consequently, people's approaches to actions, preventions and treatment of disease and illness also vary. As Hiroshi Nakajima, former Director General of WHO, and Federico Mayor, former Director-General of UNESCO put it in their Editorial in *World Health* (1996): "Procreation, childbirth, weaning, sexuality, death, disease and suffering are not just private experiences but all have an intrinsic social dimension. The health conditions in which they take place are often determined as much as by cultural practices as by biological and environmental factors." Traditional practices, such as food taboos during pregnancy and childbirth or lifestyle behaviour, can have serious consequences for people's health. All will agree that healthy lifestyle is as much a product of health consciousness as the attitude towards life. Attitudes and feelings are difficult to modify, particularly when they are deeply rooted in cultural myths and beliefs. That's why, 'cultural' causes may not always be easily separated from 'medical' causes. Cultural sphere also brings into focus the display of 'folk wisdom' by the tradition-minded people. As for instance, through trial and error over generations, traditional societies have developed culinary practices which enable them to prepare and eat safe food even in unhygienic conditions. Cooking meat in small pieces to facilitate heat penetration, using proper fermentation processes, developing indigenous techniques to preserve food – are all examples of folk wisdom. Still it has to be conceded that folk wisdom may not always be an infallible guide to healthy food habits. But this can certainly add an element of conservatism in people's attitude.

IV

Studies in the field of health provide the necessary scope for transdisciplinary sciences to go for an integrated mode of investigation. Health is one of the focal centres of integration of human biological and social sciences. The concern of human biology is not quite the same is that of epidemiology. Epidemiology deals with disease patterns exclusively, whereas human biology includes 'well-being' and normative variable in its research focus. Epidemiologists tend to be concerned particularly with risk factor for disease and in developing appropriate methods of intervention.

In human biology health-related variables are treated from a genetic or evolutionary perspective. Similarly, in sharp contrast to epidemiologists, human biologists are particularly concerned with confirming adaptive models, not with factors responsible for disease manifestation. The evolutionary perspective of human population biology can throw light on the environmental, cultural and genetic conditions that promote disease. This aspect has now been adequately reflected in medical anthropology. Medical anthropology, in its present form, represents an important application area in anthropology. It deals with culturally constituted treatments for the categories of illness as well as the categories of western scientific medicine, where the perspective is mainly 'biologistic'. These signify a combination of 'emic' and 'etic' categories. Medical anthropology provides an ideal platform for the integration of human biological and social sciences taking health as a variable. While medical anthropology takes in its stride both the problems of cultural variation as well as biological variation, human population biology and epidemiology concentrate on biological variation within and between population in respect of health. In medical anthropological studies the need for incorporating the methods followed by the latter has been increasingly realized. But, the biological dimension of medical anthropology tends to focus on an ecological framework, where the effects of disease and health practices are pinpointed on the culture itself. A medical anthropologist's search for socio-centric explanations validates a position that changes in the state of health are dependent more on non-medical factors than just on medical care. Needless to say, the major non-medical factors are derived mainly from the social and physical environment affecting a specific group of people. Only with the help of these it may be possible to explain why culturally and socially accepted forms of drug use, including intoxication on specified festive occasions, have been strongly defended by the community members. At the opposite end we find when safety promotion is undertaken by the community, it works much better. The Navajo safe community programme undertaken by the Navajo nation in the USA stands out as an example. If the developed sections of American population are moving from an era of 'medicine' to one of 'health', in case of developing regions the trend is probably the opposite. The people in the developing countries have been increasingly dependent on medicines, showing less concern about "the importance of cultural factors and the significance of human scale in the determination of health". But, these were once their strong points. That their values have been recognized once again at specific levels is a welcome sign.

References

Alland, A. (1970). *Adaptation in Cultural Evolution.* New York: Columbia University Press.

Brothwell, D. (1971). Disease, micro-evolution, and earlier populations: An important bridge between medical history and human biology. In Clarke, E. (Ed.), *Modern Methods in the History of Medicine*. New York: The Athlone Press.

Douki, S. and Tabbane, K. (1996). Culture and depression. In *World Health,* No. 2, March-April, World Health Organization, Geneva.

Holmes, T. and Masuda, M. (1973). Life changes and illness susceptibility, In P. Scott and E. Senay (Eds.), *Separation and Depression*. Washington, D.C.: American Association for the Advancement of Science, No. 94.

Logan, M.H. and Hunt, E.E. Jr. (Eds.) (1978). *Health and the Human Condition: Perspectives on Medical Anthropology*. North Scituate: Duxbury Press.

Mittler, Peter (1995). Intellectual disability. In *World Health*, No. 5. September-October, World Health Organization, Geneva.

Mohammad Aqbdussalam and Fritz Kaferstein (1996). Food beliefs and taboos. In *World Health*, No. 2, March-April, World Health Organization, Geneva.

Moore, G.G., Van Arsdale, Glittenberg, J.E. and Aldrich, R.A. (1987). *The Biocultural Basis of Health*. Illinois: Waveland Press Inc.

Nakajima, Hiroshi and Mayor, Federico (1996). Editorial: Culture and health. In *World Health,* No. 2, March-April, World Health Organization, Geneva.

Pelzer, Karl (1996). Psychotherapy and culture in Africa. In *World Health*, No. 2, March-April. World Health Organization, Geneva.

Sell, Helmut L. (1996). Ritual and culture. In *World Health*, No. 2 March-April. World Health Organization. Geneva.

Svanstrom, L. and Moa Sundstrom (1996). Promoting community safety. In *World Health*, No. 2, March-April, World Health Organization, Geneva.

Tonsella, Michele (1998). Gender difference in mental health. In *World Health*, No. 5, September-October. World Health Organization, Geneva.

III

Social Psychology of Health

10

Psychosocial Correlates of Health: A Review

N.R. SHARMA, A. SHARMA AND A. YADAVA

"Who is happy? Do any particular developmental period (age), gender, income level, genetically predisposed traits, supportive relationships, a spiritual perspective or the like make one happier than others?" Myers (2000) rightly commented that issues like these not only went unanswered during most of psychology's first century, they went largely unsolicited as psychologists focused on illness more than health, on fear more than courage, on aggression more than love. An electronic search of *Psychological Abstracts* since 1887 turned up 8,072 articles on anger, 57,800 on anxiety and 70,856 on depression, while only 851 abstracts mentioned joy, 2,958 happiness and 5,701 life satisfaction. In this sampling, negative emotions trounced positive emotions by a 17-to-1 ratio (even greater than the 7-to-1 margin by which *treatment* exceeded *prevention*). Even today, our search exhibits literature on sufferings more than happiness and positive health.

It is unfortunate to note that the conceptual definitions of health have themselves been faulty by defining health negatively in terms of what is present when health is absent. However, now-a-days, behavioural scientists have started taking a serious note of this flaw in the definition of health and have attempted redefining it in terms of what is present when health is present. They have been attempting to extend the scope of health, beyond the mere absence of disease or infirmity and, even beyond considering it "as a state of complete physical, mental and social well-being" (WHO, 1946).

Moreover, maintenance of health and well-being does not only mean *treatment* of physical diseases and/or psychological stress, but also *prevention* through restructuring the person's environment and *promotion* of general well-being through healthy lifestyles. The 'perfect functioning' approach to health conceptualizes the three most important ingredients: (i) *social* (emphasizing on the social conditions in which the individual's capacities for participation are optimal); (ii) *biological* (emphasizing a state in which every cell and organ is functioning at optimal capacity and in perfect harmony with the rest of the body); and (iii) *psychological* (emphasizing a state in which the individual feels a sense of 'well-being' and of mastery over his self and environment). As far as health has been considered as a state of physical, mental and social well-being, health indicators should ideally be given in terms of *positive* well-being rather than in terms of physical, mental and social pathology, morbidity, or rate of mortality (Nagpal, 1986). So, the world has started giving due importance to the concept of positive health and well-being. The psychologists all over the world have now been turning their focus of attention towards various possible 'correlates' of well-being.

However, the credit goes to Wilson (1967) for presenting the first major review of empirical evidence regarding the "correlates of avowed happiness". He reached to the conclusion that a person who is "young, healthy, well-educated, well-paid, extroverted, optimistic, worry-free, religious, married with high self-esteem, job morale, modest aspirations, of either sex, and of a wide range of intelligence" is a happy person. However, a lot of water has flown under the bridge since the time of Wilson's review. Researchers have been studying the concept extensively and with more sensitive and standardized measures. Interestingly, the review of these later researches reveals that Wilson was accurate in a number of respects in his description of the happy individual. But, some of his conclusions have also been overturned by subsequent research. Here is a brief review of some of these studies.

Age

In his review, Wilson concluded that younger people report more happiness than older people. So, youth is one of the most important demographic factors influencing well-being. Since Wilson's review, other behavioural scientists researched the question of age and well-being on large, representative, international samples and using sophisticated methodologies. Interviews with representative samples of people of all ages reveal that *no time of life is notably happier or unhappier than others* (Inglehart, 1990).

Happiness, however, is only a single dimension of well-being. Research suggests that well-being is a multidimensional construct and for a complete understanding of the phenomenon, the researchers recommend examining various dimensions. Recently, a study was conducted by Sharma, Sharma and Yadava (2002) to examine, in sufficient details, the effect of age, gender and level of income on various well-being dimensions. For this purpose, they prepared a battery of well-being measures to include most of the important dimensions of well-being. Measures included were Subjective Well-Being Inventory (SUBI) (Sell and Nagpal, 1992), Satisfaction with Life Scale (SWLS) (Diener, Emmons, Larson and Griffin, 1985) and General Health Questionnaire-12 (Goldberg and Hillier, 1979).

SUBI is a 40-item inventory that assesses the subjective well-being of the subjects on 11 factorial dimensions. These dimensions are general well-being-positive affect (GWB-PA), expectation-achievement congruence (EAC), confidence in coping (CC), transcendence (Trans), family group support (FGS), social support (SS), primary group concern (PGC), inadequate mental mastery (IMM), perceived ill-health (PI-H), deficiency in social contacts (DSC), and general well-being – negative affect (GWB-NA). The total scores on these 11 dimensions provide a total subjective well-being score (SWBS). SWLS contains five items requiring a general and cognitive evaluation of the respondent's life as a whole on a 7-point scale ranging from strongly disagree to strongly agree. As part of mental health surveillance, the General Health Questionnaire-12 or as popularly known GHQ-12 (Goldberg and Hillier, 1979) was also included in the study. This is a short screening test for non-psychiatric disorders. The GHQ-12 is a self-administered screening test, designed to identify short-term changes in mental health (depression, anxiety, social dysfunction and somatic symptoms). Thus, the battery provided 14 well-being scores in total.

These tools were administered on a sample of 300 educated adults selected from the general population on the basis of non-random purposive sampling procedures. The age range of the subjects was 20-50 years, with a median of 36 and a SD of 7.68. The sample was divided into two age groups on the basis of median split. The N of the first group (G1) was 154 (with age range of 36 to 50 years) and the second group (G2) consisted of 146 subjects (with age range of 20 to 35 years). Total 14 t-tests were worked out to find out the significance of difference between their means on 13 well-being dimensions. Variables showing the significant mean differences are presented below:

Table 1

Mean, SD and t-values for Well-being Dimensions (df = 298)

Well-being dimensions	*Mean*	*SD*	*t-value*	*Sig. level*
FGS	G1= 8.42 G2= 8.20	G1= 0.86 G2= 1.08	1.99	.05
PI-H	G1= 13.90 G2= 14.72	G1= 2.46 G2= 2.58	-2.827	.005
Total score on SUBI	G1= 94.66 G2= 91.32	G1= 7.96 G2= 10.09	3.19	.002
General health	G1= 7.72 G2= 8.85	G1= 4.73 G2= 4.59	-2.1	.05

Major results reveal that out of 14 comparisons, four t-values proved to be significant which imply that the older subjects experienced better well-being than the younger ones. The discrepancy of the present findings from those reviewed by Wilson may be due to the fact that older people are now healthier and stay involved in more life domains than did previous generations. Secondly, the predictors of happiness also change with age. Satisfaction with social relations and health become more important in later life. Thirdly and most importantly, in the present-day scenario, with population explosion, there is a scarcity of resources and employment. Hence, the younger people, being the most needy of jobs, have to struggle a lot but have to face problems and frustrations at every front of life – be it long queues for jobs, social gatherings or even at home. This might be a prominent source of their lower well-being on some dimensions. However, this also seems true that someone's age can give no clue to his/her average sense of well-being (Myers and Diener, 1995).

Gender

Regarding sex differences in well-being, Wilson (1967) discussed only one study, i.e., Gurin, Veroff and Feld's (1960) survey that revealed no sex differences in happiness. In a meta-analysis of 146 studies, Haring, Stock and Okun (1984) found that men were slightly happier than women, although the magnitude of this difference was very small (mean $r = .04$). Inglehart (1990), on the basis of the data collected from 169,776 people in the 1980s collaborative survey of 16 nations, reported that an equal number (80%) of men and women said that they were at least 'fairly satisfied' with life.

In the same study discussed above, conducted by Sharma, Sharma and Yadava (2002), the effect of gender on various well-being dimensions was also studied. The sample consisted of 187 males (G1) and 113 females (G2). Variables showing the significant mean differences are presented below:

Table 2

Mean, SD, t-values for Other Well-being Dimensions (df = 298)

Well-being dimensions	*Mean*	*SD*	*t-value*	*Sig. level*
GWB-PA	G1 = 7.27 G2 = 7.69	G1 = 1.44 G2 = 1.28	-2.54	.01
Trans	G1 = 5.4 G2 = 6.1	G1 = 2.08 G2 = 2.08	-2.74	.01
PI-H	G1 = 14.67 G2 = 13.68	G1 = 2.43 G2 = 2.64	3.30	.01
DSC	G1 = 7.61 G2 = 7.11	G1 = 1.73 G2 = 1.77	2.45	.05

Although females have shown better on four well-being dimensions, they do not differ from the males in global well-being. Some earlier studies have also concluded that sometimes women report slightly greater happiness and sometimes men but the net result is roughly equal hedonic balance for men and women. Wilson also concluded that person of either sex can experience happiness and well-being, and sex has nothing much to do with this.

Level of Income

Income certainly plays a role in the determination of well-being, though this relation is not always right. Argyle (1999) reported that in poor countries like India, people with low income find it difficult to satisfy even their basic human needs. Hence, being relatively well-off and in somewhat better position results in greater well-being. Sharma, Sharma and Yadava (2002) also reported that lower income group generally suffers from 'deficiency in social contacts (DSC)' and 'general well-being – negative affect (GWB-NA)', whereas higher income group is on the advantageous position and experiences greater levels of well-being. However, wealth seems to be just like health: its absence can breed misery, yet having it is no guarantee of happiness. In support of this observation, Diener, Horwitz and Emmons (1985) reported one survey in which wealthiest Americans on *Forbes'* list reported only slightly greater happiness than other Americans; alarmingly 37 percent reported less happiness than the average American. So, money in itself cannot bring all happiness.

Educational Standard

Some researchers (Campbell, Converse and Rogers, 1976; Diener, Sandvik, Seidlitz and Diener, 1993) have reported small but significant correlations between education and well-being. Education may result in both ends. On the one hand, education may contribute to well-being by allowing individuals to make progress towards their goals or to adapt to changes in the world around them. On the other hand, education may raise aspirations which, if unfulfilled, might result in dissatisfactions. In a comparative study, conducted on unemployed people, Clark and Oswald (1994) found that the highly educated were more distressed than less educated persons. So, education may lead to ill-being also if it generates expectations that cannot be fulfilled.

Level of Intelligence

As Wilson (1967) observed, intelligence *per se* is probably not directly related to well-being. A great need is felt to study minutely the relation between well-being and other types of intelligence such as social intelligence and emotional intelligence. It seems likely that the relation of intelligence to well-being will depend on the degree to which intelligent people share higher expectations that counter-balance their advantages.

Religion

Various researches reveal that well-being correlates significantly with religious certainty (Ellison, 1991), strength of one's relationship with the divine (Pollner, 1989), prayer experiences (Poloma and Pendlenton, 1991), and devotional and participatory aspects of religiosity (Ellison, Gay and Glass, 1989), even after controlling for demographic variable such as age, income and marital status. The reason behind this is that religion might provide not only psychological but also social benefits: *psychological benefits* by providing the person a sense of meaning in daily life as well as at the times of major life crises; and *social benefits* by offering a collective identity and reliable social networks consisting of people who share similar social values and attitudes.

Marital Status

Wilson (1967) seems to be right in his conclusions about the positive relation between marriage and well-being, which has been consistently replicated across cultures. Literature reveals that married people report greater happiness than those who were never married or are divorced, separated or widowed. This is because marriage provides greater benefits in terms of emotional, social (and economic) support.

Race, Social Class and Culture

Race in itself seems to have no effect on one's well-being. It is the racial discrimination that might result in lower well-being.

However, despite discrimination, people in disadvantaged groups are found to maintain their self-esteem by valuing the things at which they excel, by making comparisons within their own groups, and by attributing problems to external sources such as prejudice (Crocker and Major, 1989). As far as the cultures are concerned, nations differ strikingly in happiness. Diener and Diener (1995) reported a greater well-being in individualistic cultures than in collectivistic nations because the former place great emphasis on autonomy and internal feelings.

Employment Status

Unemployment is perhaps the biggest evil in the present-day world. We should not take the problem of unemployment as an economic issue only because it also has its own social, psychological and medical consequences. Socio-psychological research on unemployment generally reveals lowered life satisfaction, self-esteem, psychological well-being, or increased psychological distress and cognitive problems in the unemployed persons (Mohal, 1991). Sharma, Sharma and Sharma (2002), in a recent study on the mental health status of career and non-career women, observed that non-career women languish in the state of poor mental health than their counterparts.

Social Support

Social support has repeatedly been found to be related to health and well-being. Indeed, people report happier feelings when they are with others (Pavot, Diener and Fujita, 1990). Those who enjoy close relationships cope better with various stresses, including bereavement, rape, job loss and illness (Perlman and Rook, 1987), as a result, experience better well-being.

Life Events

As far as the situational/environmental effects on well-being are concerned, Suh, Diener and Fujita (1996) reported that only life events during the previous three months influenced well-being. So, only recent life events influence well-being, old life events have no deteriorating effect on well-being since people adapt to these. It has been observed that individuals have their own personal baseline of happiness and people labor on 'hedonic treadmill'. Gains and losses, however, have a strong but temporary effect, thereby, people soon adapt to the changed circumstances.

However, due to the demographic variables' failure in determining significantly people's well-being (Diener, 1984) and due to their lack of predictive power, researchers focused on internal influences on well-being such as personality variables. Many researchers have reported that well-being is primarily determined by enduring individual characteristics rather than by external life circumstances (Costa and McRae, 1980; Diener, Sandvik, Pavot and Fujita, 1992).

Personality Traits and Types

Extraversion and neuroticism are the personality traits that have received the most theoretical and empirical attention in relation to well-being. Costa and McRae (1980) reported that extraversion influences positive affect, whereas neuroticism influences negative affect. Lucas, Diener, Grob, Suh and Shao (2000) replicated the strong extraversion-pleasant affect relation. However, Diener, Suh and Oishi (1997) state, "what is not yet clear is whether extraversion predicts pleasant affect to the same extent in different cultures such as in India or Nepal".

In India, recently, such a study was conducted by Sharma (2002) to investigate the personality correlates of well-being. In order to assess the personality, 16 Personality Factor (PF) test was used while well-being was measured with the help of a battery used by Sharma, Sharma and Yadava (2002). In a sample of 300 subjects, he found that person who are outgoing, intelligent, emotionally stable, happy-go-lucky, conscientious, venturesome, and having high self-concept control experience more positive affect. Persons, who are aggressive, tender minded, suspicious, bohemian, shrewd, worrying, tense and having high anxiety, experience more negative affect. And, as far as life satisfaction is concerned, persons having higher ego strength, happy-go-lucky, conscientious, venturesome, liberal, socially precise and extraverts are more satisfied with their life whereas tender-minded, bohemian, apprehensive, tense and incisive persons experience less life satisfaction. Separate stepwise multiple regressions and factor analysis confirmed that self-esteem, extraversion and anxiety traits of personality are significantly correlated with various studied well-being dimensions of the Subjective Well-Being Inventory (Sell and Nagpal, 1992), GHQ-12 score and life satisfaction. The findings are shown in the following two tables:

Table 3

Multiple Regression Analyses Taking 16 PF Test and Self-esteem as Predictors

Sr. No.	*Well-being dimensions*	*Most significant contributing predictor*	*Direction of relationship*	*R*	*R2*	*F*	*P*
1	GWB-PA	Self-esteem	Positive	.390	.152	53.60	<.001
2	EAC	Self-esteem	Positive	.343	.118	39.86	<.001
3	CC	Self-esteem	Positive	.248	.062	19.57	<.001
4	Trans	Conscien-tiousness (G)	Positive	.451	.204	76.26	<.001
5	FGS	Self-esteem	Positive	.266	.071	22.74	<.001
6	SS	Self-esteem	Positive	.191	.037	11.31	<.001
7	PGC	Surgency (F)	Positive	.245	.060	19.05	<.001
8	IMM	Tender-mindedness(I)	Positive	.252	.063	20.15	<.001
9	PIH	Assertiveness (E)	Positive	.289	.083	27.10	<.001
10	DSC	Self-esteem	Negative	.390	.152	17.68	<.001
11	GWB-NA	Social-boldness (H)	Negative	.317	.100	33.24	<.001
12	GHQ	Self-esteem	Negative	.408	.167	59.67	<.001
13	LS	Self-esteem	Positive	.339	.115	38.72	<.001

Entries in parentheses are 16 PF test's factor designations.

Table 4
Multiple Regression Analyses Taking Predictors of Various Well-being Dimensions from Four Secondary Factors of 16 PF Test

Sr. No.	Well-being dimensions	Most significant contributing predictor	Direction of relationship	R	R2	F	P
1	GWB-PA	Anxiety(QII)	Negative	.224	.050	15.77	<.001
2	EAC	Anxiety(QII)	Negative	.263	.069	22.09	<.001
3	CC	Extraversion (QI)	Positive	.137	.019	05.66	<.018
4	Trans	Tough Poise (QIII)	Negative	.368	.136	23.31	<.001
5	FGS	—	—	—	—	—	—
6	SS	—	—	—	—	—	—
7	PGC	Extraversion (QI)	Positive	.200	.040	12.41	<.001
8	IMM	Extraversion (QI)	Negative	.172	.029	9.05	<.003
9	PIH	Extraversion (QI)	Negative	.264	.070	22.29	<.001
10	DSC	Extraversion (QI)	Negative	.266	.071	22.69	<.001
11	GWB-NA	Extraversion (QI)	Negative	.278	.077	25.02	<.001
12	GHQ	Anxiety(QII)	Positive	.303	.092	30.12	<.001
13	LS	Extraversion (QI)	Positive	.235	.055	17.43	<.001

Entries in parentheses are 16 PF test's secondary factor designations.

So, extraversion and neuroticism are clearly not the only traits that relate to well-being. Self-esteem also is significantly related to various dimensions of well-being (Sharma, Sharma and Yadava, 2004).

In a very recent and interesting review article, Richardson (2003) also reports the gist of Diener's researches that "social relationships, temperament, having long-term goals that are congruent with one another, and that are pleasurable to work for" are crucial factors for one's well-being.

As everyone of us might have experienced, "we (all) are inclined towards happiness". Despite having physical and/or mental disabilities and less money, we are mostly happy with our lives. What could be the main reason behind this? Scientific explanations to this question have been provided by Walker and associates. *Hindustan*

Times (2003) quoted research findings of Walker *et al.*, who reported that "human memory is biased toward happiness". They have elucidated two reasons for one's recollection of the past to be positively biased: "pleasant events do outnumber unpleasant events because people seek out positive experiences and avoid negative ones" and "our memory system treats pleasant emotions differently from unpleasant emotions". Seven studies reviewed by the researchers provide support for a fading affect for negative emotions. Pleasant emotions have been found to fade more slowly from our memory than unpleasant emotions.

A very careful reader might have noted that majority of the studies quoted in this paper are by foreign authors, the major reason being not much empirical work in this direction (as such) has been conducted in India and there is a lot of potential for health psychologists, counselling psychologists and mental health researchers/ practitioners in taking up research on this issue for clear and minute understanding of the concept of well-being. However, in one early (but timely) paper, Sinha (1990) reviewed intensively as well as extensively the concept of psychosocial well-being from the western and Indian perspectives. In this review, he elucidated the concepts of adjustment, health, adaptation, homeostasis, competence and quality of life as associated with psychosocial well-being stressing Indian perspective.

He derived and enlisted a number of psychological qualities from *Bhagavad Gita* (an Indian scripture) which are believed to be essential for well-being. Sinha (1990) writes: "The characteristics that have been emphasized are that a calm man is the same in pain and pleasure; he is equipoise in success and failure; he is content with what comes to him without effort, is unaffected by conflict, and is free from envy; he is even minded in success and failure and is not bound even while acting. Further, he hates no creatures and is friendly and compassionate towards all, and who is free from the feelings of 'I' and 'mine', even-minded in pleasure and pain, forbearing, ever content, steady in mediation, self-controlled and possessed of firm conviction; he is such as cannot be agitated by the world or is free from joy, envy, fear and anxiety; he is free from dependence, pure and prompt, unconcerned and untroubled, renouncing every undertaking (page 8)." His present paper provides new insights in this issue and a whole new series of research can be generated on the Indian perspective of well-being he has offered.

In his writings, Dalal (2001) also commented that social and family support have been neglected variables and must be given due attention, especially in the light of deteriorating health care services in our country. He recommended that systematic research is highly required on Indian scriptures like the *Bhagavad Gita,* the *Yoga Sutra,* and the *Charak Samhita* that offer highly developed strategies to manage tragic life experiences, to alleviate sufferings, and to promote well-being. Thus, Sinha (1990) and Dalal (2001) open up new avenues for research studies to be done from Indian perspective in the field of well-being. Moreover, other less researched variables (particularly in Indian settings) like adjustment, social and family support, hope, optimism, and temperament etc., exploring the direction of relationship/effect is also another pertinent issue, i.e., to find out whether adjustment leads to well-being or vice versa. Future research in this direction can widen our understanding of the concept.

Conclusion

The above review of the literature suggests that very few demographic factors have strong relationship with well-being. The knowledge of someone's age, gender, income level and race hardly indicate his/her level of well-being. Although external situations and circumstances matter, they have short-term impacts. What then is important in the prediction of one's well-being? It appears, however, that individual reactions to these circumstances are more important in determining well-being. It is in these individual reactions to events that personality plays its significant role. Better clues to one's levels of well-being are provided by one's personality traits, whether he/she enjoys close relationships, supportive network, or whether he/she has a faith, hope and purpose in life. There is an unfortunate dearth of Indian studies in this field and western viewpoints might not be relevant as per Indian culture. There is a great need of scientific and systematic studies to understand happiness and well-being from Indian perspective. Only then, effective psychological strategies to promote mental health and well-being could be designed and implemented.

References

Argyle, M. (1999). Causes and correlates of happiness. In D. Kahneman, E. Diener and N. Schwartz (Eds.), *Well-being: The Foundations of Hedonic Psychology*. New York: Russell Sage Foundation.

Campbell, A., Converse, P.E. and Rogers, W.L. (1976). *The Quality of American Life*. New York: Sage.

Clark, A.E. and Oswald, A.J. (1994). Unhappiness and unemployment. *Economic Journal, 104*, 648-659.

Costa, P.T. and McRae, R.R. (1980). Influence of extraversion and neuroticism on subjective well-being: Happy and unhappy people. *Journal of Personality and Social Psychology, 38*, 668-678.

Crocker, J. and Major, B. (1989). Social stigma and self-esteem: The self-protective properties of stigma. *Psychological Review, 96*, 608-630.

Dalal, A.K. (2001). Health psychology. In Janak Pandey (Ed.), *Psychology in India Revisited: Developments in the Discipline*, Vol. 2 (pp. 356-411). New Delhi: Sage Publications.

Diener, E. (1984). Subjective well-being. *Psychological Bulletin, 95*, 542-575.

Diener, E. and Diener, M. (1995). Cross-cultural correlates of life satisfaction and self-esteem. *Journal of Personality and Social Psychology, 68*, 653-663.

Diener, E., Emmons, R.A., Larsen, R.J. and Griffin, S. (1985). The satisfaction with life scale. *Journal of Personality Assessment, 49*, 71-75.

Diener, E., Horwitz, J. and Emmons, R.A. (1985). Happiness of the very wealthy. *Social Indicators Research, 16*, 263-274.

Diener, E., Sandvik, E., Pavot, W. and Fujita, F. (1992). Extraversion and subjective well-being in a U.S. national probability sample. *Journal of Research in Personality, 26*, 205-215.

Diener, E., Sandvik, E., Seidlitz, L. and Diener, M. (1993). The relationship between income and subjective well-being: Relative or absolute? *Social Indicators Research, 28*, 195-223.

Diener, E., Suh, E.M. and Oishi, S. (1997). Recent findings of subjective well-being. *Indian Journal of Clinical Psychology, 24*, 25-41.

Ellison, C.G. (1991). Religious involvement and subjective well-being. *Journal of Health and Social Behaviour, 32*, 80-99.

Ellison, C.G., Gay, D.A. and Glass, T.A. (1989). Does religious commitment contribute to individual life satisfaction? *Social Forces, 68*, 100-123.

Goldberg, D.P. and Hillier, V.F. (1979). A scaled version of the general health questionnaire. *Psychological Medicine, 9*, 139-145.

Gurin, G., Veroff, J. and Feld, S. (1960). *Americans View their Mental Health*. New York: Basic Books.

Haring, M.J., Stock, W.A. and Okun, M.A. (1984). A research synthesis of gender and social class as correlates of subjective well-being. *Human Relations, 37*, 645-657.

Hindustan Times (2003). People are made to be happy, June 10, 2003, p. 14.

Inglehart, R. (1990). *Culture Shift in Advanced Industrial Society*. Princeton, NJ: Princeton University Press.

Lucas, R.E., Diener, E., Grob, A., Suh, E.M. and Shao, L. (2000). Cross-cultural evidence for the fundamental features of extraversion. *Journal of Personality and Social Psychology, 79*, 452-468.

Lucas, R.E., Diener, E. and Suh, E. (1996). Discriminant validity of well-being measures. *Journal of Personality and Social Psychology, 71*, 616-628.

Mohal, K.S. (1991). *A Study of the Effect of Unemployment on Attributional Style, Self-Esteem, and Depression Among Educated Youth*. Unpublished doctoral thesis, Kurukshetra University, Kurukshetra.

Myers, D.G. (2000). The funds, friends, and faith of happy people. *American Psychologist, 55*, 56-67.

Myers, D.G. and Diener, E. (1995). Who is happy? *Psychological Science, 6*, 10-19.

Nagpal, R. (1986). Indicators of mental health as expressed by subjective well-being and quality of family life. Paper presented at the National Planning Workshop for Work on Indicators of Mental Health at Jakarta (Indonesia).

Okun, M.A., Stock, W.A., Haring, M.J. and Witter, R.A. (1984). Health and subjective well-being: A meta-analysis. *International Journal of Aging and Human Development, 19*, 111-132.

Pavot, W., Diener, E. and Fujita, F. (1990). Extraversion and happiness. *Personality and Individual Differences, 11*, 1299-1306.

Perlman, D. and Rook, K.S. (1987). Social support, social de-cits, and the family: Toward the enhancement of well-being. In S. Oskamp (Ed.), *Family Processes and Problems: Social Psychological Aspects*. Newbury Park, CA: Sage.

Pollner, M. (1989). Divine relations, social relations and well-being. *Journal of Health and Social Behaviour, 30*, 92-104.

Poloma, M.M. and Pendleton, B.F. (1991). The effects of prayer and prayer experiences on measures of general well-being. *Journal of Psychology and Theology, 29*, 71-83.

Richardson, J.H. (2003). Ed Diener studies that "elusive state" we all strive for Dr Happy. *Reader's Digest*, June 2003 issue, 108-114.

Sell, H. and Nagpal, R. (1992). *Assessment of Subjective Well-being: The Subjective Well-being Inventory (SUBI)* (Regional Health Paper, SEARO, No. 24). New Delhi: WHO Regional Office for South-East Asia.

Sharma, A. (2002). *Personality Correlates of Well-Being*. Unpublished doctoral thesis. M.D. University, Rohtak.

Sharma, A., Sharma, N.R. and Yadava, A. (2002). Study of well-being in relation to age, gender and level of income. Paper presented in the Inaugural Conference of the Indian Psychiatric Society (NZ), Haryana Branch, 7-8 September.

Sharma, N.R., Sharma, A. and Sharma, R.C. (2002). Employment status and frustration level of Indian housewives. *Journal of Personality and Clinical Studies, 18*, 109-113.

Sharma, A., Sharma, N.R. and Yadava, A. (2004). Self-Esteem as a determinant of well-being. In Rajbir Singh et al (Eds.), *Psychology of Individual Differences*, (pp. 97-105). Delhi: Wisdom Publications.

Sinha, D. (1990). Concept of psycho-social well-being: Western and Indian perspective. *NIMHANS Journal, 8,* 1-11.

Suh, E.M., Diener, E. and Fujita, F. (1996). Events and subjective well-being: Only recent events matter. *Journal of Personality and Social Psychology, 70*, 1091-1102.

Wilson, W. (1967). Correlates of avowed happiness. *Psychological Bulletin, 67*, 294-306.

World Health Organization (1946). *Constitution of the WHO.* New York: World Health Organization.

11

Socialization, Personal Control and Psychosocial Competence in Relation to Subjective Well-being of Educated Indian Women

RUCHIKA VARMA AND NISHA DHAWAN

The change in the social scenario has also brought about a change in the status of women. The year 2001 was declared as the *year for women's empowerment*. The education of women was and is the most important issue in developing countries like India. During the last two decades, a dramatic change has occurred in the nature of roles performed by educated Indian women. The women have exposed themselves in all spheres of life. They are now addressed more by the terms like, modern, thinking, educated and contemporary women. The woman is now changing with times adding all potentials and competencies in her. But, from day-to-day experiences with some employed and unemployed women, it was realized that although the present woman is educated, she is still in a state of flux and is also not comfortable with their newly defined roles in relation to herself, her family and her society.

The health and prosperity is meant for all human beings but it is sad that it has always been neglected in the case of women. In India, although women are held in high esteem in theory and their high status is also well documented in various epics and scriptures, the real picture is deplorable. A closer look on the history of women in India shows that they occupy a subservient and passive role in the society. In the male-dominated patriarchal structure of the society, a woman is not supposed to express her independent ideology. It is in the irony of the fate that as compared to the male members of the family (father, husband, brother and son), women remain passive and always play a second fiddle. According to Gupta and Sharma (2003), in the traditional patrifocal structure women were associated with the 'private sphere', and a preoccupation with family chastity led to social practices to control women through seclusion, segregation, early marriage, denial of public spaces and rigid notions of 'male' and 'female' work spheres. This resulted in the lack of education among women. An 'ideal Hindu' woman is a householder and this image dominates and co-exists with other images even now. Indian reformers of the 19th century advocated education for women, but this was mainly to ensure that they would be better housewives and mothers.

The physical and mental health of an individual is largely affected by the various psychosocial factors operating in his or her environment. The term 'psychosocial' refers to the factors pertaining to personal and social. The literature has been reviewed on the various psychosocial factors and their relationships with the subjective well-being are seen. The various variables are discussed on the basis of the definition, operational definition, theoretical framework and related review of literature.

Socialization

Socialization may be defined as a process, which focuses upon the development of an individual as a social being, and as the member of a society. It teaches the child the ways and norms of the society and moulds him in his early stages of development, thus determining to a large extent his later personality structure and style of functioning. An individual's cultural heritage provides the child with certain norms and values that are internalized in the individual's superego during the course of development. The superego constitutes the categorical conscience that represents the rights and wrongs, the prohibitions and mores of a given social milieu. The internalization of cultural traditions and values takes place by means of the process of socialization. The development of such a sense is important for cultural survival and it has been generally defined as "the internalization of moral values and rules of moral action from external imposition to internal acceptance of these rules" (Saraswati *et al.*, 1977).

In the traditional Indian society a girl child is subjected to a different kind of socialization process than a boy child. A girl child is exposed to an environment where she learns to behave in a responsible, caring and submissive manner. As Davar (1990) points out that guilt is built in the Indian women's psyche. The socialization process is so much ingrained that it provides a platform for the formation of this guilt and often it is difficult for the young men and women to come out of this traditional mould. For decades, women have been facing the problem because of their oversubmissive, subservient position in the society. Although the women have changed in terms of their roles but there are some core traditional traits, which affect their state of well-being. Research shows that girls and boys are treated differently by parents, teachers and other adults. Early gender and sex role socialization fails to equip girls with skills and competence and hence undermines self-confidence, thus lays a foundation for the development of mental health problems in adulthood. Crandall (1965) found that girls not only show less positive self-concepts than boys from early elementary school to college, they also rate their intellectual abilities lower than boys. Links have also been found between the role of socialization in the development of personal control. On the basis of the literature reviewed in this area, it was realized that there is a need to explore the relationship between the role of socialization and the subjective well-being of educated Indian women.

Personal Control

The boundaries of the control are very difficult to define because of the number of constructs, which could be included in the definition. The variety of constructs included in the term 'personal control' is helplessness, effectiveness, autonomy, self-determination, decisional control, competence, responsibility etc. There are many others but the work of Rothbaum *et al.* (1982) divided control as a two-process construct consisting of primary and secondary control. Primary controls involve the attempts to change the environment so that it fits the needs and desires of the individual. Secondary control is an attempt to fit in with the world and flow with the current. Decades of research in sociology and psychology have demonstrated that sense of control is a robust predictor of physical and mental well-being (Baltes and Baltes, 1986; Rodin, 1986; Thompson and Spacapan, 1991), and even longevity (Langer and Rodin, 1976; Selingman, 1975).

The most remarkable contribution to this field was the notion of internal-external (I-E) control of reinforcement, popularly known as locus of control, by Rotter (1966). He explicated the significant role of generalized expectancies of reinforcement outcomes in relation to factors within the person and external to him. The studies generally show that internal control is healthy and adaptive while external control is handicapping, dysfunctional and often limits one's success.

Another tradition of control research deals with Bandura's (1977) concept of self-efficacy. Rooted in the notion of personal agency and experiences of mastery this concept gives priority to a person's judgement about competence to undertake a given course of action (e.g., solving a problem, performing a task.)

Weisz (1986; 1990) has approached the problem of self-efficacy/ control in a developmental perspective. He has shown that control belief has two distinct components, namely, contingency judgement (i.e., the degree to which the intended events are contingent upon variations in people's attributes and behaviour) and competence judgement (i.e., the capacity of individuals to manifest attributes or behaviours on which intended outcomes are contingent). Finally, real control is assumed to be a function of an integration of control and competence judgements.

The study of control has also received attention in the field of stress and health (Peterson and Stunkard, 1989; Rodin, Timko and Harris, 1986). Control is also considered as coping (Lazarus and Folkman, 1984) and a distinction has been made between primary control and secondary control. The former involves changing the situation or the existing reality while the latter refers to changing the self to accommodate to the existing reality and leaving it unchanged but exerting control over its personal psychological impact. The evidence available evinces that primary control is more effective than secondary control.

The notion of personal control is new within the context of contemporary Indian women. The concept includes freedom, choice, autonomy, influencebility as subjectively felt or perceived by a person who is thoroughly self-centred. In contemporary psychological discourse, it is generally held that exercising control is healthy, adaptive and absolutely positive for optimal functioning, lack of which is pathological, distressing and harmful. Current interest in control greatly owes to White's (1959) proposition that human beings have an in-born tendency to influence their environments. As DeCharms (1968) has put: "Man's primary motivational propensity is to be effective in producing changes in his environment". Man strives to be a causal agent. His nature commits him to this path and his very life depends on it. In the traditional Indian society, the generally accepted norms are that women should have a subservient role in the family. The position of the women has always been eulogized for the sacrifices they make for the welfare of their menfolk but they have always been denied an independent status. According to the notions of control, as posed by White, women were not supposed to exercise any control on the their environment. With the change in the socio-economic structure, however, the status of the woman has changed dramatically.

Psychosocial Competence

The study has focussed on the concept of competence as proposed by Robert White (1959) who argues that human beings are characterized by a basic motivation to be competent, and interact effectively with the environment. It is the basic human need that is channelled into particular forms through the physical and social environment.

It is important that the distinction between competence and autonomy should be clearly demarcated. The need for self-determination or autonomy is the desire to be the origin of one's own behaviour, to be free, to choose one's course of action for oneself (DeCharms, 1968; Deci, 1975; Deci and Ryan, 1985). Although both are sources of motivation, they are conceptually and empirically distinct (DeCharms, 1981). Competence refers to the connection between behaviours and outcomes; it is the extent to which a person feels capable of producing desired and preventing undesired outcomes. Autonomy refers to the connection between volition and action; it is the extent to which a person feels free to show the behaviour of his choice (Patrick, Skinner and Connell, 1993). Information processing, a cognitive activity which involves some form of competence, is important for the survival of human beings and is innately motivated and inherently pleasurable (White, 1959). Within the context of educated Indian women, the housewives experience such state of cognitive deprivation and the absence of opportunities to exercise and prove their skills creates boredom and frustration and ultimately depression that inhibits the growth of competence.

In the present study, the psychosocial competence of the women has been studied. The Indian adaptation of behavioural attributes of psychosocial competence (BAPC), developed by Tyler, Dhawan and Sinha (1984), was used. Tyler (1978) has described behavioural attributes of psychosocial competence as energizing, tempering and guiding qualities of human behaviour as 'mastery-oriented' and not necessarily 'fit-oriented'. The person functioning competently is characterized by a more active coping orientation, high initiative, realistic goal setting substantial planning, forbearance and effort in the service of attaining goals and a capacity for enjoying success and failure and learning from both. Research reviewed in the area of competence has shown varied results in relation to academic achievement, etc., but there was a lack of evidence in the area of mental health and the linkages between competence and well-being needs exploration. So, an attempt has been made to study the relationship between psychosocial competence and subjective well-being of educated Indian women.

Mental Health

It is one of the areas where there is lack of research on women. There is also lack of awareness among the Indian women regarding their mental health needs. Most of the research available in the area of health focuses on the physical aspects. There is paucity of research concentrating on the mental health aspect of women and the factors affecting it. Subjective well-being is one of the aspects of the mental health that focuses on the experiences of the individual. The individual is considered the best judge of his or her state of well-being. The definition of health by WHO converges on complete physical, social and mental well-being. This definition is very close to that provided in the ayurvedic literature. Sushrut, a leading proponent of the traditional system of Indian medicine, defines it as a state characterized by a feeling of spiritual, physical and mental well-being (*Prasana Atam Indriaya Mann*). This mental well-being is nothing but a state of stable mind body existence. Within the context of educated women, there is a conflict regarding the values, roles, their self-definition and even with respect to their competence. In the Indian setting, the mental health aspect of women's well-being has not been considered as a serious issue. While the linkage between women's reproductive functions has received professional attention, it is only in the 1990s that a need was realized for a more pragmatic attention on women's mental health (Davar, 1995ab). Discussions on violence have had a slightly longer history, but their mental health connections have remained unexplored.

Well-being

The concept of mental health is nearer to that of psychological well-being. The former is often defined in terms of adaptation to the environment and internal equipoise or equilibrium. Wolman (1973) defines it as "a state of relatively good adjustment, feelings of well-being and actualization of one's potentialities and capacities".

All indicators of psychological well-being of an individual have objective and subjective components. The objective components relate to such concerns as are generally known by the term 'standard of living', with things such as level of education, employment status etc. These objective characteristics are believed to influence human behaviour and well-being. However, an individual's satisfaction or happiness with objective reality depends not only on the access to goods and services that are available to the community but also on his expectations and perceived reality. It is this subjective component which links the concept of life to subjective well-being, that is, "as experienced by the individual". The individual is considered as the best judge of his situation and his state of well-being. An interesting study by Andrews and Whitney (1976) shows that subjective well-being consists of three primary components, viz., life satisfaction, positive effect and negative effect. Positive effect refers to pleasant emotions or feelings such as joy and happiness, whereas negative effect consists of unpleasant emotions or feelings such as sadness and fear. Life satisfaction refers to a cognitive judgmental process, a global assessment of one's life as a whole (Diener, 1984). This study is designed to understand the relationship between the various psychosocial factors and the subjective well-being of educated Indian women.

Method

Sample

One hundred young (in the age group of 25-35 years), urban (living in the city of Delhi), educated, married women were randomly selected. Of these, 50 were teachers (employed) and the remaining 50 were housewives (unemployed). Their mean age was 31.06 years. Out of the total sample, 35 percent of the women were in the category of undergraduate with some professional qualifications, 31 percent were educated upto postgraduate level and 33 percent had still higher qualifications. The mean total monthly income of the respondents' families was Rs. 22,120. Overall, the respondents were found to belong to the middle and higher-middle classes.

Measures

The study used a structured interview schedule comprising a total of 108 questions. To assess the major areas of study, the questionnaire was divided into following four parts:

1. Socialization refers to development of autonomy, choice and freedom in decision-making. To assess this aspect of educated Indian women, a sub-scale comprising 14 items was developed. This scale assesses the amount of freedom and autonomy the parents of these women have given them during their school and university/college days. This part also assesses the role of

parents in the development of autonomy and discrimination they faced in the childhood with their sibling brother.

2. Personal control was assessed by using a sub-scale comprising 15 items and it assesses the control actually exercised by the women in their important domains of life such as children, household, self and their reproductive health.
3. This part of the questionnaire was related to the subjective well-being of the respondents and was assessed using subjective well-being inventory (SUBI) developed by Nagpal and Sell (1992). This inventory assesses the subjective well-being on 11 factors. They are subjective well-being-positive affect, subjective well-being-negative affect, inadequate mental mastery, expectation achievement congruency, confidence in coping, transcendence, family group support, social support, primary group concern, perceived ill-health and deficiency in social contacts.
4. The Indian adaptation of Behavioural Attributes of Psychosocial Competence (BAPC) by Tyler, Dhawan and Sinha (1984) was used in the study. It has 39 forced choice items (36 are scored and 3 are filler) with two alternatives (a&b). Thc scale assesses the behavioural attributes as energizing, tempering and guiding qualities of human behaviour as 'mastery-oriented' and not necessarily 'fit-oriented'. The person functioning competently is characterized by a more active coping orientation, high initiative, realistic goal setting, substantial planning, forbearance and effort in the service of attaining goals.

Procedure

Both the categories of respondents, i.e., teachers and housewives, were individually interviewed on the 108 item questionnaire consisting of four sub-scales (socialization, personal control, subjective well-being and behavioural attributes of psychosocial competence). A prior appointment was taken from most of the employed women during working hours. The housewives were interviewed at home. Face-to-face individual interviews were conducted.

Results

The main findings are presented in Tables 1, 2 and 3. Table 1 shows the means and standard deviation (sd) of the four variables in the study.

Table 1

Means and Standard Deviation on Psychological Variables

Variables	*Mean*	*sd*
Personal control	65.21	14.99
Socialization	102.64	15.63
BAPC	23.46	5.55
Subjective well-being	92.12	14.50

In socialization the maximum possible score is 140. Thus, it can be said that the score for socialization is above average. An above average score indicates that these women have experienced freedom in their school and college life, which helped them in the development of autonomy and in taking decisions independently. The maximum score possible on the personal control scale is 90. From Table 1 it can be seen that educated women have scored above average score on this scale. Personal control in the study is actual control behaviourally exercised by these women in four major areas of their lives, i.e., children, household, career, and their reproductive health. The above average score indicates that the present educated women exercise control in their major domains of life. The maximum possible score on behavioural attributes of psychosocial competence is 36. The above average score on this scale also gives an indication that educated Indian women have an active coping orientation, which is more 'mastery-oriented'. They are able to cope with their problems in lives, are planned, and have forbearance in the effort for attaining goals. The maximum score possible on the subjective well-being scale is 120. The mean score on this scale is above average indicating that the educated Indian women enjoy a good sense of well-being.

The paired sample 't' test was applied to compare the means of employed and unemployed women on the four variables. Table 2 shows the means, sds and 't' values for socialization, personal control, psychosocial competence and subjective well-being.

Table 2

Mean Comparison between Teachers and Housewives on Psychological Variables

Variables	*Mean (teachers)*	*Mean (housewives)*	*t*
Socialization	86.78	86.06	0.27
Personal control	71.60	63.06	2.95*
BAPC	23.50	23.54	-1.49
Subjective well-being	86.44	91.70	-0.33

* $p<.05$

From the above table it can be observed that the employed and unemployed women differ significantly only on the personal control exercised by them in their lives. No significant difference was found in the means of behavioural attributes of psychosocial competence, socialization and subjective well-being. These results indicate that employed (teachers) women are exercising more control than unemployed (housewives).

Table 3

Intervariable Correlation Matrix

Variables	*Socialization*	*Personal control*	*BAPC*
Personal control	.07		
BAPC	.16	.45*	
Subjective well-being	.47*	.40	-.15

* $p<.01$

Correlation coefficients were also calculated to explore the strength of relationship among the four variables, i.e., socialization, personal control, psychosocial competence and subjective well-being.

From the Table 3, it can be seen that there is a significant positive relationship between socialization and subjective well-being. It implies that more the girl child is socialized for the development of autonomy, choice, freedom and decision-making, better will be her sense of well-being. Moreover, there is a significant positive correlation between personal control and behavioural attributes of psychosocial competence. This implies that a woman with mastery-oriented, active coping style can exercise control over their major domains of lives.

Discussion

The primary objective of the study was to explore the relationship between socialization, personal control and psychosocial competence in relation to the subjective well-being of educated Indian women.

From the mean scores it can be seen that the educated Indian women scored an above average score in all the four areas, viz., socialization, personal control, behavioural attributes of psychosocial competence (BAPC) and subjective well-being. An above average score on socialization indicates that these women have experienced freedom in their school and college life, which helped them in the development of autonomy and hence in taking decisions independently. As a result, it can be inferred that the present educated Indian women are socialized in a way that helped them in the development of autonomy, choice and freedom in their lives. An above average score on personal control scale implies that educated women exercise control in four major areas of their lives, i.e., children, household, career and reproductive health. Likewise, an above average score on BAPC scale gives an indication that educated Indian women have an active coping orientation which is more 'mastery-oriented'. They are able to actively cope with their problems in lives and are moderately planned with forbearance in the effort for attaining goals. And, finally, an above average score on the subjective well-being scale shows that the present educated Indian women enjoy a good sense of well-being. The term 'subjective' refers to the perception of the individual that is as experienced by the individual.

The study has also looked upon the differential effect of personal control, socialization and BAPC on the subjective well-being of employed (teachers) and unemployed (housewives) women. The scores were compared using paired sample t test. The findings show a significant difference between the personal control scores of employed and unemployed women. No significant difference is found between the scores of socialization, psychosocial competence and subjective well-being. This indicates that employment significantly affects the amount of personal control behaviourally exercised by the educated Indian women on the major domains of their lives. From the results it can be inferred that teachers exhibit more control than housewives. Similarly, no significant difference is observed between the subjective well-being scores of housewives and teachers. A review of literature shows that there is a lack of agreement on whether the employment has an effect on the mental health of women. For example, studies by Rice and Cugliani (1980), and Kessler and McRae (1981) have shown that there is no increase either in the physical or mental health symptomatology of women despite their increasing work involvement. Hence, these studies indicate that the working women can manage well with the expectations associated with their multiple roles and thus supporting positive conceptions of mental health. Another group of studies has reported a positive association between work and both physical and mental health indicators (Gove and Gerken, 1977; Baruch, Barnett and Rivers, 1983; Wheeler, Lee and Loe, 1983). While others have shown that women who have a career are more mature and happy (Gump, 1972; Putnam and Hansen, 1972). Bhattacharya and Bhatt (1983) reported that married working women are better adjusted, more stable and experience less psychological conflicts in comparison to unemployed married women. As posed by White (1959), human beings have an innate tendency to interact effectively with the environment - a basic human need that is channelled through the physical and social environment. Information processing, a cognitive activity and involves some form of competence, is important for the survival of human beings and is innately motivating (White, 1959). Within the context of educated Indian women, the significant difference between the personal control scores of employed and unemployed supports this finding. The housewives experience a state of cognitive deprivation and the absence of opportunities to exercise and prove their skills creates boredom and frustration, which ultimately led to depression, and inhibits the growth of competence.

The study also explores the linkages between socialization, personal control and psychosocial competence in relation to subjective well-being of educated Indian women. The results show that there is a significant positive correlation between socialization and subjective well-being of educated Indian women. So, it can be inferred that socialization plays an important role in the subjective well-being of these women. Socialization in the present study is restricted to the role of parents in the development of autonomy, choice and freedom in taking a decision in life. From the findings obtained, it can be said that the educated Indian women have been socialized in a manner so that they can control their lives. Socialization seems to play an important role in the subjective well-being. It is a process by which the norms and values of a culture are transmitted from one generation to another. Within the context of educated Indian women it can be stated that the socialization process is such that it is helping to develop a sense of personal control in their present lives.

The results also show that there is a positive correlation between psychosocial competence and personal control which means that competence and control are going together and is indirectly enhancing the sense of well-being. However, from an overall analysis of the findings, it can be said that psychosocial competence and personal control are moderating the process. In the case of the women, where education has been channelled in employment, there is a significant difference between the personal control scores. We can say that although personal control is not directly related to subjective well-being but it is acting as a moderating variable in enhancing the well-being through socialization. It can be concluded that educated Indian women although being socialized for development of autonomy, it is the opportunity to exercise control, which is enhancing their sense of subjective well-being.

References

Andrews, F.M. and Whitney, S.B. (1976). *Social Indicators of Well-being: American Perspectives on Quality Life.* New York: Plenum.

Baltes, M.M. and Baltes, P.B. (1986). *The Psychology of Control and Aging.* Hisllsdale, NJ: Lawrence Erlbaum.

Bandura, A. (1977). Self-efficacy: Toward a unified theory of behavioral change. *Psychological Review, 84,* 191-215.

Baruch, G., Barnett, R. and Rivers, C. (1983). *Life Prints: New Patterns of Love and Work for Today's Women.* New York: McGraw-Hill.

Bhattacharya, P. and Bhatt, K.K. (1983). Family adjustment of married working and non-working women. *Indian Journal of Clinical Psychology, 10,* 497-501.

Crandall, V.C., Kathovsky, W. and Crandall, V.J. (1965). Children's beliefs in their control of reinforcement in intellectual academic achievement behaviors. *Child Development, 36,* 91-109.

Davar, B.V. (1995a). Mental illness among Indian women. *Economic and Political Weekly, 30(45),* 2879-86.

— (1995b). *The mental health aspects of socialization from the gender perspective.* Paper presented at the Symposium on Socialization, Theory and research. Department of HDFS, MS University of Baroda, Baroda.

DeCharms, R. (1968). *Personal Causation.* New York: Academic Press.

Deci, E.L. (1975). *Intrinsic Motivation,* New York: Plenum.

Deci, E.L. and Ryan, R.M. (1985). *Intrinsic Motivation and Self-determination in Human Behaviour.* New York: Plenum.

Diener, E. (1984). Subjective well-being. *Psychological Bulletin, 95,* 542-575.

Gove, W.R. and Gerken, M. (1977). The effect of children and employment on the mental health of married men and women. *Social Forces, 56(1),* 66-76.

Gump, J.P. (1972). Sex role attitudes and psychological well-being. *Journal of Social Issues, 28,* 79-91.

Gupta, N. and Sharma, A.K. (2003). Parrifocal concerns in the lives of women in academic science: Continuity of tradition and emerging challenges, *Indian Journal of Gender Studies, 10:2,* Sage Publication.

Kessler, R. and McRae, J. (1981). Trends in the relationship between sex and psychological distress: 1957-1976. *American Sociological Review,* 46, (August) 443-452.

Langer, E.J. and Rodin, J. (1976). The effects of choice and enhanced personal responsibility for the aged: A field experiment in an institutional setting. *Journal of Personality and Social Psychology, 34,* 191-198.

Lazarus, R.S. and Folkman, S.(1984). *Stress, Appraisal and Coping.* New York: Springer Verlag.

Misra, G. (1994). Psychology of control: Cross-cultural considerations. *Journal of Indian Psychology, 12,* 1&2.

— (1999). *Psychological Perspectives on Stress and Health*. New Delhi: Concept Publishing House.

Nagpal, A. and Sell, P. (1992). *Assessment of Subjective Well-being*. New Delhi: WHO Regional Office for South-East Asia.

Pandey, J. (2003). *Psychology in India Revisited: Developments in the Discipline.* Vol.2: Personality and Health Psychology. Sage Publications.

Patrick, B.C., Skinner, E.A. and Connell, J.P. (1993). What motivates children's behaviour and emotion? The joint effects of perceived control and autonomy in the academic domain. *Journal of Personality and Social Psychology, 65(4),* 781-791.

Peterson, C., Seligman, M.E. and Valliant G.E. (1988). Pessimistic explanatory style is a risk factor for physical illness: A thirty-five year longitudinal study. *Journal of Personality and Social Psychology, 55,* 23-27.

Peterson, C. and Stunkard, A.J. (1989). Personal control and health Promotion. *Social Science and Medicine, 28,* 819-828.

Putnam, B.A. and Hansen, J.C. (1972). Relationship of self-concept and feminine role concept to vocational maturity in young women. *Journal of Counseling Psychology, 19,* 436-440.

Rice, D. and Cugliani, A. (1980). Health status of American women. *Women and Health, 5(1),* 5-22.

Rodin, J. Timko, C. and Harris, S. (1985). The construct of control: Biological and psychological correlates. In M.P. Lawton and G.L. Maddox (Eds.), *Annual Review of Gerontology and Geriatrics* (pp. 3-55). New York: Springer.

Rothbaum, F., Weisz, J.R. and Snyder, S.S. (1982). Changing the world and changing the self: A two-process model of perceived control. *Journal of Consulting and Clinical Psychology, 43,* 56-57.

Rotter, J.B. (1966). Generalized expectancies for internal versus external control of reinforcement. *Psychological Monographs, 80* (1 whole no: 609).

Saraswati, T.S. (1999). Applied social and developmental psychology: A viable interface for preventive mental health. In G. Misra (Ed.), *Psychological Perspectives on Stress and Health.* New Delhi: Concept Publishing Company.

Seligman, M.E.P. (1975). *Helplessness: On Depression, Development and Death.* San Francisco: Freeman.

Sinha, D. (1990). Concept of psychosocial well-being: Western and Indian perspectives. *NIMHANS Journal, 8,* 1-11.

Skinner, E.A. (1995). *Perceived Control, Motivation and Coping. Individual and Developmental Series* (Vol.8). Thousand Oaks: Sage Publications.

Tyler, F.B. (1992). Psychosocial competence and developing countries. *Psychology and Developing Societies, 3,* 171-192.

Thampson, S.C. and Spacapan, S. (1991). Perceptions of control in vulnerable populations. *Journal of Social Issues, 47(4),* 1-21.

Weisz, J.R. (1986). Understanding the development of control. In M. Permutter (Ed.), *Social Cognition: Minnesota Symposium on Child Psychology* (Vol.18, pp. 219-278). Hillsdale, N.J.: Lawrence Earlbaum.

Weisz, J.R. and Stipek, D.J. (1982). Competence, contingency, and the development of perceived control. *Human Development, 25,* 250-281.

Wheeler, A., Lee, E.S. and Loe, H. (1983). Employment, senses of well-being, and use of professional services among women. *American Journal of Public Health, 73(8),* 908-911.

White, R.W. (1959). Motivation reconsidered. The concept of competence. *Psychological Review, 66,* 297-333.

12

Sociobiology of Health and Disease

S.P.K. JENA

Health and disease are the two significant dimensions of behaviour. If the former is characterized by a sense of well-being, the latter, by a feeling of distress. During the life-time, every individual traverses through health and disease. It is not an all-or-none type of phenomenon but a relative position that explains whether the individual is healthy or unhealthy. The individual perception of health status is largely a psychological phenomenon. In spite of the onset of disease process, an individual may not even perceive it at a point of time. An organic disorder may not at all affect an individual until it is perceptible. Conversely, without any organic disorder, an individual may report himself to be unhealthy. Thus, logically, disease and health may co-exist in the same individual. These two are not just mutually exclusive entities. This position is illustrated in Figure 1. Now, it is well established that stressful events of people's lives contribute to the risk of their succumbing to a wide range of illness. The impact of such events is moderated by genetic factors. How a healthy person enters into the disease process and how this pathological process can be reversed, has been a question of immense significance. The sociobiological dimension of this process has still remained relatively unexplored area of research.

Figure 1

Co-existence model: Health and disease may co-exist in the same individual. At an early stage of disease, if the pathological process is at a sub-threshold level, it may not be incapacitating or distressing at all, while at the advanced stage, it may be highly distressing and incapacitating for the individual.

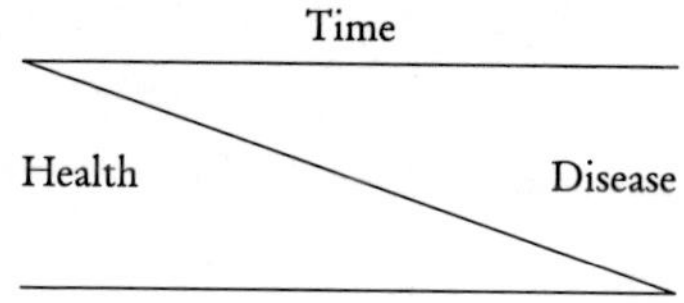

Human Health: A Creative Response

We start with the fundamental assumption that every human being is a creative social being, well equipped with a wide range of adaptive responses to the changing environment. Some of them are phylogenetically designed and shaped by learning. The major response categories include homeostasis, inhibitory and excitatory neural responses, visceral and immunological responses, assimilation and use of vital intelligence pertaining to survival, management of reinforcing and punitive contingencies, the perceptual and metacognitive processes that detect finer signals of pathological activity and activate elaborate voluntary behaviour to correct them. A wide range of social responses; like co-operation and interpersonal communication also come into play. From a boarder perspective, these responses help to maintain the well-being of the individual, protecting him against a disease. Health-maintaining behaviour involves a good deal of creativity, as it requires divergent and convergent use of alternative survival skills. Divergent skills include a variety of adaptive responses or treatment methods for the same disease. Convergent form of creativity is required where the same method of adaptive behaviour or treatment is used for a wide range of diseases. This is illustrated in Figure 2. Creative ways of living keep an individual healthy and blissful. The disease process starts victimizing the individual when these adaptive responses are either exhausted, their access is denied or underdeveloped due to congenital, and acquired deficiencies.

Figure 2

Divergent and convergent relationship between disease and treatment: (a) one disease may be treated by using several alternative methods of treatment, and (b) several diseases may also respond to a single treatment method or adaptive response. Here, D represents disease and T represents the methods of treatment.

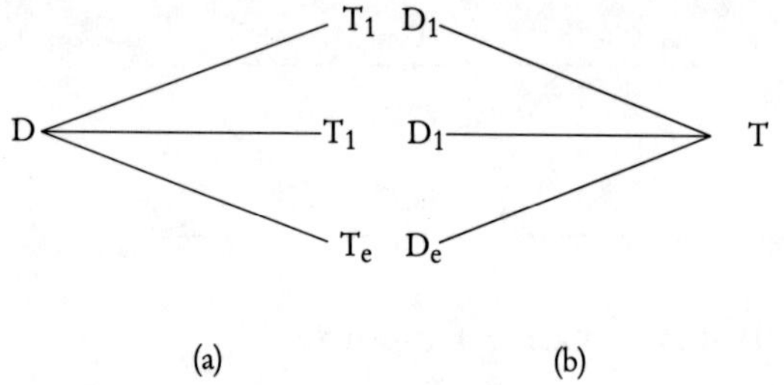

Signal Detection in the Disease Process

Before the core symptoms of a disease start manifesting, the early 'signals' keep appearing in the form of increasing psychological distress and interpersonal disorganization. Autocorrective responses, required to block the progress of a disorder, are required to begin at this level. Failure to perceive early signals complicates the pathological process. Many diseases of insidious and acute onset may be distinguished on the basis of signal detection capacity of the individual. Failure to detect it early results in acute manifestation although intensity of pathological process itself is important. Even the serious accidents, broadly conceptualized as 'human error', are often triggered by socio-psychological distress. Lesser the sensitivity to these signals, higher the chance of morbidity. Poor sensitivity reduces the chances of activating the corrective mechanism for adaptive change.

At microscopic level, most diseases of the body cause damage to the cells, altering their normal functioning. This is preceded either by a single or multiple social, as well as, intrapsychic events or a single traumatic event. Karus *et al.* (1977) studied 30 cases suffering from ulcerative colitis. In at least 18 cases, there was identifiable psychosocial trauma, such as loss of significant persons through death, separation from parents or parental surrogate, overwhelming sense of despair and hopelessness, anxiety regarding marriage, and in some cases, even anxiety regarding the wife's pregnancy. In one case, the disease was precipitated by bombing of the patient's house during the World War II, although the patient was not directly affected by the bombing. In children, this causal relationship is much more perceptible than what we see in adults, who have access to a multiple number of alternatives to cope with the trauma.

There is substantial individual difference in perception of the disease process. Even, the same individual exhibits different levels of sensitivity in different situations. Diminished vigilance to the pathological process enhances the chance of morbidity as the individual fails to make corrective adjustment to combat against the disease before it causes substantial damage. This is true for the mental disorders too. People undergoing severe psychosocial disturbances, having neurotic fixation with certain traumatic life events, ideas or activities, or suffering from free-floating anxiety, tend to be more susceptible to disease. This is for the reason that they are less vigilant about the pathological changes. The 'neurotic' traits and pathological response patterns are shaped by series of social conditioning. Some of these habits start from the early childhood and ingrained in the child rearing practice itself.

Organic vs. Functional Disorders

Classically, diseases are put under two broad groups: organic and functional. Organic diseases are those that cause identifiable physical damage as 'consequences' of certain events. These are caused by multiple sources, for instance, infections (invasion of the micro-organisms), intoxication (effects of toxic substances), allergies (effects of allergens) or trauma (accidents). Functional disorders are conceptualized as those having no known organic basis. These are of psychological nature. Some disorders are given 'functional' status, as the disturbance is quite abstract and not clearly identifiable. The biological changes that occur in these disorders are not specific.

Social Conditioning

How social events affect health of the humans was explained by Egeren (1984) in an elaborate stimulus response model, symbolically stated as S-R_m-R_d (where S represents social situation, R_m

momentary physiological response and R_d permanently dysfunctional or diseased response). A social situation triggers momentary, short-lasting responses leading to adaptive responding. When the response is abnormally longer and intense, it causes significant psychobiological changes. Why such responses are prolonged or become intense, has been explained by both psychoanalysts using constructs like fixation, regression, and behaviourists using concepts like contingencies of reinforcement, conflict and higher order conditioning of traumatic events.

The stimulus condition (S) has a special significance in this context. It represents both actual social situations, i.e., unconditional events like a high intensity stimulus or conditioned ones, remotely associated with an original stimulus, thus, almost have the same significance as the original ones. Thus, functionally, the model may be restated as $S\text{-}S_1\text{-}S_2....S_n\text{-}R_m\text{-}R_d$. Manifestation of certain symptoms depends on the genetic predisposition, like strength of nervous system (Pavlov, 1927) or structural deficit of the organ. Therefore, the model may be further extended and stated as $S\text{-}S_1\text{-}S_2\text{-}S_n\text{-}R_m\text{-}X\text{-}R_d$, where X represents the genotype, i.e., genetic predisposition as a mediating variable.

The Balancing Act

Life is a complicated balancing act. Everything alive leans on everything else alive, in one way or the other. Elements within and between various levels of organization must remain in harmony. This harmony provides a sense of well-being. A disharmony at one level of organization influences the other. A serious and irreparable disharmony at biological, social or psychological level leads to cumulative degree of disorganization at other levels. Thus, disease is the manifestation of a state of disorganization, or a failure to orchestrate different levels of organization. A symptom is just tip of an iceberg. Beneath it submerged a wide range of disorganization at various levels.

Human body plays the role of a 'comptroller' in face of the competitive investment of energy in different vital activities like feeding, reproduction, defence against micro-organisms or maintenance of social status and so on. Investment of energy in repair of one system requires equitable withdrawal of energy maintaining other systems. It is a complicated balancing act.

Levels of Organization

There are different levels of organization of the organism: (1) intracellular, (2) cell to cell, (3) organism to micro-organism, (4) organism to environment, and (5) organism to organism (Egeren, 1984). Social events, whether actual or symbolic, causing dysfunctional response, affect the organism at all these levels.

Intracellular Organization

The cells in the human body have small number of gene-controlled basic programmes such as self-maintenance, cell division and generation of specific proteins required by other cells. First two are the 'internal' functions and the third one is the 'external' function. These are conveniently named as 'programme 1', 'programme 2' and 'programme 3' (Bullough, 1965). Epinephrine plays a key role in causing cells to switch from one programme to the other by combining with tissue-specific chemicals called 'chalones'. When the local concentration of epinephrine-chalone complex is high, cells in that area do not divide. As a result of which retardation of growth occurs. In extreme cases, it leads to psychological dwarfism. When the individual is exposed to severe psychosocial stress, the adrenal hormone keeps the body constantly on high alert, signalling a majority of cells to perform their tissue-specific functions instead of engaging in mitotic cell division. As a result, there is a shift of energy utilization from 'growth and repair' to 'work'. After the stressful situation is passed, the individual takes rest or goes to sleep. It provides chance for growth (Bullough, 1965). The normal process of growth continues.

Cell to Cell Organization

Health of the organism is determined by the extent of balance between the internal and external functions of the cells (i.e., programme 3). Failure to carry out these functions leads to the onset of disease process. The intercellular communication occurs primarily through the naturally secreting hormones. When the stress-related hormones and a variety of chemical agents block this 'social' communication, it leads to many disorders of the nervous, endocrine and immune system.

Even the programme 2 is affected. Theories of tumerogenesis indicate that it is initiated by a mutant cell (Potter, 1980; Trosko and Chang, 1978). Promotion of mutant cells in coronary arteries, pancreas and other body tissues leads to atherosclerosis, diabetes and cancer, respectively. 'Failure to thrive' and 'deprivation dwarfism' are two syndromes, which caused by 'social' disturbance at the intercellular level. Conversely, it is also noted that when such children are removed from deprived home environment and placed in stimulating hospital environment, they show significant improvement. Dramatic growth spurts were demonstrated without chemical intervention (Gardner, 1972; Powell, Hopwood and Barrett, 1973). Social variables like crowding may also affect the growth (Christian, 1971).

Organism to Micro-Organism Organization

Relationship between human body and the micro-organism living on it is like that of a landlord and his tenant. This 'social' relation is open to negotiation. When the body fails to do so, micro-organisms thriving on the body turn violent, destroying the body and ultimately themselves in the process. Infections and neoplastic diseases (morbid new growth of tissues) are some of the examples (Potter, 1980). There is a 'social' relationship between the domestic and foreign cells, the former acting as host and the latter as symbiont. By 'reading' the body chemistry (e.g., in aging and stressful situation), they estimate the survivorship. In the face of stress they sacrifice themselves for the kin. By eliminating the non-viable resource-using cells, the more viable kins are benefited. This is explained through 'reciprocal altruism theory' (Trivers, 1971).

Organism to Environment Organization

Most defensive processes, such as body's response to bacteria, virus (i.e., microbial defense), control of body weight and size, response to injuries (growth and recovery process) determine body's susceptibility to a variety of diseases (infections, neoplasia, allergic hypersensitivities and autoimmune diseases). It is interesting enough to note that these responses, which seem to be 'autonomous', are controlled by the brain (particularly by the hypothalamus), and not by the gene-coded information system. Why is it so? This is because of the fact that they are largely influenced by the behavioural ecology (Morse, 1980) and life history tactics (Stearns, 1976). Perception of the finer variations in the behavioural ecology plays a significant role in survival. Apart from the immunity and growth functions, the brain has to play a very significant role in developing elaborate behavioural responses, which may be called 'survival skills' (such as migration, reproduction, health-related behaviour and social organization). The energy need of the organism to maintain, regenerate or defend itself exists outside and there is intense competition to avail it (e.g., food, shelter, social rank, etc.). Brain is the executive organ to make decisions about the behaviour in response to the fluctuations of these sources of energy. Thus, the social forces come into play in disease, health and survival at large.

The most extensively studied social variable is population density (i.e., crowding). Increased population causes density-dependent stress, leading to activation of the hypothalamic-pituitary-adrenal and sympathetic-adrenal axes. It also leads to decreased production of sex cells, decreased replacement of damaged cells, increased mortality (e.g., due to elevated susceptibility to infection, deficiency in lactation) and decreased natality rates (e.g., due to inhibition of sexual maturation) as a result of which population shrinks. Reduced stress drops the level of stress-related adrenal hormones. This entire chain of reaction restores the normal rate of growth in normal conditions.

Organism to Organism Organization

Earlier, we started with a fundamental proposition that man is a creative and social being. Being social as well as creative has a special significance for survival itself. Most animals live in groups because it pays them biologically (Allee, 1943), for instance, in food seeking, defending against enemies, rearing the young. Even for planning future survival the organism depends on the 'collective' (social) intelligence and social learning (Bandura, 1969). The important social variables that affect human health are social bonds, ranks in social hierarchy, social obligations, competition and co-operation. *Social bonds* are those behaviours, which promote physical proximity and attachment behaviour. They signal an individual's interest in contact. Of all relationships, the mother-child relationship is the most important. In a study on rodent neonates (pups), Hofer (1981) observed that body heat and nutrition provided by the mother increase the ornithine decarboxylase (ODC) – a critical enzyme required for protein synthesis. ODC concentration in heart and brain tissue was found almost 50 percent less in the unhandled pups. Thus, one may conclude that a negligent mother prepares the 'soil' for future disease for her offspring. A rupture in social bonds (bereavement) leads to a variety of illnesses as it affects the immune system. Bartrup *et al.* (1977), in a study, reported that bereavement causes sub-normal T cell lymphocyte response to mitogen (an antigen that normally multiplies these cells) injection in adults. Crying that occurs during bereavements has a special significance for health. Under normal conditions, the mucous membrane of the nose protects the body from air-borne bacteria. This is because of the bactericidal effects of lysozyme on the mucous membrane. During distress, the mucous membrane dries up weakening this effect. Intact relations may be protective during this period because not only psychologically it helps in catharsis, but also facilitates weeping – a sympathy response to tragedy.

Human tear, which is rich in lysozyme bathes and humidifies the mucosa during weeping, restores bactericidal elevating the immunological defense (Montagu, 1981). What causes diseases is quite complex. Its causal attribution to genetic, microbial or physical elements only would be incomplete. The exclusive emphasis on the immediate antecedents too provides a myopic orientation. The causal analysis requires to be broad-based. For instance, the values of the society, strong achievement need, high degree of change and competitive spirit internalized by us impose considerable anxiety and stress. When the chance of either 'fight or flight' is blocked, it causes dysfunction or damage to the body either directly (e.g., accidents) or indirectly (e.g., by hyperactivation of adreno-cortical axis). Despite the excellent adaptive abilities human beings have a finite biosystem. It cannot change this system beyond its limits (Athos and Gabarro, 1978). Therefore, in order to avoid this 'wear and tear' of the body (disease), one has to concentrate on alternative styles of living, enjoying pleasurable events, establishing reasonable life goals, changing stressful roles, accepting incompleteness of life and establishing new interests.

The Healing Process

How social processes help to recover from disease has been an interesting area of discourse. Adequate understanding of this intricate process of recovery would help to unravel many mysteries of psychosocial and self-regulatory process. Psychotherapy is used as a method of intervention. It is basically a social process in which influence of one person upon another relieves mental suffering and neutralizes the pathogenic sources of a disorder (Karus *et al.*, 1977). How do the words of the mouth used in psychotherapy reverses or blocks the pathological process of the disease? The Pavlovian school advanced the proposition that word is as a real conditioned stimulus like any other stimulus but in addition to that, by virtue of its physiological and social significance, the verbal stimulus plays a unique role in man's higher nervous activity. It reflects, replaces and generalizes meaning of the concrete stimuli coming, both from external as well as internal environment (Platanov, 1959). Therefore, it has high potential to act as a psychprophylaxis against disease. It is possible to influence many physiological processes such as water or carbohydrate metabolism, secretion in the gastrointestinal tract, thermoregulation and vasomotor activity (Platanov, 1959). In an early study, Mittelemann, Wolff and Scharf (1942) demonstrated how feeling of resentment during the interview can increase peristaltic activity and discussion on feeling of security can induce measurable decrease in this physiological activity.

However, recently, there has been an observable change in therapeutic style. The emphasis is expanding from the individual to the social processes. In a critical review of research into psychotherapeutic processes, Gendlin and Rychlak (1970) reported that the place of intrapsychic conflicts is largely taken by interactional concepts such as roles, games, interpersonal attitudes, family systems, community and institutional structures. This is considered as an extension of the purview of psychotherapy itself. Involvement of social agents in therapy has become a frequent event in behaviour therapy too. Tharp and Wetzel (1969) suggested a 'triadic model' of behavioural intervention. It involves the therapist, mediator and the client. Our concern is not only to develop health-maintenance behaviour, but also to maintain it in the natural environment. In this context, the role of the mediators is important as dispensers of reinforcement and punishment.

There is more pragmatic interest in changing patient's style of living. Research on use of self-monitoring and biofeedback techniques has opened up new dimensions in health care. Many disorders so far considered to be disorders of autonomic regulation such as systolic and diastolic blood pressure (Benson *et al.*, 1971; Shapiro *et al.*, 1970), cardiac arrhythmias (Weiss and Engel, 1971), Raynaud's disease (Blanchard and Epstein, 1978) and stomach acidity (Welgen, 1974; Whitehead *et al.*, 1975), or asthma (Feldman, 1976) are now treated through biofeedback and self-monitoring techniques.

Instead of looking into the cause of distress, now, the focus is more on positive behavioural change at individual and community levels. For instance, many dietary habits in the society promote disease and early deaths. Consumption of 'junk' food, i.e., fast food, low fibre, high sugar, high fat food (Battle and Brownell, 1996) increases such possibilities. Apart from individual control of diet, social incentives like reduced cost of healthy food (e.g., fruits and vegetables) and increase in the price of junk food would reduce the prevalence of food-related diseases and death rate, without affecting the disease process itself. Statutory warning on the cigarette packets and legal action has already brought substantial change in the prevalence of smoking.

Involvement of larger government and non-government agencies has made the process of change faster and easier. The preventive efforts are required to gear and activate the larger social machinery in order to invigorate social change. Today, this is one of the most challenging social dimensions of public health.

References

Allee, W. (1943). Where angels fear to tread: A contribution from general sociology to human ethics. *Science, 97,* 517-525.

Athos, A.G. and Gabarro, S. (1978). *Interpersonal Behaviour.* Prentice-Hall: New Jersey.

Bandura, A. (1969) *Principles of Behaviour Modification.* New York: Holt, Rinehart and Winston.

Battle, E.K. and Brownell, K.D. (1996). Confronting rising tide of eating disorders and obesity: Treatment vs. prevention and policy. *Addictive Behaviour, 21,* 75-765.

Benson, H., Shapiro, D., Tursky, B. and Schwartz, G.E. (1971). Decreased systolic blood pressure through operant conditioning techniques. *Science, 173,* 740-742.

Blanchard, B.E. and Epstein, L.H. (1978). *A Biofeedback Premier.* Massachusetts: Addison-Wesley.

Bullough, W. (1965). Mitotic and functional homeostasis: A speculative view. *Cancer Research, 25,* 1683-1727.

Christian, J. (1971). Population density and production efficiency. *Biology of Reproduction, 4,* 248.

Feldman, G.M. (1976). The effects of biofeedback training on respiratory resistance of asthmatic children. *Psychosomatic Medicine, 38,* 27-34.

Gardner, L. (1972). Deprivation dwarfism. *Scientific American, 227,* 76-82.

Gendlin, E.T. and Rychlak, J.F. (1970). Psychotherapeutic processes. *Annual Psychological Review, 21,* 155.

Hofer, M. (1981). Towards a developmental basis for disease predisposition. In H. Weiner, M. Hofer and A. Stumkard (Eds.) *Brain, Behaviour and Bodily Disease.* New York: Raven.

Iacobelli, S., King, R. Lindner, H. and Lipman, M. (1980). *Hormones and Cancer.* New York: Raven.

Karus, A., Daniels, G.E., Flood, C.A. and O' Conner, J.F. (1977). *Psychotherapy in Ulcerative Colitis.* Philadelphia: Saunders Co.

Mittelemann, B., Wolff, H.G. and Scharf, J. (1942). Emotions and gastroduodenal function. *Psychosomatic Medicine, 4,* 5-16.

Montagu, A. (1981). *Growing Young.* New York.: McGraw-Hill

Morse, D. (1980). *Behavioural Mechanisms in Ecology.* Cambridge: Harvard University Press

Pavlov, I.P. (1927). *Conditioned Reflex* (Translated by V. Arrep). London:. Oxford University Press.

Platanov, K. (1959). *The Word as a Physiological and Therapeutic Factor* (translated by David A. Myshne). Moscow: Foreign Language Publishing House.

Powell, G., Hopwood, N. and Barrett, E. (1973). Growth hormone studies before and during catch up growth in a child with emotional deprivation, and short stature. *Journal of Endocrinology and Metabolism*, *37*, 674-679.

Shapiro, D., Tursky, E. and Schwartz, G.E. (1970). Differentiation of heart rate and systolic blood pressure in man by operant conditioning. *Psychosomatic Medicine, 32*, 417-423.

Stearns, S. (1976). Life history tactics: A review of ideas. *The Quarterly Review of Biology, 51*, 3-47.

Tharp, R.G. and Wetzel, R.J. (1969). *Behaviour Modification in Natural Environment.* New York: Academic Press

Trosko, J. and Chang, C. (1978). Genes, pollutants and human disease. *Quarterly Review of Biophysics II*, *4*, 603-427.

Trivers, R. (1971). Solution of reciprocal altruism. *Quarterly Review of Biology, 46*, 35-57.

van Egeren, L.F. (1984). Social processes, biology and disease. In William M. Waid (Ed.), *Sociophysiology.* New York: Springer-Verlag.

Weiss, T. and Engel, B. (1971). Operant conditioning of heart rate in patients with premature ventricular contractions. *Psychosomatic Medicine, 3*, 1-25.

Welgen, P.R. (1974). Learned control of gastric acid secretions in ulcer patients. *Psychosomatic Medicine, 36*, 411-419.

Whitehead, W.E., Renault, P.F. and Goldiamond, I. (1975). Modification of human gastric acid secretion with operant conditioning procedures. *Journal of Applied Behaviour Analysis, 8*, 147-156.

13

Role Strain of Mothers of Physically Disabled Daughters

NISHI TRIPATHI AND DEEPA PUNETHA

The major objective of this study is to examine the role strain of mothers of the physically disabled daughters and the psychosocial barriers faced by them. It also inquires into the social and family support which these mothers have and the type of rehabilitation services available to them.

Disability is essentially a childhood problem in India, as 50 percent of the population with disability is below 18 years of age. It not only affects the well-being of the person with disability but the whole family. Care of persons with a disability in India is largely conducted in the home and is primarily the responsibility of mothers. Childcare is a natural skill for mothers. The mother is the first person to observe the child's development from stage to stage in the growth and maturation process. Mothers are often the first to detect the symptoms, decide when and whom to consult, and bear the responsibility of treatment. Mothers are also primary consumers of indigenous health methods that can be reached more effectively through traditional health channels (Pearson, 1987; MacCormack, 1988). Mothers are viewed as the main providers of childcare and feel guilty and anxious if unable to do so.

If a girl is disabled, then her situation in the family and society is even worse. The family members do not want to disclose to others that they have a disabled girl amongst them. Her disability is often neglected by other family members. Then, the responsibility of the mother increases by quantum proportions, as she has to take the care of the disabled daughter, along with other responsibilities of the household. It becomes a 'double disability' because girls who are disabled are unacceptable for marriage and considered to be a 'burden' on the family and society. Considering the status of women in India, being disabled and female can be considered to be a 'double misfortune' (COPOH, 1989).

Attitude and Disability

One of the more important subjects for study in the relationship between psychological variables and physical disability is that of attitudes. One factor that is important to take into account in considering attitudes towards people with disability is perceptions of the causes of the disability. It has been shown that more stigmas are attached to people with disabilities when they are seen as responsible for their disability (Jones *et al.*, 1984). Weiner, Perry and Magnusson (1988) have found that mental-behavioural disabilities are perceived as more onset-controllable than are physical disabilities. There is a vast body of research, which suggests that such attributions have consequences for our perception of persons with disability, their dispositions, our affective reaction and expectations. Such attributions have a complex relationship with the attitudes we hold towards the people with disability.

One important factor that is ignored in most of the western studies is attributing their misfortune to cosmic factors. The work of Dalal and Pande (1988) on accident victims with temporary and permanent disability shows that people quite often attribute their misfortune to cosmic factors. Such attributions strongly suggest medical, interpersonal and psychological implications. There is a greater degree of acceptance and rationalization in terms of the theory of *karma*, where people look for justification in something wrong they might have done in their previous birth. Depression is a common and often disabling reaction to a chronic illness. Although the correlations between life events and depression are typically quite small, some life events have been shown to relate to depression. One such life event is the experience of chronic disease, either as a person with the disease or as caregiver.

A central reason why many girls/women with disabilities are unable to do more to improve their own situation is their lack of self-esteem. Shown from birth either through neglect or overprotection, that they have little value or are unable to do much, girls with disabilities grow up with the burden of that stigma and expect little of themselves. Such attributions have a complex relationship with the attitudes we hold towards the people with disability. A disabled girl is not considered 'marriageable' because her disability is seen as 'defect' and there is fear that her disability could passed on to her children. This is why, the incidence for disabled girls is lower than for that of disabled boys.

Beliefs and Disability

Causal Beliefs

The manner in which people make attributions for others' illness is found to have significant implications for their well-being. The relationship of adjustment to the existence of an attribution, the frequency of attributions and content of attributions is important. Investigators have also examined the association between adjustment and attributional content.

Attribution theory (Kelley, 1967; Fiske and Taylor, 1984) maintains that when one encounters a sudden threat or change in one's environment, he/she will initiate a causal search in an effort to understand the reasons for that threat or change. Attributional search is thought to be initiated to understand, predict and control threat (Kelley, 1967). Central to all attribution theories is the assumption that in all our social interaction we tend to draw inferences of a cause-effect nature. There is enough research evidence to suggest that people spontaneously engage in causal search in their everyday life.

Control Beliefs

Perceptions of control and mastery are important ways in which individuals differ. Moreover, they have implications for performance, physical health and mental health (Thompson and Spacapan,

1991). People can control the course of their illness in numerous ways, though all types of controlling may not be equally adaptive.

Caregivers not only develop explanations about where, why and how the disability was perceived and how the well-being of the disabled can be improved, they may also develop beliefs about whether they can control it or not. The view, supported by many researches, was that perceived control is a crucial psychological factor mediating appraisal and response to life stresses (Cohen, Glass and Phillips, 1979: 142).

Perceived causality is a perception for attributed responsibility. We do not usually blame or credit people for things they did not do. Accordingly, attributed control is also important in responsibility attributions. One will be perceived as responsible for events that one control as well as those that one thought to be able to control. The greater the perceived control over an occurrence, the greater responsibility one bears for it in the eyes of others. Thus, attributions of causality, control and responsibility are intertwined. Control beliefs not only help in reducing caregivers' stress and strain but also promote their own physical/mental health and well-being.

Role Strain of Mothers as Primary Caregiver

The stresses of caregiving are tremendous. Caregivers experience them everyday. Caring is a complex process, determined by social and economic characteristics of the family, nature and magnitude of the care required, workload including interpersonal conflicts, coping style and social support (Julie, 1995). The effects of caregiver's stress may directly or indirectly influence the family functioning. Disability of a family member may be perceived as aggravating the already difficult situation, putting additional burden on the parents (Gandorta, 1984; 1991). One source of stress is that women's roles include supplying nurturance to other family members. Women's role obligates them to respond to others, and these demands are an important cause for women's problems in mental health. In addition, women usually perform the majority of family work but their duties have more flexibility and thus less structure, which may add to rather than reduce their stress. The duties must be done, and finding time to do them adds to the stress.

Women showed higher levels of psychological distress, and these were related to childcare inequity and childcare difficulties at home. This may lead to role overload. Role overload may cause fatigue. Fatigue may cause the woman to become impatient with her husband. Her impatience may precipitate marital conflict not experienced before in her relationship. It was also noted that if the mother spent all her time for caring her disabled daughter, she could not pay attention to the household activities. This would create tension in the family and increase role strain of mother. The severity of stress is gauged by the degree of disruption in the human system that will occur if the individual fails to cope with the adjustive demands. Several objective factors influence stress severity. One factor, which is often crucial in determining the severity of stress, is the individual's own evaluation of the stress situation.

Caregivers' Stress

Any stress reaction, of course, reflects the interplay of a combination of inner and outer determinants – some may more influential than others, but all working together to make the individual react as one does. On a psychological and interpersonal level therc are learned coping patterns and self-defences. The failure of coping efforts at any of these levels may seriously impair a caregiver's adjustment. If caregiving stress is severe, it may cause negative physical, psychological and behavioural consequences (Jamuna, 1996; 1997b). The stress and coping framework in caregiving and family research defines stressors as challenging conditions that threaten the well-being of family members (Pearlin *et al.*, 1990). The framework suggests that the care recepient's deficits in functional ability and the involvement of the caregiver in other caregiving roles are source of stress that affects caregivers' well-being.

Coping with Stress

In coping with stress, a caregiver is confronted with two problems: (a) to meet the requirements of the adjustive demand, and (b) to protect the self from psychological damage and disorganization. Coping is the process of managing demands (external or internal) that are appraised as taxing or exceeding the coping resources of the person (Lazarus and Folkman, 1984). Coping consists of efforts, both action-oriented and intrapsychic, to manage (that is, to master, tolerate, reduce, minimize) environmental and internal demands and conflicts among them (Cohen, 1987; Cohen and Lazarus, 1979; Lazarus and Launier, 1978). Coping processes can generally be divided into problem-focused or emotion-focused copings. Problem-focused coping strategies involve changes in the situation to reduce aversive impact whereas emotion-focused coping strategies alter individual's responses. In other words, problem-focused coping efforts are attempts to do something constructive about the stressful condition. Emotion-focused coping involves efforts to regulate the emotional consequences of the stressful events. The way in which the person copes with stressful events and whether or not his/her coping efforts are successful in reducing stress are important for his/her health and well-being. The fact that individuals vary in the degree of stress experienced from the same stressful events as also the same individual may experience different degree of stress from the same stressful events in a different situation has made the stress research more complex. This variability in the stress experience is due to many factors and moderates the impacts of stressors. It requires a lot of efforts to cope with stressors, especially uncontrollable ones.

Cultural beliefs play an important role in shaping coping responses to tragic events in one's life. In each society, there are beliefs about illness/disability, choices of treatment alternatives, sick roles and practitioner roles and institutions organized in a cultural system. The way an individual experiences and understands the cultural background largely determines his or her own condition. The Indian scenario is different in many ways. In traditional Indian society, metaphysical beliefs, that is, belief in *karma*, God and spirit, are presumed to be important determinants of many events in one's life, including illness and suffering. The theory of *karma* is the cornerstone of Hindu religion and philosophy (Gokhale, 1961; Radhakrishna, 1926). Such attributions strongly suggest medical, interpersonal and psychological implications in coping with disabilities. For example, belief in *karma* results in a greater degree of acceptance and rationalization in terms of the theory of *karma*, where people look for justification in something wrong they might have done in their previous birth. Dalal and his colleagues (2000) found that *karmaphala*, in fate, provides a commencing and socially acceptable explanation for their illness.

Social Support

The term 'social support' refers to a variety of material and emotional support a person receives from others. Social support appears to be an important resource for those suffering from chronic illness. According to Krause (2001: 273), social support is best defined operationally as a measure of "social embeddedness (e.g., indicators assessing the frequency of contact with others), received support (e.g., measure of amount of tangible help actually provided by social network members), and perceived support (e.g., subjective evaluations of supportive exchanges)".

The notion that social support can affect physical and psychological well-being has gained currency in the past decade. Social support may affect caregivers' well-being positively and negatively (La Gaipa,1990). Some conceptualize social support as an individual's degree of social integration or social embeddedness (Rook, 1984; Barrera, 1986), while others define it in terms of a sense of assurance which an individual receives from his environment, that he is loved and cared for. That is, social support is associated with good physical health regardless of whether an individual is under stress or not. When social support is assessed more qualitatively, such as the degree to which a person feels that there are others available to him or her if needed, buffering effects of social support have been found (Cohen and Wills 1985; House, Umberson and Landis, 1988; Kessler and McLeod, 1985; Wrotman and Dunkel-Schetter, 1987). Experience in India shows that social support provided in various forms to the individuals helps them in adherence to medical regimens, faster recovery and more effective rehabilitation.

Family Support

Disability is essentially a family problem in India. The family is required to mobilize its external and internal resources to share additional demands and responsibility of caregiver. More often than not, emotional support, as well as physical health, extra-medical expenses and a myriad of special needs, depending on the disability, need to be handled. Interruption or distortion of the normal developmental process of the child is liable to be noticed first by the family. A typical Indian family comprising kith and kin from many generations. Despite economic hardships and limited resources, Indian families have shown enough resilience to provide long-term, often life-long, care to their disabled members. Family has an important part to play in identifying caregivers' problems and providing support to caregivers (Cohen, 2000). The family in most cases makes all decisions for the person with disability and these decisions are guided by the belief system of the larger community. Studies have shown that cultural beliefs about disability play an important role in determining the way in which the family perceives disability and the kind of measures it takes regarding prevention, treatment and rehabilitation (Chaturvedi and Malhotra, 1984; Sen, 1988; Kashyap, 1991). It was found in these studies that parental expectations were mostly negative and unrealistic. These parents often needed encouragement to believe in the possible achievements of their handicapped children. Susman (1994) argued the ways disabilities are cognized and responded to or/experienced depends primarily on perceptions, which are generated, sustained, or changed in the course of everyday life.

The Study

Objectives

The objectives of the study were to study mothers' reaction to their daughters' disability, perception of future possibilities, beliefs, attitude and the family support because all these variables would have an impact on the role strain of mothers.

Method

The sample comprised of 54 mothers having physically disabled daughters. Their age, education, perceived socio-economic status, family income, occupation and family structure were recorded using a demographic data sheet.

Instruments and Procedure

Mothers were interviewed regarding the nature and causes of their daughters' disability, first advice taken from, places gone for help, hope for improvement, perceived severity of disability, perception of disability, worries and problems, and future possibilities of their disabled daughters.

Two attitude measures (semantic differential attitude and relational attitude) were used to assess the attitude of the mothers towards their disabled daughters. Both these measures were taken from the research work of Dalal *et al.* (2000) and were further modified and tested in the context of present study.

Belief measures dealt with two aspects: causal beliefs, to what factors mothers attribute the occurrence of disability; and control beliefs, to determine the control strategy used by mothers of the disabled girls when confronted with a crises situation. Both these measures were also taken from the research work of Dalal *et al.* (2000) and were further modified and tested in the context of present study.

Pilot Study

In pilot work, five mothers having physically disabled daughters were interviewed. It was observed that these mothers found no difficulty in understanding the questionnaire. So, there was no ambiguity in framing of the questions. These mothers also reported that the questionnaire was relevant to tap the difficulties and problems faced by them in the process of adjustment. They felt that the questions were relevant.

Main Study

Each respondent was interviewed at her home. Effort was made to ensure that only mothers should give the answers, as in most cases it became difficult to separate mothers from other family members. Mothers were told that the purpose was to learn from their experiences in dealing with their disabled daughters. They were asked questions about their disabled daughters, other children, family members and their own interests, likes, dislikes etc. A good rapport was established. Then, they were informed about the objective of the study and assured that their responses will be used only for research purposes.

Results

Descriptive Characteristics of the Respondents

The average age of mothers having physically disabled daughters was around 42 years, while their disabled daughters' average age was 17 years. All mothers were literate. Among them, 50 percent had 8th-10th grade education, 7.4 percent had 11th-12th grade education, 14.8 percent were graduate and 27.8 percent were post-graduate. A total of 35.2 percent were working women and 64.8 percent were non-working women. In all, 68.5 percent mothers were from joint family whereas 31.5 percent were from nuclear family. While 74.1 percent mothers perceived themselves as belonging to higher-middle class and 22.2 percent to lower middle class, only 3.7 percent mothers discerned themselves as belonging to lower class. Their average family income per month was Rs. 5,507.

Causes and Types of Disability

The main cause of disability was polio (89%). Most of the mothers (64.8%) revealed that their daughters had become disabled at the age of one year due to polio. There were also 11 percent mothers who reported the reason of their daughters becoming disabled was accident within 10 years of age. Only 24.2 percent mothers stated that the disability was congenital.

Table 1

Mothers' First Reaction to Daughters' Disability

Category	*Frequency*	%
Assistance from family	2	3.7
It was God's will	3	5.5
With pain and sorrow	28	51.9
Deeds of past life	2	3.7
Accepted that they had become disabled now	2	3.7
With the help of medical treatment	17	31.5

Chi-square $=67.55$, df$=5$, $p < .0001$

The findings documented in Table 1 suggest that most of the mothers (51.9%) face their daughters' disability with a lot of pain and sorrow and those who took the help of medical treatment were only 31.5 percent.

Places Gone for Help

For their daughters' treatment mothers had gone different places like doctors (both allopathic and ayurvedic), local healers, family members, health workers, holy places, government hospitals as well as rehabilitation centre. Most (64.8%) of the mothers reported that they had taken the first advice from the medical doctor.

At the time of interview, most of the mothers revealed that they were taking help from more than one kind of doctors (medical or ayurvedic) and hospitals (government/private/PHC) and were offering prayers and worships. Only 3.7 percent mothers had hope for improvement in their daughters' disability.

What Disabled Daughters Can Do/Cannot Do?

Most of the mothers (92.6%) stated that their disabled daughters had maximum difficulties in those activities which involved physical use of the affected body parts as wiping floor (63%), lifting heavy things like furniture, water bucket (18.5%), and walking and climbing steps (11.1%). Very few mothers narrated difficulty in reading/writing (3.7%) and doing any work (3.7%).

Likewise, two-third (66.7%) mothers reported that their daughters did not need help in their daily routine activities. However, a few said that their daughters required help in specific activities such as going to school, function or for shopping (29.6%), and lifting water bucket during bath (3.7%). They further said that their disabled daughters were able to perform some unskilled work. Mothers were also asked whether they felt that they did not give proper time and attention to other children and family members because of the care of their disabled daughters. All mothers (100%) replied in the negative as they were paying equal attention to all family members.

Table 2
Mothers' Perception of Daughters' Disability

Category	*Frequency*	%
Dependent on others due to physical incompetence	2	3.7
Physically weak	17	31.5
No difference between disabled and non-disabled	12	22.2
Inferior to others	4	7.4
Lonely, emotional, sad, shy and unhappy	17	31.5
No future	4	7.4

Chi-square=28.89, df=5,P<.0001

The data in Table 2 indicate that most of the mothers perceived their daughters as physically weak, lonely, emotional, shy and sad. Similarly, the findings reported in Table 3 reveal that most of the mothers were worried about the marriage (44.4%) and future (33.3%) of their disabled daughters and had mental tension and stress (63%) regarding their well-being.

Table 3
Worries and Problems of Mothers

Worries of Mothers	*Frequency*	%
Regarding future of their daughter	18	33.3
Regarding marriage of their daughter	24	44.4
Regarding job of their daughter	6	11.1
Regarding education of their daughter	4	7.4
No worries	2	3.7

Chi-square = 34.52, df = 4, P<2.001

Problems of Mothers	*Frequency*	%
Thinking a lot	12	22.2
Tension and stress	34	63
Physical manifestations	8	14.8

Chi-square = 21.78, df =2, p<.0001

Then, findings of Table 4 suggest that most of the mothers were anxious for their disabled daughters' future. They wanted them to have jobs (44.4%) so that they could become independent and they also wanted to settle them through their marriage (29.6%).

Table 4

Mothers' Perception of Future Possibilities

Category	*Frequency*	%
To get job for their daughters	24	44.4
To get married their daughters	16	29.6
To educate their daughters	2	3.7
To leave their future on God's will	5	9.3
No future plans	7	13

Chi-square=30.26, df=4, p<. 0001

Routine Activities of the Mothers

Daily Routine Care

Almost all mothers (100%) reported that they needed no extra time for their disabled daughters' care and they paid equal attention to all family members. Most of the mothers (66.7%) stated that care of their disabled daughters did not increase their workload. Only 33.3 percent mothers reported increase in their workload. It suggests that mothers who felt no increase in their workload would have less strain.

Periodical Care

Most of the mothers disclosed that they needed help for physical exercise of their daughters (70.4%), going to hospital (59.3%), check-up from doctor (61.1%) and for religious activities and rites (20.4%) of their disabled daughters.

Family Support

An overwhelming majority (92.6%) the mothers revealed that their family members helped them. While 66.7 percent mothers received maximum help from their in-laws, children and other family members, 25.9 percent mothers reported that only their husbands helped them and 7.4 percent said that none of the family members helped them in the daily routine care of their disabled daughters.

Financial Support

About 92.6 percent mothers expressed that they got financial help from their husbands. Most of the mothers solved their problems with the help of their husbands (66.5%) and other family members (18.5%). Only 13 percent mothers reported that they solved their problems individually.

Emotional Support

More than half of the mothers said that their disabled daughters got emotional support from their grandparents (55.6%), followed by fathers (25.9%) and siblings (14.8%). Only 3.7 percent mothers reported no such emotional support.

Most of the mothers also stated that their husbands (77.8%), in-laws (14.8%) and other children (7.4%) also helped them during festivals and functions where their disabled daughters had to participate.

Help in Household Activities

Most (96.3%) of the mothers reported that their family members (husband 46.3%, children 3.7%, in-laws 46.3%) also helped them, and according to only 3.7 percent mothers, nobody helped them in their daily household activities.

Care during Emergency

While a total of 48.2 percent mothers were of the view that in all conditions/circumstances their disabled daughters were given 'full' attention and proper care, 40.7 percent revealed that their disabled daughters were paid 'some' attention and care and only 11.1 percent expressed that 'no' care was given to their daughters.

Leisure Time Activities of Mothers

All mothers spent their leisure time in different types of activities like other household activities except cooking (61.1%), knitting, sewing and embroidery (5.6%) and teaching their children (1.9%). Only 13 percent mothers reported that they had no extra time and 18.5 percent mothers revealed that they were worried and anxious regarding the disability of their daughters.

Table 5
Adjustment of Mothers

Category	*Frequency*	*%*
Mothers became habitual of these problems	22	40.7
It was God's will	2	3.7
With the help of family members	10	18.5
Adjusted for the sake of disabled daughters	12	22.2
Diverting their attention to other activities	8	14.8

Chi-square $=19.70$, df$=4$, $P<.0006$

The findings shown in Table 5 indicate that while 40.7 percent mothers have become habitual with their problems, 22.2 percent have adjusted themselves to support their disabled daughters with the help of their family members.

Tension Reduction by Mothers

More than half of the mothers (59.2%) kept themselves busy in the family activities, while 11.1 percent mothers reduced their tension by weeping and crying. Some of them read magazines (7.4%), performed religious activities (7.4%) and by being courageous (7.4%) reduced their tension. Only 7.4 percent mothers revealed that they were always tensed. All mothers were aware and had given suggestions for the care of the disabled child.

Table 6
Correlations of Attitude Measures with Control and Causal Beliefs for the Mothers of Disabled Daughters (N=54)

Attitude Measures	*Overall Control Beliefs*	*Causal Belief*		
		Internal	*External*	*Cosmic*
Attitude scale	.26	-.28*	.22	-.14
Relational attitude scale				
Assimilation	-.09	-.43**	.48***	.14
Integration	-.04	-.23	.30*	.36*
Segregation	-.17	-.12	.14	.41*
Marginalization	-.20	-.18	.22	.11

* $p<.05$, ** $p<.01$, *** $p<.001$

Table 6 indicates that mothers having positive attitude reported less internal causal belief. Mothers, who perceived their disabled daughters more assimilated, had attributed less internal causal beliefs and more external causal beliefs, whereas mothers who discerned their disabled daughters more integrated reported more external and cosmic beliefs. And, mothers, who perceived their disabled daughters more segregated, reported more cosmic beliefs.

Discussion

The responses, reactions, talks and perception of mothers of the disabled daughters clearly show that how mothers undergo a lot of role strain in taking care of their disabled daughters. Mothers visited different places for the cure of their daughters' disability but failed to get full support. It suggests that mothers who reported that they received little support or no support had to face additional stress. At the time of interview, most of the mothers still continued to visit to doctors or hospitals for their daughters' treatment and also offering prayers and worships. It appears that this practice resulted in a reduction of stress and tension of mothers. In Indian culture, one of the traditional methods of releasing tension and anxiety is by hoping for divine intervention in the form of a miracle.

One notable finding was that an overwhelming majority of the mothers perceived their daughters' disability as being more severe. It was a shocking experience for them but for the well-being of their daughters most of them controlled their emotions and used different types of coping strategies to face their daughters' disability as God's will, deeds of past life, with the help of medical treatment and family support and by accepting the reality (disability) that their daughters were disabled now and they had to bear it throughout.

Mothers' major worries were regarding their daughters' marriage to ensure their future. In Hindu society, it is parents' duty to settle their daughters by getting them married. It was found that girls who are disabled are most often unacceptable for marriage and are considered to be a burden on the family. This is one of the reasons why mothers were very much worried. This shows that because of these worries the mothers were tensed and were undergoing a lot of problems such as mental tension and stress, thinking problems and psychosomatic manifestations like headache, fatigue, restlessness, sleep disturbance, etc. These problems are highly associated with stress and stressful events. Similar findings were also obtained from investigations in the west on caregiving burden that caregivers with extreme stress suffer from fatigue, insomania, depression and excessive irritability (Montgomery, Goneya and Hooman, 1985; Rabins, Mace and Lucas, 1982; Anthony, Zarit and Gatz, 1988). This indeed is an indicator of severe role strain of the mothers.

The findings further reveal that most of the mothers solved their worries and problems with the help of their husbands and other family members and only a few had to deal by themselves. It seems that mothers who had no family support and tried to solve their daughters' problems by themselves would undergo more strain than those who got full support of the family.

The mothers were of the view that getting a job and marriage would secure their daughters' future and also solve their problems. It appears that still these mothers were very shocked and were not adjusted with their daughter's disability; this is the reason, they were not in the condition to think or make future plans for their disabled daughters.

Since the disabled daughters needed constant help from their mothers in carrying out physical activities, the mothers perceived their daughters as physically weak. As a consequence of this, the mothers experienced more strain. It seems that mothers, who had not accepted their daughters' disability, did not make any differentiation between or comparison with the non-disabled offspring. Such a defensive attitude on the part of mothers would lead to temporary tension reduction but it makes negative impact on their well-being. Coleman (1982) suggested that denial of any reality (disability) would be an indicator of unsatisfactory adjustment.

It is clear from findings that regarding their daughters' disability most of the mothers' perception was negative; this would also contribute role strain. How these mothers cope and adjust themselves with these strains is an important area of investigation. It was assumed that daily routine activities of mothers regarding their disabled daughters, periodical care given by mothers, financial/ emotional support given to mothers by their family members regarding the care of their disabled daughters would also have an impact on role strain of the mothers.

The other significant finding is that most of the mothers reported that their disabled daughters did not need help in their daily routine activities. They also revealed that they obtained help and assistance from their family members and husbands. It seems that the help and support obtained from family members is one of the ways of sharing the tension and additional burden. This is the reason according to most of the mothers that the care of their disabled daughters did not increase their workload. It has also been found that the Indian extended family fulfils the emotional and social needs of its members (Basa, 1978; Gore, 1978; Kakar, 1978). It also appears that help provided by family members helped mothers to reduce their strain and they were able to perform different leisure time activities such as other household activities except cooking, knitting, sewing and embroidery, and teaching their children. These mothers had learned to adjust and cope with the problems of their disabled daughters. Mothers reduced their tension by keeping themselves busy in their family. They also obtained emotional relief by crying and weeping, being courageous, reading magazines, and performing religious activities. It is important to note that disability caused tension, frustration and distress in both daughters and mothers and they have tried to deal with them by using different strategies.

The findings also reveal that education is an important determinant, which is good for both: in the care of the disabled daughters and also facilitating good health for mothers. Educated mothers have shown realistic attitude because of their broader perspective. They know that the cause of their daughters' disability is polio/ accident, which is controllable but not fully curable. This is why, these mothers have not underestimated the help they received. The findings further reveal that mothers who perceived their social status higher overestimated their economic condition but in reality they were not able to earn extra money for the well-being of their disabled daughters and hence were dissatisfied by the result of their caring. This shows the negative self-perception of the mothers.

The mothers were trying to reduce their tension by believing in God or deeds of past life. It seems that they have evaluated the disability in such a manner as does not deny the reality. It also strengthens them by accepting the fact that it was because of fever and it might be God's will and so how anyone could else be responsible or control it. The combination of these three attribution patterns helps them in easing their adjustment and tolerating the pain of disability. It is a sort of defence-oriented approach used by mothers for tension reduction (Coleman, 1982). Mothers having a positive attitude did not blame themselves for their daughters' disability. This suggests that those mothers who are more prone to evaluate event externally and tried to denial of reality, are maladjusted. Mothers whose daughters had been disabled since long period were not hopeful for their daughters' future improvement.

The family structure is also an important aspect to the lives of persons with a disability. Children who are disabled are cared by their families in their homes. The present research also suggests that mothers from nuclear family perceived that their disabled daughters required more caring as compared to joint family mothers. It shows the importance of family as a good source of social support.

From all these findings it is clear that despite their daughters' disability and their own worries and anxieties, mothers were willing to work hard to help their disabled daughters. It seems that they recognized that it was a difficult and painful endeavour but in spite of these problems they attempted to cope with the situation. It also appears that these mothers were alert and were task-oriented in their efforts. They were not defensive. Using the task-oriented approach (Coleman, 1982), they tried to solve problems in a realistic manner. Some mothers accepted the situation as God's will and they were more withdrawn. Few mothers used denial of disability as a coping mechanism.

To sum up, it must be noted that the role strain of the mothers of disabled daughters was great but they were caring, concerned and conscious of their duties and their family was supportive, so the stress was tolerated. It may be because the Hindu family system that gives more emphasis on strong familial bonds and clearly defines the primary duties of parents, so that even without outside support, the mothers and the other family members of the disabled girls were able to achieve a satisfactory level of adjustment.

References

Anthony, C.R., Zarit, S.H. and Gatz, M. (1988). Symptoms of psychological distress among caregivers of dementia patient. *Psychology of Aging, 3*, 245-248.

Basa, D.M. (1978). From the traditional to the modern: Some observations on the changes in the Indian childrearing and parental attitudes, with special reference to identity formation. In E.J. Antony and C.L. Chiland (Eds.), *The Child in His Family: Children and Their Parents in a Changing World* (Vol. 5). New York: Wiley.

Barreara, M. (1986). Distinctions between social support concepts, measures and models. *American Journal of Community Psychology, 14*, 413-445.

Chaturvedi, S.K. and Malhotra, S. (1984). A follow up study of mental retardation focusing on parental attitudes. *Indian Journal of Psychiatry, 26*, 370-376.

Cohen, C.A. (2000). Caregivers for people with dementia: What is the family physician role? *Canadian Family Physician, 46*, 376-380.

Cohen, F. and Lazarus, R. (1979). Coping with the stresses of illness. In G.C. Stone, F. Cohen and N.E. Adler (Eds.), *A Handbook Health Psychology*. San Francisco: Jossey-Bass.

Cohen, F. (1987). Measurement of coping. In S.V. Kasi and C.L. Cooper (Eds.), *Stress and Health Issues in Research Methodology.* New York: Wiley.

Cohen. S. and Wills, T.A. (1985). Stress, social support and the buffering hypothesis. *Psychological Bulletin*, 98, 310-357.

Cohen, S., Glass, D.C. and Phillips, S. (1979). Environment and health. In H.E. Freeman, S. Levine and L.G. Reeder (Eds.), *Handbook of Medical Sociology*. Englewood Cliffs, New Jersey: Prentice Hall.

Coleman, J.C. (1982). *Abnormal Psychology and Modern Life*. Bombay: D.B. Taraporevala Sons and Co.

COPOH (1989). *Women, Development and Disability*. Winnipeg, Canada: COPOH Bulletin.

Dalal, A.K. and Pande, N. (1988). Psychological recovery of the accident victims with temporary and permanent disability. *International Journal of Psychology*, *23*, 25-40.

Dalal, A.K., Pandey, N., Dhawan, N. and Dwijendra, D. (2000). *The Mind Matters: Disability, Attitudes and Community-based Rehabilitation.* Allahabad: University of Allahabad Publication.

Fiske, S.T. and Taylor, S.E. (1984). *Social Cognition*. New York: Random House.

Gandotra, V. (1984). Management problems and practices of home-makers with a disabled member in the family. *Indian Journal of Social Work, 45*, 485-490.

— (1991). A comparative analysis of time management by mothers of orthopedically handicapped and mentally retarded children. In M. Desai (Ed.), *Research on Families with Problems in India: Issues and Implications.* Bombay: Tata Institute of Social Sciences Publications.

Gokhale, B.G. (1961). *Indian Thoughts Throughout the Ages: A Study of Some Dominant Concepts*. Bombay: Asia Publishing House.

Gore, M.S. (1978). Changes in the family and the process of socialization in India. In E.J. Antony and Chiland (Eds.), *The Child in his Family: Children and Their Parents in a Changing World, 5,* New York: Wiley.

House, J.S., Umberson, D. and Landis, K.R. (1988). Structures and processes of social support. *American Review of Sociology, 14,* 293-318.

Jamuna, D. (1996). Psychological dimensions of caregiver's stress. In Vinod Kumar (Ed.), *Aging: Indian Perspective and Global Scenario*. New Delhi: Vinod Kumar.

— (1997b). Stress dimensions among caregivers of the elderly. *Indian Journal of Medical Research,* 381-387.

Jones, E.E. *et al.*, (1984). *Social Stigma*. San Francisco: Freeman.

Julie, S.M.C. (1995). Current provision of effectiveness of day care services for people with dementia. *Reviews in Clinical Gerontology, 5,* 313-320.

Kakar, S. (1978). *The Inner World: A Psychoanalytic Study of Childhood and Society in India*. Delhi: Oxford University Press.

Kashyap, L. (1991). Research on families with disabled individuals: Review and implications. In M. Desai (Ed.), *Research on Families with Problems in India: Issues and Implications.* Bombay: Tata Institute of Social Sciences Publications

Kelley, H.H. (1967). Attribution theory in social psychology. In D. Levine (Ed.), *Nebraska Symposium on Motivation*. Lincoln: University of Nebraska Press.

Kessler, R.C. and McLeod, J.D. (1985). Social support and mental health in community samples. In S. Cohen and S.L. Syme (Eds.), *Social Support and Health*. Orlando, FL: Academic Press.

Krause, N. (2001). Social support. In R.H. Binstock and I.K. George (Eds.), *Handbook of Aging and Social Sciences.* San Diego. CA: Academic Press.

La Gapia, J.J. (1990). The negative effects of informal support systems. In S. Duck (Ed.), *Personal Relationship and Social Support.* New York: Sage.

Lazarus, R.S. and Folkman, S. (1984). *Stress, Appraisal and Coping*. New York: Springer.

Lazarus, R.S. and Launier, R. (1978). Stress-related transactions between person and environment. In L.A. Pervin and M. Lewis (Eds.), *Perspectives in Interactional Psychology*. New York: Plenum.

MacCormack, C.P. (1988). Health and the social power of women. *Social Science and Medicine, 26*, 677-683.

Montgomery, R.T.V., Goneya, J.C. and Hooman, N.R. (1985). Caregiving and the experience of subjective-objective burden. *Family Relations, 34*, 19-26.

Pearlin, L.I. *et al.*, (1990). Caregiving and the stress process: An overview of concepts and their measures. *The Gerontologist, 30*, 583-594.

Pearson, M. (1987). Old wives or young midwives? Women as caretakers of health: the case of Nepal. In J. Henshall Momson and G. Townsend (Eds.), *Geography of Gender in the Third World*. London: State University of New York Press.

Rabins, P.V., Mace, N.L. and Lucas, M.J. (1982). The impact of dementia and the family. *Journal of Medical Association, 24*, 333-325.

Radhakrishnan, S. (1926). *The Hindu View of Life*. Bombay: Blackie.

Rook, K.S. (1984). The negative side of social interaction: Impact on psychological well-being. *Journal of Personality and Social Psychology, 46(5)*, 1097-1108.

Sen, A. 1988). *Psychosocial Integration of Handicapped: A Challenge to the Society*. New Delhi: Mittal Publications.

Susman, J. (1994). *Perceptions of Disability of the Long-term Caregivers*. Unpublished manuscript, University of Michigan, Ann Arbor.

Thompson, S.C. and Spacapan, S. (1991). Perceptions of control in vulnerable populations. *Journal of Social Issues, 47 (4)*, 1-21.

Weiner, B.J., Perry, R.P. and Magnusson, J. (1988). An attributional analysis of reactions to stigma. *Journal of Personality and Social Psychology, 55*, 738-748.

Wortman, C.B. and Dunkel-Schetter, C. (1987). Conceptual and methodological issues in the study of social support. In A. Baum and J.E. Singer (Eds.), *Handbook of Psychology and Health, 5*. Hillsdale, NJ: Erlbaum.

IV

Indian Health Scenario

14

Social Virus of Female Foeticide More Dangerous than HIV/AIDS

ASHISH BOSE

The public health scenario in India is, of late, dominated by the spectre of HIV/AIDS, largely because of the aggressive advocacy of AIDS control programmes supported by World Bank and foreign donor agencies. To our mind, the spread of female foeticide is a far greater threat than HIV/AIDS. To control this sinister virus, social scientists, particularly sociologists and psychologists, must give high priority to research on the causes and consequences of sex-selective abortion in different regions of India. The Centre for Behavioural and Cognitive Sciences of the University of Allahabad has taken lead in this direction by organizing a national seminar on "Social Dimensions of Health" in April 2003 successfully. The Supreme Court, while giving a ruling on the implementation of the PNDT Act, has recently observed that "the Court would not be able to change the mindset of the population" (*Times of India*, September 11, 2003). We should not forget that the son complex is a deep-rooted phenomenon in Indian society and it cannot be wished away by passing resolutions or enacting laws.

It should be more than obvious that legal enactments like the PNDT Act of 1994 and the amendments in 2002 will not be able to contain the epidemic of female foeticide unless we know how to change the mindset of the people. The unholy alliance between tradition and technology must be frontally attacked and gender balance restored. A distorted sex composition of the population will create serious social problems like increasing violence against women, abduction and rape, apart from the disastrous impact on the physical and mental health of women undergoing repeated abortions to get rid of the female foetus. Health, medical ethics, gender, reproductive and human rights issues must be tackled simultaneously while drawing up action plans to combat female foeticide.

Declining Child Sex Ratio: Evidence from 2001 Census

The interpretation of declining child sex ratio (females per 1,000 males in 0-6 age group) calls for considerable demographic expertise. Consider, for example, the contradictory trends revealed by the censuses of 1991 and 2001. In 1991, the overall sex ratio declined and so also the child sex ratio, while in 2001, the overall sex ratio increased but the child sex ratio declined. How do we explain this phenomenon? The first point to consider is the quality of census enumeration. Suppose, the quality of enumeration worsened in 2001 compared to 1991, and the extent of under-enumeration of girls increased, the sex ratio will tend to decline. Likewise, if the 2001 enumeration is better than that of 1991 and the extent of under-enumeration of females is of a lesser degree, the sex ratio will tend to increase. It is too early to make a firm comment on this aspect – one must wait for the results of the post-census enumeration survey of 2001 census and compare the results with those of the 1991 census. In a recent census publication (*Census of India 2001, Series 1, Paper 1 of 2001 Supplement: District Tables*), the Census Commissioner hints that the increase in the sex ratio of seven-plus population in several districts of India may be the result of better enumeration of women. To quote him at length: "It is interesting to note that 477 districts consisting of over 82 percent of the districts register an increase in sex ratio of the population in the age group of seven-plus. Of these, 215 districts have recorded substantial gain of over twenty points. The possibility of some positive impact on the enumeration of adult female population in many parts of the country during the current census due to various factors such as gender-sensitive approach in training and publicity measures also cannot be ruled out. Majority of the districts recording gains of above 20 points are from Uttar Pradesh, Uttaranchal, Bihar, Rajasthan, Assam, Madhya Pradesh, Tamil Nadu and Arunachal Pradesh. It is noteworthy to mention that all the districts of Uttaranchal, West Bengal, Jharkhand, Kerala, and Andaman and Nicobar Islands show an improvement in the sex ratio age seven-plus at the *Census of India, 2001* as compared to the 1991 census. Among these, nine districts of Arunachal Pradesh, seven districts of Uttaranchal and four districts of Uttar Pradesh have recorded an increase of 50 or more points in the sex ratio age seven-plus" (p.56). One can argue that if the 2001 census has been more gender sensitive than before, there should have been an improvement in the child sex ratio as well but this has not happened. It seems that a real decline in the child sex ratio must have wiped out the gains of better enumeration of the girl child. There is convincing evidence in the district-wise analysis of 2001 census data that the decline in the child sex ratio is all pervasive and has occurred throughout India, while it is more pronounced in Punjab, Haryana, parts of Himachal Pradesh and Gujarat, apart from cities like Chandigarh, Delhi, Surat, Mumbai and Kolkata. *Census Paper No. 1 Supplement* provides comparable data for 1991 and 2001 on the child sex ratio in 577 districts of India (this excludes 14 districts of Jammu and Kashmir where the 1991 census was not conducted and Kachchh district of Gujarat and Kinnaur district of Himachal Pradesh where the 2001 census was not conducted). As many as 456 districts out of 577 record a decline in the child sex ratio in 2001 compared to 1991. In 70 districts, the decline is in the order of 50 points. In several districts, the decline is more than 100 points. Regardless of the quality of census enumeration in the censuses of 1991 and 2001, one can conclude that the decline in the child sex ratio is a real phenomenon and not a statistical aberration. The Census Commissioner observes: "The decline in child sex ratio is assuming an alarming proportion in certain districts of Punjab, Haryana,

Himachal Pradesh and the decline in majority of the districts in other states and union territories across the country (Uttar Pradesh, Madhya Pradesh, Chhatisgarh, Orissa, Karnataka, Assam, Delhi, etc.) is rather intriguing. The social cultural bias against the girl child might have been possibly aggravated by recent medical support in terms of sex determination tests and requires further field investigation. Before arriving at any definite conclusion among other details we have to wait for single year age-wise desaggregated population data for the 2001 Census" (*Census Paper 1 Supplement: 53*).

In passing, it may be pointed out that the term 'child sex ratio' is somewhat misleading. The definition of child is not restricted to six years. Usually, the cut off point is 14 years. Indian census presents data in five-yearly age groups like 0-4, 5-9, 10-14, and so on. The sex ratio data for the 0-6 age group is a by-product of the literacy data. Literacy rate is calculated in the Indian census since 1991 for the age group seven-plus. The 0-6 age group population is subtracted from the total population. For a proper study of the child sex ratio, one needs data on sex ratio at birth and also at ages one, two, three, four and five, but single year age data are not very reliable. SRS data present figures for the 0-4 and 5-9 age groups. These data have to be analyzed both for 1991 and 2001. The most comprehensive study of juvenile sex ratio (JSR) for the age group 0-9 years was done by Satish Agnihotri (2000), based on 1961-1981 census data. His book *Sex Ratio Patterns in the Indian Population: A Fresh Exploration* gives a valuable insight into this complex phenomenon. It was published much before the 2001 census results were available. Nevertheless, his simulation exercise does lead him to the right conclusion. Commenting on sex-selective abortions and female infanticide, Agnihotri says: "The rise in sex-selective abortions and emergence of female infanticide in various parts of the country are two serious aspects of excess child mortality" (2000: 302). Agnihotri brings out the close linkage between female foeticide and female infanticide. He argues: "Prenatal selection is a new technological tool which has gained acceptability as something scientific, neutral and performed by the 'professionals' concerned. It has accorded legitimacy to the elimination of a child on the basis of its sex. Where money and facility are available, it is resorted to by the social superstratum. Those who do not have the access to this facility look for 'affordable' alternatives since the process has been 'sanctified' anyway. This 'affordable' alternative is infanticide. As the incidence of infanticide spreads, those who practise prenatal selection occupy a 'holier' pedestal. After all, they are not resorting to the 'barbaric' or the 'cruel' practice of killing a new born infant. So, the doctor who goes around the countryside with this 'mobile facility' in his new luxury car can claim to be doing social service. The verdict is now passed not on whether the elimination on the basis of sex is acceptable or otherwise but on which method is more acceptable – sex-selective abortion or infanticide. The technological alternative gets legitimized in comparison with infanticide while sanctifying the idea of elimination of the child on the basis of sex. This in turn spreads the practice of infanticide further among those who do not have access to the facility, e.g., high castes in rural Bihar, or those who cannot afford it, e.g., the rural poor in Salem district of Tamil Nadu. Notwithstanding the spread in the 'facilities' for prenatal selection, it will continue to remain beyond the reach of a large number of people in foreseeable future. The two processes will therefore, feed on each other" (ibid.: 303). The Centre for Women's Development Studies (CWDS), under the leadership of Vina Mazumdar, who is well known for her pioneering contribution to gender issues, has brought out a useful volume, *Enduring Conundrum: India's Sex Ratio: Essays in Honour of Asok Mitra* (Mazumdar and Krishnaji, 2001). This book, however, was published before the detailed data from 2001 census were available.

In the light of the census detailed data, which are now available, we have classified various districts of India as follows:

D1: child sex ratio between 850-900
(females per thousand males)

D2: child sex ratio between 800-850

D3: child sex ratio between 750-800

The worst category, obviously, is D3.

Our analysis reveals the black holes in India's demographic transition. We have coined an acronym, "DEMARU" which stands for daughter eliminating male aspiring rage for ultrasound. The three worst states are Punjab, Haryana and Himachal Pradesh as indicated below (the child sex ratio in 2001 is given in brackets):

1. PUNJAB: Overall rating - D3 (793)
   Districts:
   D1: nil.
   D2: Faridkot (805), Muktsar (807), Hoshiarpur (810), Nawanshahr (810), Ludhiana (814), Moga (819), Ferozpur (819)
   D3: Fatehgarh Sahib (754), Patiala (770), Kapurthala (775), Gurdaspur (775), Bhatinda (779), Mansa (779), Amritsar (783), Sangrur (784), Roopnagar (791), Jalandhar (797).
   Note: all the 17 districts of Punjab are in D category.

2. HARYANA: Overall rating - D2 (820)
   Districts:
   D1: Faridabad (856), Gurgaon (863).
   D2: Jhajjar (805), Yamuna Nagar (807), Panipat (807), Karnal (808), Mahendragarh (814), Rewari (814), Jind (818), Sirsa (818), Hissar (830), Fatehbad (830), Panchkula (837), Bhiwani (838).
   D3: Kurakshetra (770), Sonipat (783), Ambala (784), Kaithal (789), Rohtak (796).
   Note: all the 19 districts of Haryana are in D category.

3. HIMACHAL PRADESH: Overall rating - D1 (897)
   Districts:
   D1: Hamirpur (864), Bilaspur (884), Solan (900).
   D2: Kangra (836), Una (839).
   Note: Five out of 12 districts of Himachal Pradesh are in D category.

4. UNION TERRITORY OF CHANDIGARH: Overall rating - D2 (845)

5. GUJARAT: Overall rating - D1 (878)
   Districts:
   D1: Surendranagar (861), Patan (862), Anand (873), Vadodara (873), Surat (873), Sabarkantha (876), Kheda (880), Porbandar (886), Bhavnagar (886), Jamnagar (894), Amreli (894), Junagadh (898).
   D2: Ahmedabad (814), Gandhinagar (816), Rajkot (844).
   D3: Mahesana (798).
   Note: 16 out of 25 districts in Gujarat are in D category.

6. DELHI: Overall rating - D1(865)
   Space does not permit us to give detailed figures for all the districts in India, except to say that in the most progressive state, Kerala there was not a single district belonging to the D category whereas in Tamil Nadu, another demographically progressive state, there were four districts in D category:

7. TAMIL NADU
   Districts
   D1: Dharmapuri (878), Theni (893), Namakkal (895).
   D2: Salem (826).
   Note: Four out of 30 districts are D category.

In Table 1 we give the sex ratio for two categories – 0-6 and 7+ population. It may be noted that 7+ category is influenced by migration. One can infer from this table that 0-6 girls have fared badly while the situation has improved in the 7+ category. The overall increase in the sex ratio in India during 1991-2001 (from 927 to 933) conceals the fact that the child sex ratio during this period has gone down from 945 to 927.

Haryana's 'Unwanted' Generation: Fallout of Population Explosion, Unemployment and Corruption

It would be incorrect to say that female foeticide is just a social phenomenon. The economic factors are no less important. To illustrate this point I give below some observations based on my recent fieldwork in Haryana. I realized how unwanted the new generation was in Haryana. The girls are not wanted because of the increasing

Table 1
Child Sex Ratio (0-6 Age and Seven-Plus Age Group)
State/UTs Ranked According to Decline in Sex Ratio of 0-6 Population

Rank	*India/ States/ UTs*	*Sex ratio (0-6 age group)*			*Sex ratio (7+ age group)*		
		1991	*2001*	*Difference points*	*1991*	*2001*	*Difference points*
	INDIA	945	927	-18	923	935	12
1	Punjab	875	793	-82	883	886	3
2	Haryana	879	820	-59	862	869	7
3	Himachal Pradesh	951	897	-54	980	981	1
4	Chandigarh	899	845	-54	772	763	-9
5	Gujarat	928	878	-50	936	927	-9
6	Delhi	915	865	-50	810	813	3
7	(Uttaranchal)	948	906	-42	933	976	43
8	Dadra and Nagar Haveli	1,013	973	-40	936	779	-157
9	Daman and Diu	958	925	-33	971	682	-289
10	Goa	964	933	-31	967	964	-3
11	Maharashtra	946	917	-29	931	923	-8
12	Arunachal Pradesh	982	961	-21	829	888	59
13	Nagaland	993	975	-18	865	899	34
14	Orissa	967	950	-17	972	976	4
15	Bihar	953	938	-15	895	916	21
16	Manipur	974	961	-13	955	981	26
17	(Jharkhand)	979	966	-13	908	936	28
18	Madhya Pradesh	941	929	-12	905	918	13
19	Meghalaya	986	975	-11	947	974	27
20	Uttar Pradesh	927	916	-11	863	895	32
21	Assam	975	964	-11	910	926	16
22	Karnataka	960	949	-11	960	966	6
23	Andhra Pradesh	975	964	-11	972	980	8
24	(Chhatisgarh)	984	975	-9	986	992	6
25	Tamil Nadu	948	939	-9	978	992	14
26	Andaman and Nicobar Islands	973	965	-8	790	830	40
27	Rajasthan	916	909	-7	908	925	17
28	Pondicherry	963	958	-5	982	1007	25
29	West Bengal	967	963	-4	907	929	22
30	Mizoram	969	971	2	911	932	21
31	Kerala	958	963	5	1049	1071	22
32	Tripura	967	975	8	940	947	7
33	Sikkim	965	986	21	860	858	-2
34	Lakshadweep	941	974	33	943	943	0
35	Jammu and Kashmir	NA	937	—	NA	894	—

Source: Ashish Bose, *India's Billion Plus People*, 2001.

Table 2

Distribution of Districts by Ranges of Child Sex Ratio in Age Group 0-6 – India: 1991 and 2001

Sex Ratio (0-6)	*1991*			*2001*		
	Number of districts	*Population (million)*	*Percent*	*Number of districts*	*Population (million)*	*Percent*
1000-1049	21	8.67	1.04	8	3.87	0.38
950-999	306	454.01	54.27	242	403.83	39.38
900-949	181	287.91	34.41	208	381.36	37.59
850-899	68	83.49	9.98	71	155.66	15.34
800-849	1	2.57	0.31	32	47.85	4.72
Less than 800	–	-	-	16	22.08	2.18
Total	577	836.65	100.00	577	1,041.65	100.00

Source: Census of India 2001 Paper I of 2001, Supplement.

Table 3

Distribution of Districts by Ranges of Sex Ratio of Seven-Plus Population – India: 1991 and 2001

Sex Ratio (7+)	*1991*			*2001*		
	Number of districts	*Population (million)*	*Percent*	*Number of districts*	*Population (million)*	*Percent*
1050+	18	21.2	2.53	26	40.32	3.97
1000-1049	47	67.76	8.09	65	90.77	8.95
950-999	139	209.45	25.03	152	277.91	27.29
900-949	162	243.4	29.09	170	315.49	31.09
850-899	115	171.28	20.47	108	194.35	19.15
800-849	73	97.86	11.70	46	86.92	8.57
Less than 800	23	25.7	3.07	10	8.89	0.88

Source: Census of India 2001 Paper I of 2001, Supplement.

demand for dowry, fuelled by mindless consumerism, especially on TV (there is a craze for TV everywhere). The boys have become a burden on parents because they do not get jobs, partly because there are too many applicants for jobs in the organized sector while employment is shrinking, thanks to globalization! The worst part of the story is that almost everybody is convinced that without a hefty bribe directly or through the middlemen, one cannot get a job, say, in the police force or the army (the traditional vocations of the youth in Haryana, especially of the Jats and Ahirs). The net result is devaluation of youth. The adolescent girl feels unwanted and guilty of being a burden on the parents and the adolescent boys feel the same way. In short, their self-image is that they belong to an 'unwanted' generation.

I was going round the village with an ex-policeman. I stopped near a pond where little children were playing marbles under a tree. Nearby a tall well-built young man was standing with a vacant look. I asked him about his studies. He had passed Class X examination and wanted to take up a job. He was 19 when he tried for a job in the police and the army but did not succeed though he was medically cleared. With an angry look he told me: "How can I pay two lakh rupees to get into the police force? And for army recruitment, the agent wants one lakh rupees. I tried again the next year but the story was the same. They want bribe. I have only one more chance." The ex-policeman informed me that new recruits must be below 21 years. What about other jobs, say in some factory? There are no jobs going. In fact, factories in Faridabad (a part of Haryana) are being closed down. The social worker accompanying me lives in Faridabad and she told me that factory after factory is being closed down under the adverse impact of globalization. The village people also confirmed that there are hardly any new jobs in the industrial sector. What about government jobs? The level of corruption is even higher in most government departments. There is also a ban on new recruitment. What do the young people do then? Migrate to other places, go abroad? The professor of sociology, who accompanied me, told me: "Mobility is very restricted here. People are attached to land." I was surprised to find that there was nobody from the biggish village I visited who went abroad for employment. This is in sharp contrast to the situation in Punjab where during my fieldwork, I would come across numerous families with their sons working abroad, not only in UK and USA, Canada and the Gulf countries but also in countries like Sweden, Italy and New Zealand.

Haryana has a high per capita income and the level of poverty is low. The Human Development Index is high for Haryana, according to Planning Commission's National Report on Human Development, 2001. But I am not convinced that 'human' development is indeed high in this state. High population growth rates for three decades, rising unemployment and galloping corruption make a deadly mixture and pave the way for increase in crime, violence against women (widespread female foeticide and the shortage of girls will add to the misery of women who survive), anti-social activities and even terrorism. I remember an ex-Governor of Punjab telling me: "Terrorism in Punjab is the result of unemployment among youth."

Will Haryana women be driven to male foeticide in future? Some elderly people in the village told me: "The stage is soon coming when boys will not be valued any more. They are loitering about and the prospects of getting employment in the government is nil. Who will marry them? Unlike the general impression that Haryana farmers have a lot of land, most people have very little land and the land cannot sustain them." In the village I visited, some unemployed young men in desperation started English medium schools for little children as there is a craze for sending children to such schools. But, these are hardly schools. These are not even teaching shops! Charge high fees and make some money in the name of English medium. But, the sponsors of these schools hardly know any English! It seems such schools are mushrooming in Haryana. Nobody bothers about registration. It is a pathetic picture of the plight of the robust young men of Haryana. Why not join sports, go to Rai, I asked the young men. "This is easier said than done", was the answer. One needs influence, apart from money. The picture is much worse when one thinks of the young men belonging to scheduled castes. They belong to landless families, by and large. They could work on the farms but Bihari and UP migrants are preferred by the big farmers: these workers will not demand minimum wage or agitate like local labour.

There is no denying the fact that relentless population growth in Haryana over the last five decades has meant increasing population pressure on land. In a state like Haryana, which is primarily agricultural, obviously, land is of paramount importance. The young men of Haryana do not see any prospects of their getting involved in agriculture, given the size of average landholding.

Let us have a look at the population growth figures for Haryana. The decadal growth rate was 33.8 percent during 1951-61, 32.2 percent in 1961-71, 28.8 percent in 1971-81, 27.4 percent in 1981-91 and 28.1 percent in 1991-2001. The growth rate has increased during the last decade. The annual exponential growth rate was as high as 2.5 percent during the last decade.

It is difficult to produce data on corruption but I believe that the rate of growth of corruption during the last five decades has been higher than the rate of growth of population! I believe that this is true of the whole country and not only of Haryana. Does this not make the young generation feel doomed? If you cannot bribe, you cannot get a job was the refrain of all the young people I talked to during my field visit. It does not follow, however, that if the rate of population growth comes down, the level of corruption will also come down. Take, for example, Kerala, where the rate of population growth is low; in fact, the total fertility rate is below replacement level but corruption is on the increase in Kerala. You cannot blame population growth *per se* in explaining the sharp increase in the level of corruption all over India. If at all, the rate of population growth is slowing down. But, there is no doubt that relentless population growth over the decades has meant an increase in the size of the labour force. In the absence of commensurate employment opportunities, unemployment is increasing and new entrants to the labour are the most affected persons in the labour market. As already mentioned, globalization has added to their miseries and has very often meant discarding labour. In such a situation, corruption is inevitable.

A pathetic aspect of this scenario is parents with sons capitalizing the situation by marrying off their sons after taking a hefty dowry. Even if the young man is unemployed, he can get married merely because his family has some agricultural land. Then, there is the emerging phenomenon of bride burning and dowry deaths. As some of the village women argue that if girls are to be treated like this after marriage, it is better not to produce girls at all.

It would be wrong to assume that the women are always pushed by their husbands and in-laws to go for the ultrasound test and abortion of the female foetus. Most of the women themselves want to avoid having daughters at least in Haryana and Punjab. I recall the advertisements for pre-birth sex determination tests till the PNDT Act prohibiting such tests was passed. The message was: Save five lakh rupees in dowry and marriage of your daughter by paying just 500 rupees.

VHAI's Study in Punjab, Haryana and Himachal Pradesh

Subsequently, I was involved in a comprehensive study of female foeticide in the three worst states of India, namely, Punjab, Haryana and Himachal Pradesh, launched by the Voluntary Health Association of India (VHAI). The summary report titled *Darkness at Noon: Female Foeticide in India* (VHAI, 2003) prepared by Ashish Bose and Mira Shiva (2003: 44-45) says: "The intriguing question that faced us was: why the prosperous states like Punjab, Haryana and Himachal Pradesh have the highest incidence of female foeticide as inferred from the latest Census statistics? We took up in-depth field surveys in the three worst districts of these states to understand this phenomenon. We conducted perception surveys of doctors and panchayat members, focus group discussions and house to house surveys in nine villages in the three worst districts with the lowest child sex ratios. At the outset, we must note the following findings of a general nature:

- The force of son complex cuts across religion, caste, socio-economic groups and place of residence, and is strong in all the three states under study.
- It is increasing with the rise of consumerism propagated by commercial TV advertising, and the growing greed is reflected in higher and higher demands for dowry and the increasingly high cost of marriage.
- The spread of female foeticide has been facilitated by at least three factors, all of which are prevalent in Punjab, Haryana, Himachal Pradesh, namely, (i) access to medical technology (sex determination tests and abortion), (ii) capacity to pay for the test and abortion, and (iii) good transportation network

which enables women to travel to the nearest town and also the mobility of doctors who can reach villages with their equipment.

In short, female foeticide is the result of an unholy alliance between traditional preference for sons and modern medical technology, increasing greed of doctors, rising demand of dowry, making daughters a financial burden, the ineffectiveness of the PNDT Act and the liberal MTP Act and the lack of any serious involvement of civil society in fighting this social menace.

References

Agnihotri, Satish, Balram (2000). *Sex Ratio Patterns in the Indian Population: A Fresh Exploration.* New Delhi: Sage Publications.

— (2001). Rising sons and setting daughters: Provisional results of the 2001 census. In Mazumdar, Vina and Krishnaji, N. (Eds.), *Enduring Conundrum: India's Sex Ratio*. Centre for Women's Development Studies. Delhi: Rainbow Publishers.

Bose, Ashish (2001). *India's Billion Plus People, 2001 Census Highlights, Methodology and Media Coverage.* New Delhi: B.R. Publishing Corporation.

— (2001). Census of India 2001 and after. *Economic and Political Weekly*, May 19.

Bose, Ashish and Shiva Mira (2003). *Darkness at Noon: Female Foeticide in India*, Voluntary Health Association of India, New Delhi.

Census of India (2001). Paper No.1 of 2001, Registrar General and Census Commissioner, New Delhi.

— (2001). *Provisional Population Totals, Paper 1 of 2001 Supplement*, Registrar General and Census Commissioner, New Delhi.

Mazumdar, Vina and Krishnaji, N. (2001). *Enduring Conundrum: India's Sex Ratio*, Centre for Women's Development Studies. Delhi: Rainbow Publishers.

Planning Commission (2002). Human Development Report, 2001, New Delhi.

15

Future Status of Elderly in India

ABDUL MAJEED KHAN

The contemporary social, cultural, political and economic changes in the backdrop of globalization are resulting in more impersonal approach to life and relationships. A shift towards individuality from collectivity is becoming more apparent, as people are becoming more and more self-centric. The concern for others, a significant feature of Indian society, is decaying. This phenomenon is affecting family as a cohesive unit of society. In developing countries, like India, which are struggling with a population problem and having scarce resources, survival of the society hinges on the core social value of 'caring for others'. The elderly persons are gradually becoming appendage and burden on the family and are no longer remain integral members of the family. There is a breakdown of family system, structurally and functionally, and the support base for the elderly is eroding. It is anybody's guess what would be the status of an elderly in this consumer society where material values have replaced family values. How vulnerable would the elderly be in the face of the rapidly changing society? The emerging scenario of greater number of elderly people in the society will pose many serious political, administrative and environmental challenges. All these issues deserve detailed discussion. This article endeavours to deal with some of these issues.

Ancient literature in India is replete with eloquent references to the elderly. Long life was cherished, old age was viewed with respect, and the elderly used to play an important role of advisors and counsellors. The family and community looked after them regardless of their productive capacity. In the 21st century, however, all these positive values attached to the aged people and their care are changing both in rural and urban areas. Depleting emotional bondages in the new interaction pattern within the family, abysmal provision of health care facility for the aged persons, economic insecurity, growing scarcity of caregivers – all these hint that the modern Indian society is heading towards difficult times, as far as the care of elderly is concerned.

World Scenario of Elderly

In 1950, there were about 200 million persons aged 60 and above in the world (contributing 8.1%) of the total global population. By 2050, nine-fold increase (around 1.8 billion) of elderly, representing about 20 percent of the total population, is projected; at that time three-fourth of elderly will be in the developing countries. From 1999 to 2025, the elderly population in Asia will rise from 50 percent of the world elderly to 58 percent. In Africa and Latin America, the rise will be just 5 to 7 percent. In Europe, the figure will drop from 19 to 12 percent of world elderly. There would be about 604 million older women in the world by 2025: 70 percent of them are likely to be in developing countries, and bulk of them living in the rural poverty.

For the first time in human history. a majority of world's older persons would reside in Asia (53%), while the Europe will have the next largest share (25%). The percentage of older persons is currently higher in the developed region as compared to less developed region. But, the scenario is changing rapidly. In the developed countries, for example, France took 115 years for the proportion of older persons to rise from 7 to 14 percent, whereas in the countries like China, Brazil and Thailand, doubling is likely to occur in the next 20 years (Kalache, 1999). In 2000, there were 374 million people over 60 in developing countries; in 2030, there will be over a billion older people (Help Age International, 2002).

Therefore, issues such as economic, social and cultural, affecting the growing cohort of people, need to be researched, analyzed and taken into consideration (Powell and Leppard, 2002).

Indian Scenario

India has entered into an era of ageing society. As per the UN definition, the society is young if the percentage of 60+ is between 4 and 7 percent and ageing if it is above 7 percent (Surpal, 1999). The percentage of 60+ persons in the total population has been rising steadily rise from 5.1 percent in 1901 to 6.8 percent in 1991. It is expected to reach at 8.9 percent in 2016. The projection beyond 2016 made by the UN (1996 revision) has indicated that 21 percent of Indian population will be 60+ by 2050. One, out of seven elderly persons, would be from India by 2016. As per 1991 census, out of about 136 million, 52 million are 70+ (old age). Four of every five persons live in rural areas. Females outnumber males. According to 42nd round of National Sample Survey (NSS), 34 percent of rural elderly were financially independent as against 28.94 percent in urban areas. Ageing of the population in India is occurring at very fast pace, quicker than in the developed countries; and the number people above 60 years of age would swell to nearly 150 million in the next three decades.

The life expectancy at birth rose from 32.5 to 60 years for men (gain of 27.5 years) and from 31.7 to 61 years for women (gain of 29.3 years) between 1941 and 1993. Life expectancy is higher for elderly women as compared to elderly men. Between 1951 and 1960, the life expectancy was 42 years, and between 1986 and 1990, it reached to 58 years. As per 2001 census, it has reached to 66 for men and 67 for women. As per projections, between 2011 and 2016, the life expectancy would be 67 years (increase of nine years in 25 years, i.e., 1986-2016 period). And, by 2020-2025, the life expectancy for males would be 68.8 years and for females, 72.1 years.

Demographic Transition in India

The census data of 100 years in India reveal three stages of demographic transition. The first stage was till 1920, in which both birth rate and death rate were very high. The birth rate was 50.2

(1901), 49.2 (1911) and 48.1 (1921) whereas the death rate was 44.6 (1901) and 47.2 (1921). By that time, the total population of the country was 251 million. The second stage of demographic transition started immediately after 1920. The death rate declined sharply and reached at 19 per thousand by 1971. In comparison, the birth rate declined very slowly. By 1971, country's population reached at 439.2 million. In the third transition, the birth rate started declining from 1971 onward and by 2001, it reached at 23 per thousand and death rate at the low of 7.8 per thousand. According to Premi (1991), India will enter into the fourth stage of demographic transition by the year 2020.

Demographic transition in India has resulted in continuous increase in the population of elderly. It has increased from 24.7 million (1961) to 32.7 million in 1971 (25% increase during 1961-71). About 13.5 million increase was recorded during 1981-91. As per 1991 census, highest population of elderly was in Kerala (8.8%), followed by Himachal Pradesh (8.1%), Punjab (7.8%), Haryana (7.7%), Tamil Nadu (7.4%) and Goa (7%). In the remaining states, in 1991 the percentage of elderly was lower than the national figure (6.7%). The scenario of elderly women is not identical. While Kerala, Goa and Haryana have got largest population of elderly men, Punjab and Himachal Pradesh have reported highest population of elderly women. As per estimate, after 20 years from now, the proportion of elderly will increase in disproportional manner and the difference between men and women would become more glaring. Feminization of elderly phenomenon would be more visible by 2016 as elderly female population (9%) will surpass those of elderly men (8.8%) in most of the states. Changes in the fertility behaviours are affecting population under 15 years across different states. From the available trend, it is expected that Kerala and Tamil Nadu would be the first states, where population of elderly would exceed the child population. It is to be noted that 90 percent elderly come from unorganized sector (no social security at the age 60 years), 80 percent live in the urban areas and 40 percent are below poverty line, whereas 55 percent (19 million) of 60+ women are widows and 73 percent are illiterate (Helpage India, Annual Report, 1998-99).

According to the UN Secretary-General, Koffi Annan, "we need nothing less than a dramatic reorientation of attitudes and policies towards ageing". Rigid dismissal of the notions of 'age' and 'ageing' has no place in today's world. There is an emerging need to pay greater attention to ageing issues and promote holistic policy and programmes for dealing with the problems and challenges of an ageing society (*Population Headlines*, March-April 1999). In the 55th session of ESCAP, held in April 1999, representatives of governments (to which India is a partner) in the Asia and Pacific region unanimously adopted a report containing a number of resolutions, one of which called for the integration of older persons into the work of United Nations and national socio-economic programmes. It also urged all governments to pay attention to older persons in severe poverty and enable them to have access to basic health services.

Elderly represent a valuable national asset because of their experience and maturity. They have a good deal of spare time, which could be utilized for social service; and they can bring about significant changes in our country. Dr. Karan Singh (2001) has classified ageing into five categories: chronological age, physiological age, emotional age, psychological age and spiritual age. All these categories are inevitable. The lifestyle is changing fast with the breaking down of joint families, diminishing acceptance of family responsibilities towards elders, and leaving the aged often to fend for themselves.

The increase in the life expectancy and decline in fertility are two major pushing forces for phenomenal acceleration in the population of elderly and these phenomena is visible. But, unfortunately, the process to meet the basic needs, including health, social and psychological, cultural, religious and security needs, of the elderly in our country as against the developed countries has yet to take off. Our country is definitely a late starter for the health care of elderly (Bagchi, 2001); not even the Department of Gerontology has started except at one or two places. For health professionals, it is really a great challenge to design the services for elderly persons.

Recent Research Studies

The review of literature about ageing in our country highlights many special features. These features, however, are different and distinctive in nature if compared with the developed countries. For example, the pace of growth of elderly population has varied. In the developed countries, it has taken relatively a longer period for the present build-up of the elderly population. In the developing country like India, it has been much faster and posed an immediate challenge of the care of aged people. Rural-urban migration under various social and economic pressures is rampant. The situation appears grimmer when one notes that the dependency ratio is 1:2. The percentage of elderly under the poverty line is high, and 90 percent are not covered under any social security provisions or pension schemes. The data collected on economic dependence of rural elderly depict that 70.6 percent of rural aged females are fully dependent on others. The 1991 census survey report shows that life expectancy of women at 60 constitutes a larger group than that of men. As a result, there are a greater proportion of older women suffering from widowhood, economic hardship, functional impairment, disabilities and dependency on earning members (Chaudhary, 2001). The review highlights the following challenges:

Growing Scarcity of Caregivers

The scenario of caregivers is changing due to rapid migration of young population, leaving behind majority of older persons on the mercy of neighbours and culture of 'money order economy'. Changing roles and expectations of women, including privacy, career, ambition and employment outside home implies considerably reduced time for caregiving. Millions of older persons are left in the rural areas without essential care (Khan, 2001).

Constraints on Young Earners

In the urban areas, the younger generation is so much hard pressed into economic and space constraints that they are hardly able to live a good quality of life. With such constraints, how long and how much younger generation from the deprived section would retain their old age values of caring the elderly, the available literature does not speak about this.

Imbalance between Rural and Urban

The major load is shifting from rural to urban areas. The percentage of population in rural areas is declining since 1950 (82.75%). It is expected to come closer to 46.40 percent in 2025. During the same period, urban population would move up from 17.25 percent (1950) to 53.6 percent (2025). Whether the urban load would maintain essential health facilities to keep its balance, or would it tilt towards catastrophic situation, is hard to predict. Country will have literary elders more than illiterate elders in coming years and more women than men. So ignoring their needs would be more difficult than today?

Scarcity of Space and Needs

Today, those migrated in the larger cities years back and settled down in the urban slum areas have become elderly. The limited space in the house and increased number of family members over the decades basically have given a genesis of new need pattern (NNP) amongst the aged.

The list of needs, however, could be exhaustive and broadly classified into six categories. These are: nutrition needs, psychological needs, social needs, needs of special groups, economic needs, health needs, safety and security needs and spiritual needs. Under each category, there is a long list of needs to be taken up for the care of elderly population. In addition to these classified needs, the perception of elderly regarding their contribution to the society, living arrangement, family life, programmes, and expectations from the family, society and government and the life preparatory measures are also vital reflection of needs. The other needs, as identified by Chaudhary (1992), are: protection against outliving and saving; protection against being financially devastated by medical and other emergency; protection against inflation, development and maintenance of social support network; provision of opportunities for increased productive activity in a variety of ways; provision of opportunities for social and economic interaction in community control over some indoor and outdoor activities; and protection against illness and being physically assaulted. The empirical data on these issues are not available.

Case studies of older persons residing in old age homes also furnish a set of other needs. These are: need for security, counselling needs, need for consultation with specialist, need for attendant, physical aids, need for recreation, participation in cultural events, interaction inside and outside home, participation in religions activities outside home, desire for contribution to society, need to get respect, recognition, social support, and awareness about saving schemes (Sur and Khan, 2001). The healthy ageing depends a lot on nutrition care. Whether quantity and frequency of eating across different groups of older persons is same or different is also a matter of serious concern as far as nutritional care of elderly is concerned. Ghokhle (2001) remarked while calculating poverty and ageing on the consumption of 2,200-2,400 calories that we generally forget that the level of consumption changes according to the age, gender and location.

Study by Rajan, Misra and Sharma (2001) revealed that only 6.5 percent elderly (60-69 years) rated themselves unhealthy, whereas 70.6 percent fairly alright and 18.6 percent unhealthy. The self-rating, however, need to be linked with commonly found health problems reported by older persons. The study by Khan and Hussain (2001) disclosed that elderly are heavy consumers of drugs. What are these drugs? Who are they? Whether they are those who report themselves as healthy or those who report themselves unhealthy. Such picture, however, is not clear from this study.

Physical Health Problems

From morbidity viewpoint, almost 50 percent of Indian elderly suffer from chronic diseases and 5 percent from immobility. Infections take a heavy toll of elderly population apart from well-known degeneration disorder. Five County Study on elderly indicates that arthritis, high blood pressure, foot problem, heart disease and stomach ulcers are five most common elderly illnesses along with visual and hearing impairment.

The clinical profile reveals disease conditions like opthalmological, orthopaedic, cardiovascular, neurological, urogenital, gastrointestinal, metabolic, hormonal or psychiatric disorders like depression, paraphernalia, dementias, menopausal syndrome in women, and anatropous or low testosterone syndrome in males (Rao, 1999). Major health problems of ageing are associated with disability and degenerative diseases such as cataract, hearing loss, malignancies and atherosclerosis (Shah, 1999). Deterioration in vision and hearing loss along with slowness of reflexes and responses among the aged persons expose them to the risk of bone and joint injuries (Srivastava, 1999). Prostate is the most commonly diseased organ in the ageing male population (Sharma, 1999). Cancer is emerging as one of the leading causes of mortality in elderly patients, following by cardiovascular and cerebrovacular diseases (Coshic, 1999). Cardiorespiratory diseases are significant causes of morbidity and mortality in Indian society (Dye, 1999). A community-based study in South India revealed that cardiovascular and respiratory diseases were diagnosed in 17.49 percent and 16.1 percent cases respectively. Among them, 5 percent had hypertension and 4 percent COAD. An AIIMS' study revealed hypertension (40%), IHD (19%), COAD (20%) and tuberculosis (3%). In a meta-analysis of 34 Indian studies, hypertension ranged between 0.36 percent and 30.9 percent in subjects above 60 years, and between 0.52 percent and 9 percent in subjects below 60 years, showing an increasing trend. The most common health problems found are ophthalmic (48.8%), respiratory (29.5%) and musculoskeletal morbidities (10.2%). The most common chronic illnesses/symptoms reported in an NSS report are: joint pain, followed by cough, heart disease, hypertension, diabetes and physical immobility (NSS Report, 1986). ICMR Madurai study (1999) found visual handicap (65%), pain in joints (34%), vague body pain (15%), giddiness (15%), cough (10%) and sleeplessness (8%) as most prevalent problems. In India, around 4 million people who age 60 years and above are said to be suffering from mental illness, two-fifth of them are diagnosed as depressed. Health problems reported by the majority of the studies are joint pain (35%), cough (22%), visual handicapped (65%), vague body pain (15%) and giddiness (15%). Population of elderly persons with chronic illness rose from 38 percent in the 60+ group to 45 percent in 65+ group and 54 percent in the 70+ group.

Psychological Problems and Emotional Needs

Elderly men scored significantly higher on domestic anxiety, psychic anxiety, muscular tension and suspicion (Rathore and Saroj, 1991). Impaired cognitive function, poor subjective well-being and poor adjustment are all associated with negative self-concept (Patel, 1992; Natrajan *et al.*, 1992). On hopelessness, alienation and life dissatisfaction (known as psychological health) males were found better than females (Chadha *et al.*, 1995). Lower mental efficiency, reduced and general orientation and memory information are found lower in aged as compared to young. Kohli *et al.* (1992) report more score on depression in aged persons. Decline of psycholinguistics-social interaction and self-related flexibility were found significantly lower in old age group (Sharma *et al.*, 1992). Dissatisfaction with their segregated life in old age was found in the sample of elderly people in the old age houses (Misra, 1993). Positive self-regard, satisfaction with role activity, satisfaction in husband-wife relationship and subjective assessment of general health were found to be significant determinants of successful ageing (Jamuna, 1992). Cluster of psychiatric problems continuously accelerates across the age (Kanwar, *et al.*, 1995). Loneliness and hopelessness are prevalent in elderly persons (Sinha, 1999). Elderly perceived their spouses as caretakers during their own illness whereas sons and daughters-in-laws were perceived as caretaker of the elderly during illness in other households. Elderly believed that their status declined because of dependency. More positive status was found among Jat elderly (Mangal, 1994; Bhingradiya *et al.*, 1991). Aged persons do not indulge into sports and physical activities (Jaiprakash, 1999). Abuses to elderly in home for aged was reported by Ushasree *et al.* (1999). Elderly felt relieved out of perception of supportive environment. Geriatric medicine is directed to mental morbidity, psychiatric disorder and physical disorder. Morbidity is affected by a large number of factors. Higher positive effect and hopelessness and ability to maintain functional competence are reduced, and availability of social support network is reduced (Bali, 1997). Reaction in intra-aggressive direction and of ego-defensive type increased with age. (Ushasree *et al.*, 1999). Psychological distress was reported by Shirolkar and Jaiprakash (1996). Apprehension, depressive trends and tendency to underestimate them are reported by Pareek (2000). Senior women perceive their time not as something they can actively structure in ways that fulfil the classified definition of leisure. They structure the time to their in and out the household. The study revealed that pensioners faced major problems regarding health, leisure, accommodation and adjustment with family. Non-pensioners faced problems regarding finance, family and feeling of isolation. Married people experienced problems regarding health, social and family condition, leisure and fear of death, while widowers faced problems regarding finance in security adjustment and feeling of isolation (Jaiprakash, 1999; Malhotra and Chadha, 1996). Four types of problems in Indian elderly were reported by Reddy (1994). These are: income insecurity, health care insecurity, physical insecurity and emotional insecurity.

According to Ramamurti (2001), the problems of rural and urban elderly vary considerably. He observed that in the past the elderly (those in the Vanaprastha and Sanyasa Ashramas) were greatly respected for their wisdom and kept with a great care in the family fold. It is unfortunate that as a result of western influence they are becoming increasingly marginalized in our society today. What sort of economic planning for old age care is carried out by elderly is most essential to develop future plan of action. It is equally important to explore the status of elderly in the organized sector. What sort of planning elderly did for housing, education, marriage and settlement of their children? And, what sort of suggestions come from elderly for younger people? These are pertinent questions for research.

Quite often, it so happens that in the organized sector, people at the fag-end of service become tensed, and most of the pension money is lost within a few years and their subsequent life becomes vulnerable. The problem in the care of elderly runs across all the social and cultural groups, possibly in the different colours. The empirical studies are needed in this area. Which socio-economic classes of elderly are relatively more satisfied is also a matter of research.

The choice of living arrangement has many implications for the well-being of an older person. Changes in living arrangement are likely to be associated with changes in the level of care and assistance received. Living together with other family members eases situations of illness while living alone makes coping with illness harder. Under such circumstances, what kinds of living arrangement are preferred by the elderly across rural, urban, upper, lower and different cultural groups? According to Ilango (2001), 7.3 percent in rural areas and 50-54 percent in urban areas live alone outside home in the old age. The study, however, does not reveal the difference that exists between slum-dweller, middle-class and upper-class. Therefore, the picture of urban elderly has yet be ascertained. A study conducted by Chaudhary (2001) revealed that elderly face significant economic, social and health problems, particularly women in Himalayan areas lead a poor quality of life – physiologically, psychologically and socio-economically.

Most of these reported studies, however, have small samples and cannot depict the real picture of old age across different social and cultural groups in rural, urban and slum backgrounds. The studies also do not show how elderly people treat the elderly and what sort of economic planning should we have to meet their health care needs in view of changing family circumstances, and rapid migration, constraints of caregivers. There is not sufficient literature regarding what elderly people think regarding old age planning, living arrangement, economic independence? What do they expect from the government for their health care? The views of elders from different social and cultural groups are extremely essential for scientific old age planning.

Government's Mindset

Effective planning for the qualitative care of elderly has yet to take off. So far, almost all the medical colleges producing human resource for catering the health needs of people have not started departments of geriatric; so is the status of gerontology in medical colleges. People working in the area of health in different roles have hardly developed any mindset for the care of elderly. The worldwide literature reveals that science of geriatric and gerontology has grown up in the developed countries, where the population of elderly had reached to the significant level much earlier. A growing population of elderly people is hardly a concern in planning under medical model of health care.

The institutions at national and international levels, engaged in public health planning and human resource development for the health service providers also have not developed proper mindset about the care of elderly. A huge human resource, catering health and family welfare services under primary health care approach, has yet to start thinking about knowledge and learning for the purpose of providing qualitative health care to the elderly. In all, the health service planners, professionals and providers have hardly started thinking for the growing section of society, i.e., elderly, whose number is likely to cross the number of children by 2025. Possibly out of international commitment in the International Year of Old Age People in 1999, the Government of India has come with a National Policy for Older Persons in the same year. More than five years have gone and no follow-up measures have been taken.

Here, a critical evaluation of national policy for older persons is made.

Commitments under National Policy for Older Persons, 1999

Policy Commitments	*Existing Status*
Long-term Management of Illness at Home and Nursing Care (Chronic Cases)	
• Good affordable health services	• It has yet to be created.
• Heavily subsidised for poor	• Picture is not clear.
• Graded system of users charges for others	• Picture is not clear.
• Judicious mix of public health services	• It needs elaboration.
Development Health Insurance	
• Health services by non-profit organizations	• Started here and there.
• Encouraging trust, charitable society and voluntary agencies, means and grants	• Government has encouraged trust and charitable society by providing free of cost land for hospital. But these hospitals primarily catering the need of elite group and middle class people.

Contd...

Policy Commitments	Existing Status
• Private medical care facilities + tax relief + land on subsidies, medicines, treatment to poor	• Coming up.
• Involvement of private general practitioners - reasonable user change	• Not clear at the moment. Directions and guidelines are yet to be developed.
• Elderly persons are not subjected to large wait and visit to different countries for medical test and treatment	• In the hospital at some places separate queue of elderly is created. But services are not designed as par needs of the elderly.
• Private hospitals 100 bedded directed for the above	• Provisions yet to be made.
• Training to medical and para-medical personnel in primary health care	• Has yet to take a shape in case of para-medical. In case of medical, only Professor of medicines is getting orientation at AIMS.
• Secondary and tertiary health cares facilities in health care of the elderly	• Not even a debate and discussion started. We need first of all to ascertain the profile of health needs of old people.
• Facilities for specialization in geriatric medicine in medical colleges including geriatric care in the training of nursing care, problems of accessibility	• Geriatric care has yet get into on going nursing training and medical orientation.
Problem Regarding	
• Use of health services by the elderly due to distance/absence of escorts and transportation	• It is a matter of research, survey.
Mobile Health Services	
• Special camps and ambulance service	• Organized by Helpage India and other NGOs.
• Welfare fund within hospital for free treatment and medicine to poor elderly patients	• Organization has to take up initiative for such fund.
• Assistance to geriatric care societies for IEC matter on self-care, material for family care given	• Some NGOs have been given grant-in-aid project.
• Educational material on nutritional need to elders	• Some NGO bring out small leaflet and distribute among people.
• Health education programmes counselling facilities to community	• It is most urgent needed. Government has not done anything so far.
• Training of personnel for nutrition geriatric	• Nothing so far has been done.

Contd...

Policy Commitments	*Existing Status*
Shelter	
• 10% allotment of house/house site to older person under housing scheme for urban and rural lower income sequent (Indira Awas Yojna and others)	• Somewhat it is being implemented.
• Motivating earning persons to invest in housing during earning days	• No organised efforts are being done.
• Respond to the lifestyle of elderly under layout of housing colonies	• Has yet to get some shape.
• Multipurpose centre for older person in colonies, earmarking site for such centres in all housing colonies	• It has not been undertaken so far.
• Common service facilities for meals, laundry, common and rest room	• Part of Old Age Home – Strategies are poor as per evaluation. A nominal number of OAH has been established.
Education	
• Continuing educational programme incorporating material under formal and non-formal education to	• Has yet to be initiated in the existing system of education.
• Strengthen intergenerational bonds mutually supporting relationship	• Action plan on this is not developed.
• Interaction with children, young persons in the school	• Some action plan has yet to come.
• Education about ageing process	• Education mindset has to be developed.
Protection of Life and Property	
• Widow's rights of inheritance, occupancy and disposal	• Effort is on.
• Special provision in IPC to protect older persons from domestic violence	• Effort is on.
• Tenancy legislation	• Under process.
• Assistance to voluntary organizations and associations of older persons	• It is done.
• Police protection	• How many older persons could be given protection.
Non-Governmental Organizations	
• Due recognition to NGO	• A few NGOs are working in this area. However, Senior Citizen Association is gradually increasing.

Contd...

Policy Commitments	Existing Status
• Continuous dialogue and communication with NGO	• Yes – Advocacy by NGO and associates of senior citizens have started dialogue in AP and Maharashtra.
• Networking, exchange of information and interactions among NGOs	• Number of Senior Citizen Association has started networking on their own. Government support for such networking has yet to come to level of recognition.
• Grant-in-aid policy	• On a very small scale, it is being implemented.
• Involvement of trust, charities, religious and other endowments	• Gradually involvement is increasing.
• Setting of volunteer programmes for older persons	• This has to yet to take-off.
• Volunteers orientation training about care of elders	• National Institute of Social Defence has started 6-months certificate and one-year diploma courses.
Welfare	
• Trust toward vulnerable such as poor, disabled, infirm, chronically sick and those without family support	• Part of value education, no concrete scheme for it.
• Nutritional schemes by voluntary organizations	• May be, some NGOs are working.
• Grant-in-aid for construction and maintenance of old age home	• Some work is going on.
• Poor will be having subsided services	• Some work is going on.
• Welfare funds for older persons	• Yes, it has come into existence.
Other Areas of Action	
• Issue of identity cards	• Effort is on.
• Fair concessions in all modes of travel	• Effort is on.
• Preference in reservation of seats	• Effort is on.
• Earmarking of seats in local public transport	• Effort is on.
• Modifications in designs of public transport vehicles for easy entry and exit	• No such efforts are visible.
• Strict enforcement of traffic disciplining at zebra crossing to facilitate older persons to cross streets	• Effort is on.
• Priority in gas and telephone connections and in fault repairs	• Effort is on.

Contd...

Policy Commitments	*Existing Status*
• Concessions in entrance fees in entertainment facilities	• Effort is on.
• Speedy disposal of complaints	• Matter of research, survey.
• National Older Person's Day	• It is celebrated.
• National Year for Older Persons (year 2000)	• It is celebrated.
• Regular updating and compilation of facilities, concessions and relief given to older persons	• Matter of research, no comment could be recorded.
Family	
• Family support system	• Decay of support is increasing. The Government does nothing to retain old values.
• Promoting family values	• Thinking of some section has yet to start.
• Providing tax relief and rebates for medical expenses, incurred by children for their parents	• Has yet to be started.
• Short-term stayin facilities for older persons	• Day Care Centres scheme is being implemented.
• Counselling services	• Scheme has yet to be worked out.
Research	
• Centres for Gerontological Studies and Geriatrics	• Some NGOs, academic and service institutions have come out of its own.
• Funding supports to academic bodies for research project on ageing	• Provision is there.
• Interdisciplinary coordinating body on research	• Does not exist.
• Professional associations of gerontologists	• Yes
• National Institute of research, training and documentation	• Has yet to be planned and developed.
Training of Manpower	
• Specialization in geriatrics in medical colleges	• Has not started anywhere.
• Training for nurses and paramedics	• Process has started here and there.

Contd...

Policy Commitments	*Existing Status*
• Orientation courses on geriatric care	• It is available to only Professor of medicines.
• Sensitization programmes on ageing for legislative judicial and executive wings at different levels	• Need to be initiated.
Media	
• Important role to play by media in highlighting the changing situation of older person	• Media is also not highlighting the issue of old age.
• Identifying emerging issues and areas of action	• Some Professional Organizations, NGOs have started working.
• Creative use of media for promoting the concept of active aging and strengthening inter-generation bonds	• It is being debated here and there.
Implementation	
• Wide dissemination of national policy on older persons and preparation of an action	• Policy has not been disseminated. Action plan has been prepared.
• Collaborative action by apex level organizations of older persons	• Apex level organization has to be fully developed.
• Ministry of Social Justice and Empowerment will be nodal ministry to coordinate all matters relating to the implementation of the policy	• Ministry is nodal – it has started some initiatives.
• Creation of a separate bureau of older persons	• Has not been created.
• An inter-ministerial committee will coordinate matter relating to implementation and monitor its progress	• Implementation of various policy commitments has yet to start.
• Formation of separate directorates of older persons in this state for coordination and monitoring	• It is only commitment in the policy.
• Five year for annual plans by each ministry	• Annual planners need orientation and sensitization towards older persons.
• Budgetary provisions by Planning Commission and Finance Ministry	• -
• Detailed reviews by nodal ministry, states governments after every three years	• It can be done only when some of the policy commitment is converted in scheme and action.

Old Age Schemes

Under the Ministry of Social Justice and Empowerment, Government of India the old age homes started a long back. However, the number of old age homes up to 1970 were very nominal. After 1970, the number started increasing. More recently, has increased considerably particularly in the southern Indian states, possibly due to fast growing percentage of aged people in these states. For example, the percentage of elderly persons in the state of Kerala is highest and the similar trend is evident in the states of Tamil Nadu, Maharashtra and Karnataka.

The day care centres for old people have been further added as one more service possibly with a view to enhance of avenue of services and their accessibility to more people. In a country like India, where the population has already reached 1.27 billion, more than 80 million people fall in the category of old age. The services under the umbrella of day care and old age homes are just a drop in the ocean. At various forums, it is recognized that regardless of the quality required to be provided through the old age homes and day care centres, in the present era of privatization where government's concerns and commitments for the welfare of vulnerable sections of societies are continuously declining, the infrastructure for large sections of people cannot be created and, therefore, family has to remain as a best institution for the care of elderly. The challenge before the planners is how the traditional and moral obligations of family members towards elderly are to be safeguarded from the contemporary consumeristic forces that are strengthening self-centric behaviours in the society.

Thrust on Self, Family and Institution

The planners need to realize that the responsibility for providing qualitative care to the large sections of elderly cannot be left on the shoulders of family only. Care of the elderly is much affected by the structural and functional changes that are taking place in the family system. A large section of family earners are migrating and leaving their parents as well as places of birth. The migration is not only a rural-to-urban phenomenon, it is also taking place from urban-to-urban areas in search of relatively better avenues for the life. Therefore, in both the rural and urban areas, the aged parents are left to lead a vulnerable life of their own. Unlike other age groups, the aged person's care needs cannot be fulfilled by the remote control method because the aged people, like children, need physical presence of caregivers. Since phenomenon of migration cannot be reversed back, therefore, considering family as an institution for providing the quality care of elderly would prove misnomer in the future for a larger section. In these circumstances, the old age planning needs to be visualized completely different from what we are generally talking about. Every young person from the early stage of life needs to be given proper education in scientific planning for future. Economic sufficiency, sustainability and ability of buying qualitative care are the key concepts. Institutions for healthy planning for future have yet to grow in this country.

Old age planning is of great importance; and a lot of scientific and empirical literature has to be developed in order to reach to the point where the country starts advocating the concept of old age planning from the individual's point of view. Regardless of economic status, people from all class need institutional support in case their caregivers have migrated and settled elsewhere and failed to provide required support. The nature of support cannot be the same for all the sections of the society. For example, those who are economically well-off, they expect services of well-trained caregivers. But, where are the institutions to create and develop caregivers as human resource? Which institutions are venturing to start the training programme? What should be reasonable cost to shoulder the responsibility of a caregiver? What has to be done for those who are economically poor and not able to bear the cost of caregivers, or whose children have migrated to cities and are hardly able to meet out their own requirements and essential needs? The percentage of such categories of persons is increasing. Such people definitely need institutional support of the government. A large section of society is already living sub-standard life and going through the scarcity of resources throughout their life. However, they have been earning whatsoever minimum resources are available. But, whenever their bodies negate physical labour, and they start the life of vulnerability during the old age, what sort of services government need to plan? Whether the government alone can fulfil the requirement of such a large section? Or, the people need to be educated for successful old age planning. These challenges demand urgent deliberations.

References

Bali, A. (1997). Socio-economic status and its relationship to morbidity. *Indian Journal of Medical Research*, *106*, 349-306.

Bhingradiya, P. and Kamala, R. (1997). An inter-generational study on the situation of the elderly in rural Saurastra, *UG, 11* (3&4), 78-84

Bagchi, K. (1998). Some important areas of gerontological research in India, Helpage India. *Research and Development Journal, 4*, 10-15.

Chaudhary, Abha (2001). Producing ageing: A step towards socio-economic empowerment of rural elderly women in Himalayan Areas. In I. Jaiprakash (Ed.), *Ageing the Indian Experience.* Bangalore: Globe Folders.

Chadha, N.K. and Willigen, John Van (1995). The life scale: The development of a measures of successful ageing. *Indian Journal of Gerontology, 9*, 83-90.

Chaudhary, D. Paul (1992). *Ageing and the Aged.* New Delhi: Inter-India Publications.

Coshic, O. (1999). *Cancer in the Elderly Patient.* Workshop Report, NCD, ICMR, New Delhi.

Census of India (1991). Ministry of Home Affairs, Government of India, New Delhi.

Dey, A.B. (1999). A perspective of cardio-respiratory disorders in elderly Indian. Helpage India, *Annual Report* (1998-1999), New Delhi.

Government of India (1999) *National Policy for Older Persons.* Ministry of Social Justice and Empowerment, Government of India.

Gokhale, S.D. (1992). Towards a productive and participatory ageing in India. *Caring*, 5, 86-89.

Helpage India (2000). *Senior Citizens Guide.* Helpage International, New Delhi.

Helpage International (2002). *Status of World's Older People*, Helpage International, London.

Jaiprakash, Indira (2001). The ageing: The Indian experience. Report of the workshop organized on 9-10th August, Bangalore University.

— (1999). Seminar women's perception of leisure in India. *Bombay Psychologist, 24* (11), 82-85.

Jamuna, D. (1998). Challenges of changing socio-economic and psychological status of the Aged. *Help Age India Research and Development Journal, 5* No.1.

— (1992). Caring for the disabled elderly: Problems and perspectives. In S.K. Chaudhry (Ed.), *Problems of the Aged and of Old Age Homes*. Mumbai: Akshar Pratiroop.

Kalache, A. (1997). Active ageing makes the difference. *WHO Bulletin*, 77 (4).

Kanwar, Priya and Chadha, N.K. (1997). Retirement and ageing: Leisure activities and health ailments. *Indian Journal of Gerontology, 11* (1&2), 28-35.

Khan, A.M. (2001). *Health Care of Elderly*. Workshop Report, NIHFW, New Delhi.

Khan, Ghazala and Akbar Hussain. (2001). Sex differences in psycho-physical effects of psycho-tropic drugs among elderly. *Indian Journal Gerontology* (Special Issue), *15*, No.384, 381-384.

Kohli, A. (1992). Mental efficiency in elderly depressives. *Indian Journal of Gerontology, 6* (3&4), 93-97.

Malhotra, Renu and Chadha, N.K. (1996). Family relations of the elderly after retirement and widowhood. *Indian Journal of Gerontology, 10* (1&4), 30-50.

Mandal, M. (1998). The work of the NGO's for older person. *Research and Development Journal, 5* (1), 22-37.

Mangal, A.P. (1994). Changing status of the elderly in rural India. *Journal of Gerontology, 8* (3&4), 73-81.

Misra, S. (1993). Scenario of segregated seniors. *Indian Journal of Gerontology, 7*, 104-110.

Mishra, U.S. (1999). Health implications of ageing. *Medico Friend Circle Bulletin*, November-December. 2666-267.

Nandan, Deoki (1999). *An Overview of Geriatric Problems and Identifying the Research and Health Care Priorities*. Workshop Report, NCD, ICMR, New Delhi.

Natrajan, V.S. (1997). Common geriatric problems research and development. *Journal of Gerontology, 3(2)*, 3-11.

Paintal, H.K. (1992). Self-concept and successful ageing in medical men. *Indian Journal of Gerontology, 6* (3&4), 61-75.

Population Headlines (1999). UNFPA funded Newsletter March-April, United Nations Building, Rajadamnern NOK Avenue, Bangkok.

Parikh, D.R. (2000). The psyche of Indian middle-aged women. *Bombay Psychologist, 17* (1&2).

Patel, H.N. (1997). Mental problem of ageing and care of them by their family. *Research and Development Journal, 4*(1), 27-30.

Premi, M.K. (1991). *India's Population: Heading Towards a Billion*. New Delhi: B.R. Publishing Corporation.

Rajan, S., Mishra, I. and Sharma, U.S. (1999). *India's Elderly: Burden or Challenge*. New Delhi: Sage Publications.

Ruthpowell, S. and Leppard, M. (2002). *Ageing in Developing Countries: With Reference to Bangladesh, Malawi and Naizeria*. Centre for International Studies, Edinburgh, UK.

Ramamurti, P.V. (2001). Institutionalization of elderly and quality of life. *Indian Journal of Gerontology, 15*(3&4).

Rathore, S. (1991). A comparative study of problems in old age and middle-aged men. *Indian Journal of Gerontology, 5* (3&4), 92-101.

Reddy, K.N. (1994). Social security for the elderly in India: Need for reform. *Research and Development Journal, I (I)*, 8-22.

Registrar General of India (1996). *Population Projections for India: A Status Report of Technical Group on Population Projection*, RGI, New Delhi.

Sur, S. and Khan, A.M. (2000). *Perceptions of Elderly People About the Care of Their Needs: A Case Study*. Diploma Dissertation, New Delhi, NIHFW.

Sharma, R.C., Bansal, A. and Bhatt, S.C. (1992). Language loss in ageing. *Indian Journal of Gerontology, 6* (3&4), 98-105.

Sharma, K.L. (1999). Elderly women of kachi basti: A socio-psychological profile. *Indian Journal of Gerontology, 13* (1&2), 40-57.

Shah, Bela (1999). *Morbidity, Mortality and Disability in Old Age*. Workshop Report, NCD, ICMR, New Delhi.

Shirolkar, R.A. and Jaiprakash, Indira (1996). Interaction of age, sex and geographical variables in psychological distress. *Indian Journal of Clinical Psychology, 23* (1), 24-28.

Sinha, J.N. (1999). *The Pharmacokinectic Problems in Elderly: An Overview*. Workshop Report, NCD, ICMR, New Delhi.

Srivastava, R.K. (1999). *Spectrum of Orthopedic Conditions and Rehabilitation Needs Amongst the Aged*. Workshop Report, NCD, ICMR, New Delhi.

Ushasree, S. and Bdasha, S. Azmal (1999). Domestic abuse among the elderly. *Indian Journal of Gerontology, 13* (3&4), 99-104.

United Nations (1998). *The State of World's Population 1998: The New Generations*. New York: United Nations Population Fund.

16

Influence of Community Living and Environmental Stressors on Health and Well-being: A Study

DINESH NAGAR AND ASHUTOSH SHARMA

A striking factor of the urbanization process in India is the growth of metropolitan cities. The pace of urbanization has been increasing rapidly. In 1971, the urban population in India was 109 million (19.9% of the total population), and by 1991, it has increased to 217 million (25.72% of the total population). In a majority of cases the population increase in inner city areas is evident, as these areas accommodate a large number of residents, apart from being a representative hub of myriad activities, including commercial, religious and industrial. The present study was carried out in Bhopal, the capital city of the state of Madhya Pradesh. The city has undergone unusual changes in terms of social and physical transformations. Initially, in year 1856, the area was planned for only 37,539 people with a prominent mosque as the focal point and most of the roads emerging from it. The demographical profile indicates that the population of inner city areas of Bhopal, as reported in 1991 census, has touched 1.72 lakh (Sharma, 1996). To accommodate the increased population in many areas of the inner city, multi-storied buildings are on increase, thus, putting considerable pressure on the existing infrastructure. With narrow pedestrian lanes, congestion, inadequate sewage and drainage system and very few open spaces, the residential areas located in the vicinity of the inner city area are unable to provide adequate infrastructure to the increased population. Furthermore, with the increase in the population, a commensurate deterioration of environmental quality is evident. It is also observed that relative to population statistics of 1941, the population figures of 1991 reveal that Hindus and Muslims are more or less evenly distributed in most of the residential areas of Bhopal. Within this backdrop, a study was undertaken to examine how two major communities (Hindu and Muslim) living in the inner city for a prolonged period of time respond to environmental stressors (density and varied environmental quality) embedded in their primary and secondary environment and what are its social, psychological and health-related consequences.

A considerable literature on environment and behaviour referring to housing environment has focused on several demographic variables, specially housing for the single parents and their children (Anthony, Weidemann and Chin, 1990), the elderly (Lawton, 1975; Carstens, 1985) and the disabled (Anderson *et al.*, 1988). Attitudes on housing have been studied in settings ranging from single-family dwellings, apartments, high-rise developments, dormitories, prisons and mobile home parks (Dillman, Tremblay and Dillman, 1979; Newman, 1972; Rainwater, 1970; Shaly, 1985; Paulus, Nagar and Camacho, 1991). In addition, the literature on the dimensions of the housing environment is described in terms of social relationship (Gans, 1967; Nagar, 1985), physical structure (Greenfield and Lewis, 1969), management (Ahlbrandt and Brophy, 1976), ecological quality (Paulus *et al.*, 1991), crowding (Ajin, 1987; Nagar, 1998; Baum and Paulus, 1987) and residential satisfaction and health (Amerigo and Aragones, 1997; Paulus *et al.*, Nagar 1996).

Studies on residential satisfaction have noted that housing is not simply a structure with associated tenure characteristics. It also consists of external-to-house components. Housing comprises a bunch of features with extended boundaries ranging from neighbourhood characteristics, access to local amenities (e.g., shopping, school, hospital, workplace, religious places), density and size of the place, as well as ecological quality. Granted the fact that both crowding and ecological quality of the neighbourhood are stressors, the question arises why people are residing in such places for a prolonged period of time? Evidence exists that various factors may contribute to resident's choice of living in areas where the surrounding environment is stress provoking (e.g., crowding, poor ecological quality, pollution). These factors may be related to social network, place, dependence security, financial security, religion, access to facilities, and so forth. Apart from daily household routine, interaction with other people in the home was found to be an important determinant of the definition of home. Thus, it seems that people need to get out of their homes to appreciate the taken-for-granted order of life. People also need to be away to recognize that interaction with friends and neighbours is an important part of home life. Neighbours have an inescapable interdependence emanating from common local concerns, such as house, values, safety and status (Downs, 1981). There is some evidence that specific groups of people are more dependent upon local place than others. One could expect dependence upon local place to be stronger for groups which share some constraint upon their physical mobility. Evidence from other kind of ethnic areas suggests that personal network communities have corresponded with local place (Gans, 1967; Stuttles, 1976). A strong sense of community has measurable consequences for the larger life experiences. It seems that the communities are able to offer many religious facilities, shops and services which provide employment, reinforce ethnic values and constitute a framework for the traditional way of life.

The two factors that seem to be inseparably interlocked in the housing environment are crowding and environmental quality of the surrounding. Both these factors are related to residential satisfaction, feeling and health. Research studies on experiences and consequences of crowding have grown in voluminous proportion and comprehensive reviews are available in the literature (Baum and Paulus, 1987; Jain, 1987; Nagar, 1999). The review of studies conducted in a range of residential settings reveals inconsistent results regarding effects of crowding and thus any generalized conclusions cannot be drawn. However, a large number of studies have reported that crowding is a stressor and is correlated in some way or the other with health-related problems, negative mood states and psychopathological symptoms (Ruback and Pandey, 1991; Nagar, 1985; Gove, Hudges and Galle, 1979). Similarly, some studies have noted that the adverse effects of crowding are mitigated by social support, tolerance and coping (Jain, 1987; Nagar, 1998). For instance, Jain (1987) found competition tolerance as a mediator of density and its motivational and affective consequences. Furthermore, competition tolerance and social support mediate the effects of density on life stress and withdrawal. Whereas, perceived control seems to be a mediator only for withdrawal (Jain, 1987). Finally, supportive climate was found to mediate the adverse effects of density and psychosocial adjustment in the home environment.

A number of studies have indicated that the objective features of the environmental quality do influence housing satisfaction (Christensen *et al.*, 1992; Galster, 1987). It seems plausible to expect that low-quality housing may be stress inducing and should probably be related to mental and physical well-being (Christensen *et al.*, 1992; Kasl, 1974; Caspi, Bolger and Eckenrode, 1987). However, the study on army families conducted by Paulus *et al.* (1996) reported that high-quality housing was associated with positive rating of house but not with more favourable morale, harmony, health and well-being. Studies with older populations have found that they are reasonably satisfied with housing that appears deficient by objective criteria (degree of maintenance, basic plumbing, heating and electrical features (Christensen *et al.*, 1992). A study on young army families also indicated that environments that differed in observed quality did not yield large differences in residential satisfaction (Paulus *et al.*, 1991). Mobile homes and apartments were rated differently along several dimensions such as noise and attractiveness but no differences were obtained on overall housing satisfaction. However, housing that was of overall low quality was rated significantly more negatively relative to high-quality housing.

In summary, the overall objectives of this study were to examine:

(a) how residents belonging to different community groups respond to different aspects of their primary and secondary environment and how they differ on various dependent and outcome measures related to social support, tolerance, residential satisfaction, health and well-being;
(b) the effects of density and environmental quality on dependent and outcome measures related to support, tolerance, health, residential satisfaction and well-being;

(c) the relative influence of major predictors with major outcome measures related to health, well-being and residential satisfaction; and
(d) the relative influence of major predictors and dependent variables with outcome measures related to health, well-being and residential satisfaction.

It is expected that both high density and poor environmental quality would adversely affect the health and well-being. However, psychological variables like social support and tolerance will be helpful in mediating the adverse effect of density and environmental quality. With regard to community groups it is expected that Muslim respondents will derive more residential satisfaction because of better social support mechanism relative to their Hindu counterparts. One plausible reason seems to be that most of the prominent mosques are located in the inner city areas of Bhopal. Besides, because of several traditional and ethnic reasons, the minority group exhibits more cohesiveness relative to majority group.

Method

Delineation of Study Area and Pilot Study

To acquire requisite knowledge about the inner city housing, the investigators visited all the 29 wards where around 78 *mohallas* (localities) were located. Three criteria were used to select the appropriate *mohallas* wherefrom the sample was proposed to be drawn. These criteria were related to: (1) residential density of the *mohallas*, (2) the percentage of Hindus and Muslims in the *mohallas*, and (3) the environmental quality of the *mohallas*. The high and low density areas taken in this study are based on 1991 census data of the different wards. The density of *mohallas* in the inner city ranged from approximately 1,185 persons per hectare to 116 person per hectare. The *mohallas*, where the ratio of persons per hectare was less than 625, were treated in low density category. In contrast, *mohallas* having persons per hectare ratio of more than 725, were treated in high density category. Thus, with respect to density, only 18 *mohallas* were selected. Of these four *mohallas* were dropped because more than 80 percent of the households were dominated by either of the two major communities. Thus, on the basis of our initial survey, only 14 *mohallas* were selected, which met out criteria related of density and presence of reasonable percentages of two community groups.

A group of six independent judges, specializing either in architectural design or in environmental and behaviour, made an independent assessment of 14 pre-selected *mohallas* on various dimensions of environmental quality. A 16-item checklist was prepared to assess the environmental quality of the *mohallas*. The seven items on architectural features were as follows: how does the scale of *mohalla* suit the pattern of the surrounding streets; how does the scale of the *mohalla* suit the site it sits upon; do the private and public areas relate well with each other; does the land use adjacent to the *mohalla* seem to fit harmoniously with the fabric; does the building use adjacent to the *mohalla* seem to fit harmoniously with the fabric; does the appearance of the *mohalla* fit well with the type of buildings and surroundings; and is the scale and character of the *mohalla* per house identifiable distinctly. The eight items of objective environmental quality of the surrounding assessed the upkeep of the *mohalla*, upkeep of the streets, garbage condition, drainage condition, foul air circulation, congestion, noise structural condition of the *mohalla* and overall attractiveness of the *mohalla*. All the items were measured on a five-point rating scale where high score is indicative of high environmental quality. Only those *mohallas* where the ratings of the judges were found to be reasonably consistent, were selected. The total score on the quality scale ranged from 16 to 80. The score below 32 was treated low on environmental quality and score above 64 was treated as indicative of high quality. Finally, the requisite sample was drawn from 10 *mohallas*.

The pilot study was carried out on a small group of subjects belonging to Hindu and Muslim communities living in the pre-selected 14 *mohallas* located in the inner city areas. The pilot study was needed to examine the appropriateness of design, suitability of items and effectiveness of instructions. More than twenty items were either deleted or modified in order to make them easier and communicable.

Sample and Design

The sample, comprising 320 males, were owners of their house and also head of their family. The sample was drawn following a 2 x 2 x 2 factorial design with two levels of density (high and low), two levels of environmental quality (high and low) and two community groups (Hindu and Muslim). In each of the eight potential categories, there were 40 respondents. An attempt was made to select only those respondents who had been residing in the inner city areas for more than twenty years.

Measures

A ten-page questionnaire entitled "Community Living in Inner City" was used in this housing survey. The detailed instructions for each of the six sections regarding the rating of the items were given to the respondents. The first section of the questionnaire contained some personal information about the respondents. Some of the items included in this section were related to age, sex, ethnic group, income, duration of stay in the present dwelling, number of rooms in the dwelling and number of family members. The preceding sections of this questionnaire incorporated various sub-scales related to perceived crowding, tolerance, community lifestyle, assessment or neighbourhood and own home. Finally, the respondents were asked to give their response on measures related to health, well-being, feelings and residential satisfaction. A brief description of these scales is presented below:

Perceived Crowding Scale

A condensed version of the scale constructed by Nagar and Paulus (1997) was utilized. The items of this scale were related to spaciousness, space satisfaction, discomfort from insufficient space, interference, disruptive relationship, disturbance, loss of control and privacy. All the items were to be rated on a 5-point Likert type rating scale. The high score on this scale was indicative of high crowding experience. The scores on this scale ranged from 8 to 40. The reliability coefficient (Cronbach alpha) of this scale was found to be .83.

Tolerance

To assess the tolerance, a 21-item scale was developed. The items of this scale were designed after consulting the tolerance scale of Jain (1978). The respondents were asked to rate the items on a 5-point scale which ranged from 1 (almost never) to 5 (almost always). The high score was indicative of high tolerance. The factor analysis was performed after obtaining the responses from the subjects that indicated the presence of the two factors, which were labelled as *environmental tolerance* and *people tolerance.* The content of the fourteen items of the environmental sub-scale included standard of living, poorly maintained *mohallas*, adequacy of supply of electricity, uncertainty of future environmental conditions, water supply, sewage and drainage conditions, street dogs, safety and security conditions, air pollution, mosquitoes and flies and overall maintenance of *mohalla*. The scores ranged from 14 to 70. The internal consistency among the items was found to be 78. The people tolerance sub-scale comprised six items. Included in this sub-scale were items related to unpleasant people in the *mohalla*, community life in the *mohalla*, uncontrolled entry of unauthorized people, congestion and crowding. The score ranged from 6 to 30 and the internal consistency was found to be .83.

Community Lifestyle

To assess the community lifestyle, a 15-item scale was developed. The items used in this scale were simulated from the scales utilized in military studies (Paulus, Nagar and Camacho, 1991; Paulus, Nagar, Larey and Camacho, 1996). The responses obtained from the subjects were factor analyzed. The factor results indicated the presence of three distinct factors labelled as *sense of community, social support* and *socialization.* The *sense of community* sub-scale included six items. Some of them related to liking of the *mohalla*, unpleasant housing experience, probable duration of stay in the *mohalla*, proud to be part of the *mohalla*, and so on. The scores on this scale ranged from 5 to 24 and the internal consistency among items was found to be .82. The *social support* sub-scale contained four items. This scale measured the degree of social support derived in the neighbourhood, help in emergencies, taking care of children, loan of money and food, and so forth. The internal consistency among the items was found to be .87. Finally, the *socialization* sub-scale comprised six items. The items in this scale related to degree of socialization, entertaining guests outside and inside the primary and secondary environment. participation in social activities, getting along with others in the *mohalla*, and so on. The internal consistency among the items was found to be .87.

Residential Satisfaction

A three-item scale was used to assess the degree of residential satisfaction of the respondents. The items were prepared after consulting the scale used by Wandersman *et al.* (1985). The scale consisted of items related to the expected length of stay in the *mohalla*, selection of similar type of housing in case of moving out and possibility of vacating the *mohalla* if provided with an opportunity. The score ranged from 3 to 15. The internal consistency among the items was found to be .88.

Well-being

To assess the general well-being and health, a 14-item scale developed by Dupuy (1978) was used. This scale measured the extent to which individuals had experienced depression, anxiety, nervousness and various bodily ailments. Subjects were required to rate these items on a 6-point scale. The composite score was treated as index of well-being. This scale had been used successfully in the past (Martin and Iokovvic, 1987). The high score was indicative of positive well-being.

Health

A condensed version of the Hopkins Symptoms Checklist-90R (Derogatis, 1983; Derogatis *et al.*, 1974) was administered as a measure of overall health. For each of the fifteen common symptoms including watery eyes, itching or painful eyes, temporary deafness or hard hearing sensation, sneezing spells, running nose, congested nose, asthama, coughing, out of breath, chest pain, deep difficulty, toothaches, upset stomach and headaches, the subjects were asked to indicate the extent to which they had been bothered by that symptom during the preceding month. The rating of these symptoms was done on a 5-point rating scale. This checklist has been used successfully by many studies to demonstrate the health-related effects of stress (Schaeffer *et al.*, 1988). The scale scores ranged from 0 to 75 and the high score indicated less health-related problems.

Feeling

To assess the emotional state, an 8-item feeling scale was used. The items of the scale were designed to tap how often the respondents had felt confused, pressurized, alone, upset, nervous, excited, unworthy, lacking concentration on work, and so forth. The scores ranged from 8 to 40. The internal consistency among the items was found to be .80.

Procedure

After the selection of the wards, a brief one-page questionnaire was distributed to the potential 600 respondents. The major purpose was to understand some of the demographic characteristics of the respondents, like age, length of stay in the present dwelling, income, number of residents in the dwelling, ethnic group, and so on. Besides, the residents were asked whether they desired and were willing to participate in such kind of survey in future or not. A little more than 400 respondents expressed their willingness to participate in the in-depth housing survey. After a lapse of four months, the participants who had previously expressed their willingness for participation were approached after seeking appointment from them in advance. The purpose of the survey was explained to them. The instructions were read and the scoring pattern was explained to them. They were also encouraged to raise their queries, if any. They were then assured that their responses would be kept secret and would not be disclosed to anyone. In most cases, the questionnaire was completed by the respondents in about 50 minutes.

Results

Resident Characteristics

The background characteristics for residents belonging to the two community groups were similar except that Muslim residents had more members in their house and less income relative to their Hindu counterparts. There were no significant differences between Hindu and Muslim residents in terms of age, duration of stay in the dwellings, and number of rooms, courtyards and balconies in their present dwellings. The income of residents residing in high-density areas was significantly more than their counterparts living in low-density areas. Similarly, residents residing in high environmental quality areas had reported significantly more income than those residing in low environmental quality areas. No significant differences across density and environmental quality were obtained on other measures related to age, duration and length of stay, number of residents in the dwellings, and number of courtyards and balconies in the dwellings.

Analysis of Variance

To examine the mean differences across major independent variables on major dependent and outcome measures, an analysis of variance was computed. A separate 2 x 2 x 2 ANOVA was employed with two levels each of density, environmental quality and community groups for all the dependent and outcome variables. The results are presented in Table 1.

Table 1

Means and F Ratio of Dependent and Outcome Measures as a Function of Main Effects of Density Environmental Quality and Community Groups

Predictors	*Density*			*Environmental quality*			*Community groups*		
Criterion variables	*HD*	*LD*	*F*	*HEC*	*LEC*	*F*	*Hindu*	*Muslims*	*F*
Perceived crowding	31.52	25.78	7.12	25.40	26.80	.78	32.78	36.50	7.89
Environmental tolerance	50.78	44.19	12.10	34.60	39.50	8.92	50.13	57.60	17.90
People's community	23.79	20.80	4.18	36.73	37.12	2.18	20.13	24.80	5.70
Sense of community	20.10	16.42	7.40	16.90	20.40	5.82	16.40	21.70	8.19
Social support	14.10	11.92	5.60	12.80	17.40	7.20	13.40	16.80	5.13
Socialization	20.40	21.42	2.10	17.30	22.17	9.70	20.90	22.40	3.70
Residential satisfaction	11.92	12.00	.85	12.40	10.12	4.10	12.40	11.90	1.78
Home rating	18.90	22.70	5.40	20.98	16.32	5.30	24.80	19.90	5.58
Well-being	40.18	49.30	14.85	60.75	55.12	7.80	63.13	55.68	12.07
Health	39.12	47.80	13.60	56.90	50.63	9.70	58.20	50.63	14.19
Feeling	30.60	32.19	2.18	35.80	30.93	8.40	33.80	35.73	2.89

$F(1,313) = 3.92, p < .05$; $F(1,313) = 6.84, p < .01$

An analysis of Table 1 reveals that respondents residing in high-density areas significantly perceived high crowding, high tolerance, high sense of community and more social support than their counterparts residing in low-density areas. In contrast, respondents residing in low-density areas significantly reported more positive rating about their home environment, exhibited less health complaints and higher levels of psychological well-being relative to their high-density counterparts. Finally, no significant difference was found across variation of density on measures related to residential satisfaction and feeling.

The main effects of environmental quality on various dependent and outcome measures can be seen from Table 1. The results depict that respondents residing in low environmental quality areas reported significantly high environmental tolerance, high sense of community, higher social support and socialization as compared to respondents living in high environmental quality areas. However, residents residing in high quality environment reported higher residential satisfaction, positive home rating, less health problems and positive well-being than their counterparts residing in low environmental quality areas. No significant differences on environmental quality were found on measures related to perceived crowding and people's tolerance.

The mean differences between Hindu and Muslim respondents on various dependent and outcome measures are also presented in Table 1. The results show that Muslim respondents, relative to Hindu respondents, reported significantly more perceived crowding, higher degree of tolerance, higher sense of community feeling and more social support. In contrast, the Hindu respondents significantly reported positive home rating, less health problems and higher psychological well-being relative to their Muslim counterparts. No significant mean difference was obtained on measures of socialization and feeling.

A significant two-way interaction effect was found between community groups and outside density on social support [$F(1,132) = 8.26$, $p < .01$]. As can be seen from Figure 1, both Hindu and Muslim respondents residing in high-density areas reported deriving more social support relative to their counterparts residing in low-density areas. However, only marginal difference was found

Figure 1

Mean difference in social support as a function of outside density and community groups

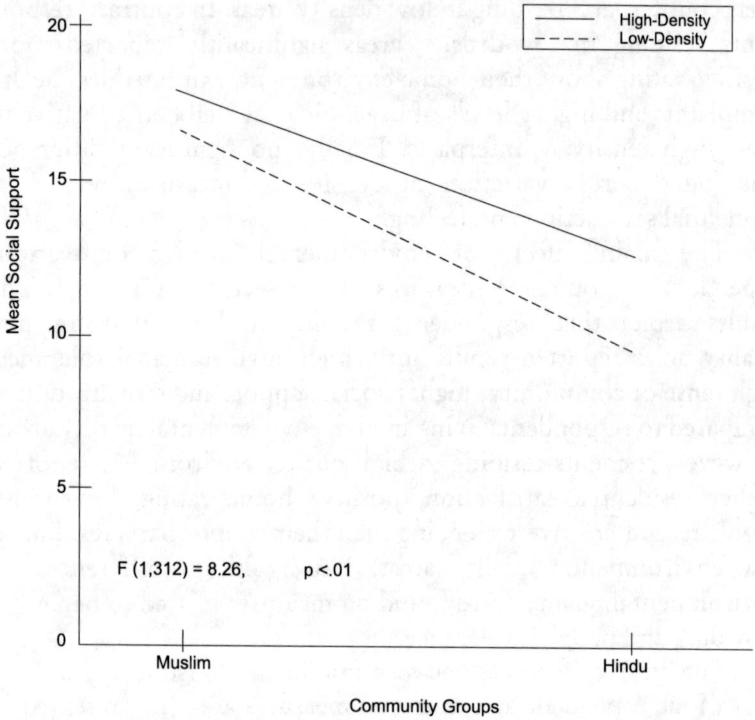

between Muslims residing in low- and high-density areas on social support. In contrast, significant difference was revealed by Hindu residents residing in varied density areas on social support measure with respondents residing in high-density areas reporting high social support than their counterparts residing in low-density areas, who reported low social support. Thus, it seems that social support may moderate the effects between density and community groups.

Another significant interaction was found between density and community groups on measure of socialization [F (1,312) = 15.84, $p < .01$]. The graph presented in Figure 2 reveals that Muslims residing in high-density areas reported higher level of socialization relative to their Hindu counterparts. However, this trend is reversed across the community groups in low-density conditions where

Figure 2

Mean difference in socialization as a function of outside density and community groups

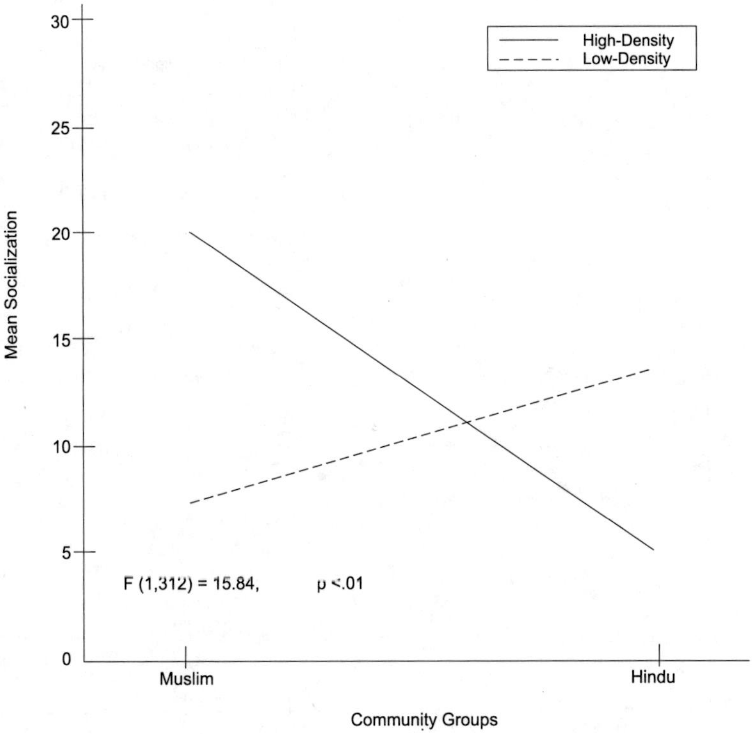

Hindus expressed more socialization relative to Muslims. There is a possibility that socialization acts as a moderator between density and community groups.

On the health measure, a three-way interaction was found significant between density, environmental quality and community groups [$F(1,312)=6.24$, $p<.01$] on symptomalogy. An analysis of Figure 3 reveals that both Hindu and Muslim respondents residing in low density and low environmental quality areas reported similar degree of health problems. However, less health complaints were reported by Hindus, relative to Muslims, in high-density and low environmental quality areas. In contrast, the health complaints by Muslims were more or less similar irrespective of density variation. Moreover, residents residing in low environmental quality areas

Figure 3

Mean difference in symptomology as a function of outside density and community groups and environmental quality

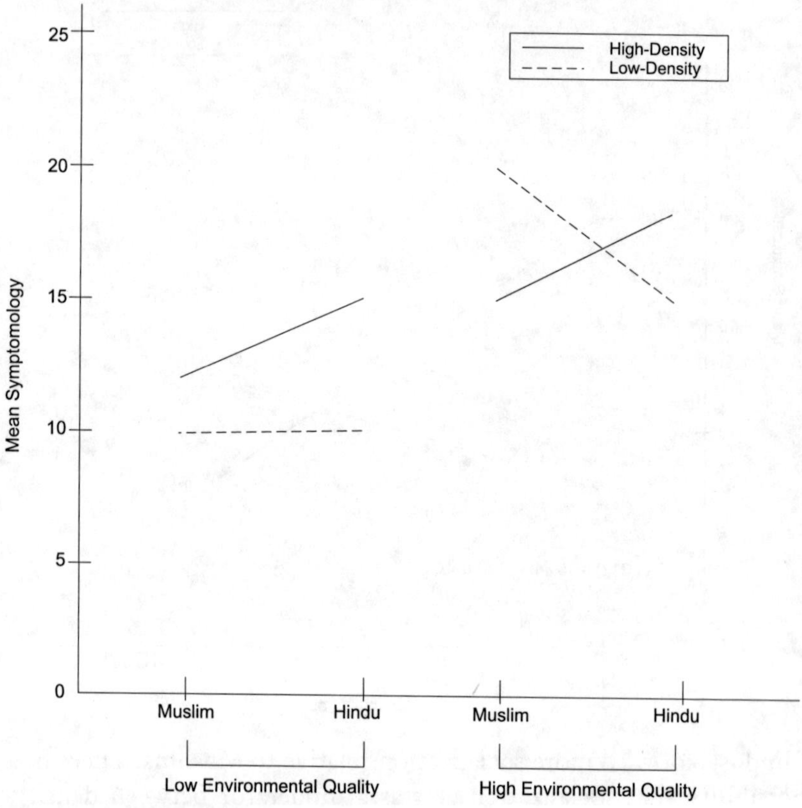

reported more health problems relative to their counterparts residing in high environmental quality areas with Muslims reporting less health problems in low-density areas relative to Hindus. This trend is reversed for Hindu respondents residing in high-density and high environmental quality areas, who reported less health problems in low-density conditions relative to high-density conditions.

Multiple Regression Results

To compare the residents' reaction to density and environmental quality on various dependent and outcome measures, step-wise regression analysis was performed. The initial analysis revealed that income and number of residents were significantly different with regard to major predictors (density, environmental quality and community groups). Thus, apart from our major predictors, these two variables were also included as predictors in the regression analysis. Analysis of Table 2 reveals that income was not able to predict any of the four dependent variables related to environmental tolerance, people's tolerance, social support and socialization. The number of residents significantly predicted environmental tolerance and socialization. Furthermore, excluding some cases, all the three major predictors significantly predicted dependent variables.

Table 2

Step-wise Regression Predicting Major Dependent and Outcomes

Predictors	*Environmental tolerance*		*People's tolerance*		*Sense of community*		*Social support*		*Socialization*	
	R^2	F	R^2	F	R^2	F	R^2	F	R^2	F
Density	.26	4.14	.08	4.15			.17	6.28		
Environmental quality	.23	5.78					.14	7.13	.19	4.76
Community groups	.20	6.14	.11	3.76			.22	5.12	.24	4.07
Number of residents	.15	7.82							.07	5.92
Income										

Predictors	*Residential satisfaction*		*Home rating*		*Health*		*Well-being*		*Feeling*	
	R^2	F	R^2	F	R^2	F	R^2	F	R^2	F
Outside density	.21	9.23			.17	8.78	.16	7.48		
Environmental quality	.18	13.91	.10	3.18	.24	5.72	.18	4.89	.18	4.91
Community groups	.23	5.97			.11	12.04	.07	9.72		
Number of residents					.06	16.78	.11	8.64	.07	8.22
Income	.14	16.42	.08	4.78	.14	13.21	.05	12.84	.13	6.18

Table 3
Results of Step-wise Regression Predicting Major Outcomes

Predictors	*Residential satisfaction*		*Home rating*		*Health*		*Well-being*		*Feeling*	
	R^2	F	R^2	F	R^2	F	R^2	F	R^2	F
Outside density	.11	14.21	.20	4.31	.09	16.31	.05	16.13	.10	9.80
Environmental quality	.24	8.06	.06	19.21	.14	13.21	.11	14.21	.26	4.84
Community groups			.11	13.21						
Number of residents										
Income										
Perceived crowding	.06	21.32	.12	9.08	.06	15.48			.07	14.78
Sense of community	.15	12.28	.15	6.12			.15	13.21	.15	7.90
Social support	.19	9.05	.18	5.13	.29	6.33	.16	10.43	.18	6.42
Socialization			.13	8.32						
People's tolerance					.18	10.41	.21	8.21	.09	12.10
Environmental tolerance					.26	6.07	.24	6.14		

The results predicting outcome measures on residential satisfaction, home rating, health, well-being and feeling are presented in Table 3. As can be seen from Table 3 the most potent predictor of residential satisfaction was environmental quality, followed by income, outside density and community groups. All the significant predictors significantly explained 23 percentage of variance. The home rating was predicted by environmental tolerance and income. All the five predictors contributed to the total of 24 percentage of variance on health measure. The most potent predictor of health was found to be number of residents in the dwelling (6%), followed by community groups, income, density and environmental quality. Similarly, all the five predictors were able to predict the psychological well-being. Of the total of 18 percent variance explained, income was found to be the most potent predictor entering the regression equation, followed by community groups, number of residents, density and quality. Finally, outside density and community groups were not able to significantly predict feeling. The number of residents, income and quality were the significant predictors of feeling, collectively explaining 18 percentage of variance.

The step-wise regression results discussed above clearly indicate that all the three major predictors (density, quality and community groups) and two background measures (number of residents, income) predicted various dependent measures and outcomes. The subsequent regression analysis was planned with the inclusion of six dependent measures (sense of community, tolerance) with three major predictors and two background variables to explain the variance for five major outcome measures pertaining to residential satisfaction, health, well-being, home rating and feeling.

Residential Satisfaction

Of the total of eleven predictors, only five were able to enter the regression equation explaining together 24 percent of variance on residential satisfaction. The most potent predictor was found to be perceived crowding, which independently explained 6 percent of the variance, followed by outside density (5%), sense of community (4%), social support (4%) and environmental quality (5%).

Home Rating

Of the total of eleven predictors, only seven were able to enter the regression equation explaining together 20 percent of variance on residential satisfaction. The most potent predictor was found to be environmental quality, which independently explained 6 percent of the variance, followed by community groups (5%), perceived crowding (1%), socialization (1%), sense of community (2%), social support (3%) and outside density (2%).

Health

A total of 27 percent variance was explained by the six predictors on health measure. The most potent predictor was found to be perceived crowding, which independently explained 6 percent of the variance, followed by outside density (3%), environmental quality (5%), people's tolerance (4%), environmental tolerance (6%) and social support (3%).

Well-being

Of the total of eleven predictors, only six were able to enter the regression equation explaining together 24 percent of variance on residential satisfaction. The most potent predictor was found to be perceived crowding, which independently explained 5 percent of the variance. In the order of priority, other significant predictors were environmental quality, sense of community, social support, people's tolerance and environmental tolerance.

Feeling

A total of five predictors entered the regression equation and together explained 26 percent of variance on feeling. The most potent predictor was found to be perceived crowding, which independently explained 7 percent of the variance, followed by people's tolerance (2%). outside density (1%), sense of community (5%) and environmental quality (11%).

On the basis of regression results, one can conclude that income, number of residents and community groups failed to independently predict most of the outcome measures. Outside density and environmental quality of the area were found to be significant predictors even after the inclusion of dependent measures like perceived crowding, sense of community and tolerance for most of the outcome measures. Furthermore, the dependent measures, when treated as predictors with other major predictors, explained significant variance on most of the outcome variables. Thus, it seems plausible to infer that all the psychological variables (perceived crowding, sense of community and tolerance) mediate in complex ways the relationship between density and environmental quality and major outcome variables.

Discussion

The major concerns of this study were to determine how Hindus and Muslims residing in high- and low-density areas having differential environmental quality conditions respond to various socio-psychological aspects of their inner city housing environment. Also, what were its likely consequences on health, well-being, residential satisfaction and feelings. A unique feature of this study was that the we were able to examine these issues for a fairly homogeneous population, who were very similar on various demographic and background characteristics like age, length of stay, number of balconies and provision of courtyards in their dwellings, and so forth. All the respondents were owners of their dwellings and belonged to the business community.

In the Indian context few studies have compared the responses of the two prominent community groups across differential density and varied environmental quality conditions. A large number of previous studies have examined the effects of objective density in a range of laboratory and field settings (Jain, 1987; Nagar, 1998). Very few studies on residential settings have incorporated both objective and subjective indices of crowding (Jain, 1997; Nagar, 1998). Attempts are also lacking to examine the independent effects of impact of both crowding and objective environmental quality prevailing in the residential areas in a single research tradition on a range of dependent and outcome measures. The present study attempts to examine all the broad dimensions of objective environmental quality and architectural features of the residential areas as suggested in the literature (Paulus *et al.*, 1996; Rapoport, 1985; Baum and Valins, 1977). In view of the above-mentioned gaps, the present research was undertaken to examine the influence of density, environmental quality and community groups on various social, psychological and health-related measures.

The initial results with respect to demographic and background characteristics reveal that only income and number of residents were found to be significantly different across all the three predictors (density, environmental quality and community groups). This trend of result is very understandable. It is very obvious that residents with high income, relative to their low-income counterparts, tend to stay in low-density areas and relatively better environmental quality places. Furthermore, empirical evidence exists that Hindus relative to Muslims have significantly higher income. In fact, a large number of Muslims, who were previously residing in the core areas of the inner city, have drifted to the peripheral areas in Bhopal across a period of time (Sharma, 1996). Finally, consistent with the national demographical statistics, it was found that the number of residents in a typical Muslim household is relatively more than that of the Hindu household.

The prominent trend obtained from the ANOVA and regression results reveals that resident residing in high-density areas perceived more crowding experience, exhibited high tolerance, high sense of community feeling and reported more negative effects on outcome measures, including health and well-being, relative to their low-density area counterparts. With minor variation the same trend was found across high and low environmental quality areas on most of the dependent and outcome measures. Looking at the major trend of analysis of variance results, one can conclude that both high-density conditions and low environmental quality of the area are perceived as stress provoking and adversely affect the health and well-being of the residents. The results obtained with regard to density effects are to a large extent consistent with those obtained by the other researchers (Baum and Paulus, 1987; Jain, 1997; Nagar, 1998). For instance, the study conducted by Gove *et al.* (1979) revealed that the perceived residential crowding is associated with a number of adverse consequences, including high psychosomatic complains and negative home evaluation. In the similar vein, studies conducted in other residential settings like prisons (Paulus, 1987), dormitories (Baum *et al.*, 1975) and homes (Baum and Paulus, 1987) reported evidence that crowding was found to be associated with ill-health, negative home evaluation and negative emotional states. A number of studies conducted in Indian cities have similarly reported correlation between crowding and its adverse effects. For example, in Varanasi, Tripathi (1988) reported positive correlation between high density and maladjustment neuroticism and anxiety. In Ahmedabad, Kulkarni (1984) found high incidence of crime in high-density areas. With regard to the dependent measures related to sense of community and tolerance, the respondents residing in high-density areas reported higher social cohesion and degree of tolerance. Evidence indicates that tolerance and sense of community sometimes mediate and sometimes moderate the relationship between crowding and its consequences (Jain, 1987; Baum and Paulus, 1987). For instance, Jain (1987) conducted a series of studies and concluded that exposure to high density increases the competition tolerance, which is helpful in dealing with aversiveness of stressors. Similar results are obtained by other scholars (e.g., Gifford, 1987).

A close similarity of results as obtained across high- and low-density areas is seen with regard to environmental quality on dependent and outcome measures. The analyses of variance and regression results reveal that respondents residing in high-quality environment reported less health-related problems, high psychological well-being and positive emotional states, in comparison to their counterparts residing in low-quality environment. Furthermore, residents residing in low environmental quality areas reported high sense of community and high level of tolerance relative to their counterparts residing in high environmental quality areas. It seems that after staying in low environmental quality areas for a prolonged period of time, the residents might have developed insensitivity to bad environmental quality on one hand and stronger community ties on the other. Our results on the effects of environmental quality are to a large extent similar with the findings obtained by other scholars (Newman, 1980; Paulus *et al.*, 1991). For instance, the study of Newman (1980) reported strong evidence that when residents, who were previously living in sub-standard environmental housing conditions, were displaced to newly constructed high-rise complexes, they felt emotionally and psychologically depressed. Across the period of time, the respondents have developed strong social ties with their neighbours. In the new high-rise complexes, the probability of social interaction was reduced, which resulted in social anomaly. Furthermore, the social support literature also provides indication that stronger social ties are seen in environment that are sub-standard and are of poor quality. Similarly, the study conducted by Paulus *et al.* (1996) revealed that residents staying in sub-standard housing reported stronger ties within their neighbourhood than residents residing in good-quality homes. In contrast, the residents staying in high-quality areas reported better health, higher well-being and more positive emotional states than their low-quality area counterparts. In a longitudinal study, conducted by Paulus *et al.* (1991), an attempt was made to examine the quality of life in mobile home parks. A survey of more than 40 parks near the army base was conducted. The researchers found that several parks had unpleasant surrounding. The trailers were poorly maintained. The area was littered and the streets were in poor conditions. The residents residing in the parks reported positive feelings about the environment and their fellow residents in particular. Evidence of strong social network was found in these parks. Evans *et al.* (1989), in their study, revealed that that the adverse effects of residential crowding on psychological health and well-being are mediated by a breakdown of social support system. They view weakening of social bonds as an unintended side-effect of a typical strategy for coping with overcrowding.

The theory of choice and self-selection posits that many individuals are willing to live in sub-standard environments. They may choose them because of convenience, proximity to facilities and friends, low expense or even because of lack of sensitivity to environmental characteristics (e.g., aesthetics, noise, sanitation, crowding). Furthermore, people living in a homogeneous neighbourhood for a prolonged period of time are likely to become interdependent and attached emotionally to the people and places of the locality. A strong attachment of place may develop through a cost/benefit analysis by residents in which they evaluate the degree of social support in present neighbourhood relative to other neighbourhood (Sarason, 1974).

The analysis of variance results across two community groups on various dependent and outcome measures reveals that Muslims, as compared to Hindus, reported high crowding experience, lower home rating, lower psychological well-being and more health-related problems. Furthermore, the Muslim residents exhibited significantly stronger sense of community and higher tolerance for people than their Hindu counterparts. In the initial regression analysis, the community group was entered in the regression equation together with other major predictors (density, quality, income and number of children) predicted most of the dependent and outcomes related to sense of community, tolerance, health, well-being and emotional states. However, when all the five major predictors and six dependent measures were together treated as predictors the community groups failed to predict any of the five outcomes related to health, well-being, residential satisfaction, feelings and home rating. The outside density, environmental quality, sense of community and tolerance were found to be major predictors, of most of the outcome variables. Thus, it seems that residents, irrespective of their different ethnic groups, react more or less similar to environmental stressors like density and environmental quality. However, because of different cultural and religious practices, some differences between Hindu and Muslim residents are evident. For example, significant interaction effect was found between outside density and community group on health measure and residential satisfaction. In addition, significant interaction effect was found between density and community group on socialization and social support measures. This reveals that Muslims, irrespective of their level of density, derive more social support in their neighbourhood than Hindus. Furthermore, Muslim residents, living in high-density areas, have, relative to their low-density counterparts, reported more socialization and social support, while the reverse is true for Hindus.

The difference between Muslim and Hindu residents on psychological measures (sense of community and tolerance) can be explained if we examine various traditions and customs. For instance, the close proximity to prominent worship places from both home and workplace may facilitate adherence to well-defined religious practices. The Muslims are supposed to offer 'Namaz' five times a day. The timings are prefixed and are of a very short duration. Besides, it is a group activity. Thus, Muslims have the opportunity to interact with their community members very frequently, which may presumably be one major reason for developing more social cohesiveness. In contrast, the Hindu prayers are not restricted to one God but depending on the caste, sub-caste and individual preference, different Gods are identified for 'puja'. In the Hindu religion, no time schedule is prescribed for prayer. A Hindu can visit the temple or can offer prayer even at home at any time of his choice. Thus, the probability of social interaction for Hindus at their worship place is limited. Furthermore, the 'purdah' system prohibits the Muslim females to interact freely. While the number of residents in a typical Muslim house is more and the 'purdah' system is practised, the adults may stay outside the house to give the desired quota of privacy to the female family members. Evidence indicates that in a supportive home climate family members living in crowded households develop various privacy regulation mechanisms to accommodate the needs, desires and aspirations of other family members (Altman and Chemers, 1980). Finally, sufficient literature on inter-group relations is available that seems to suggest that the community holding minority status often shows a high degree of cohesiveness. This reasoning may be applied to the Muslim community members, who are in minority, relative to their Hindu counterparts.

In a nutshell, the overall results seem to suggest that both environmental stressors (density and environmental quality) are potent predictors of health, well-being, residential satisfaction and feeling. Although, in the initial regression analysis, the community group emerged as a potent predictor of most of the social, psychological variables and outcomes, however, with the inclusion of dependent measures with major predictors, the effect of community group in predicting outcomes disappeared. The interaction effects suggested that social and psychological variables acted as moderators between density and community groups. Thus, density and environmental quality are perceived as stressors and affect the health and psychological well-being, irrespective of community group members of the respondents. The adverse effect on health is found to be moderated socio-psychological variables, like sense of community and tolerance which favour the Muslim community members more than their Hindu counterparts.

This study has a number of implications for policy makers. The adverse consequences of both density and environmental quality on major outcome measures, including health and well-being, are reported uniformly by Hindu and Muslim respondents. Adaptation to high density and bad environmental quality can be inferred for the Muslim respondents largely because of better community lifestyle and high tolerance. The influx of population to the inner city area is greatly disturbing the environmental quality and is increasing the density level of the inner city areas. The existing infrastructure and available resources are insufficient to meet the demand of the increased population. Some of the interventions like shifting some of the commercial activities to other places and removal of encroachments planned by the state government implemented forcibly are likely to reduce the pressure created by the influx of residents living in these areas for generations. By dislocating some of the commercial activities from the inner city areas, a sizeable population will move to the next location. This is likely to enhance the environmental quality, which at present is deteriorated. Some open areas may be created and developed to improve the environmental quality of the inner city areas. The cohesive community existing in the inner city areas may be solicited to improve the quality standard of residential areas. These efforts may be helpful in reducing the adverse effects of high density and bad environmental quality on people.

References

Ahlbrandt, R. and Brophy, P. (1976). Management: An important element of the housing environment. *Environment and Behaviour, 8*, 505-526.

Altman, I. and Chemers, M.M. (1980). Cultural aspects of environment-behaviour relationships. In H. Triandis (Eds.), *Handbook of Cross-Cultural Psychology*, Vol. 5, Boston: Allyn and Bacon.

Amerigo, M. and Aragones, J. (1997). A theoretical and methodological approach to the study of residential satisfaction. *Journal of Environmental Psychology, 17*, 47-57.

Anderson. T.R., Anthony, K., Weidemann, S., Bain, B. and Allen, L. (1988). *Housing for Disabled Adults: User Experience with Alternate Bathroom Design* (report supported by grant from the national endowment for the arts), Urbana: Housing Research and Development Programme, University of Illinois.

Anthony, K.I.I., Weidemann, S. and Chin, Y. (1990). Housing perception of low-income single parents. *Environment and Behaviour, 22*, 147-182.

Baum, A., Harpin, R.E. and Valins (1975). The role of group phenomena in the experience of crowding. *Environment and Behaviour, 7*, 185-198.

Baum, A. and Paulus, P. (1987). Crowding. In D. Stokols and I. Altman (Eds.), *Handbook of Environmental Psychology* (Vol. I, pp. 553-570). New York: John Wiley.

Baum, A. and Valins, S. (1977). *Architecture and Social Behaviour: Psychological Studies of Social Density.* Hinsdale, NJ: Erlbaum.

Carstens, D.Y. (1985). *Site Planning and Design for the Elderly: Issues, Guidelines and Alternatives.* New York: Van Nostrand Reinhold.

Caspi, A., Bolger, N. and Eckenrode, J. (1987). Linking persona and the context in the daily stress process. *Journal of Personality and Social Psychology, 52*, 184-195.

Christensen, D., Carp, F., Cranz and Wiley, I. (1982). Objective housing indicators as predictors of subjective evaluations of elderly residents. *Journal of Environmental Psychology, 12*, 225-236.

Derogatis, L.R. (1983). Misuse of the symptom checklist 90. *Archives of General Psychiatry, 40*, 1152.

Derogatis, L.R., Lipman, R.S., Rickels, K., Uhlenhuth, E.H. and Cove, L. (1974). The hopkins symptom check list (HSCL): A self-report symptom inventory. *Behavioral Science, 19*, 1-15.

Dillman, D., Tremblay, K. and Dillman, J. (1979). Influence of housing norms and personal characteristics on stated housing preferences. *Housing and Society, 6*, 2-19.

Downs, R.M. (1981). Maps and mapping as metaphors for spatial representation. In L.S. Liben, A.H. Patterson and N. Newcomb (Eds.), *Spatial Representation and Behaviour Across the Life Span.* Academic Press. New York.

Dupuy, H.J. (1978). Sell-representation of general psychological well-being of American adults. Revision of a paper presented at the meeting of the American Public Health Association, Los Angeles, CA.

Galster, G. (1987). Identifying correlates of the dwelling satisfaction: An empirical, Critique. *Environment and Behaviour, 19*, 539-568.

Gans, I.L.T. (1967). *The Levittowners.* New York: Pantheon.

Gifford, R. (1987). *Environmental Psychology: Principles and Practice.* Boston: Allyn and Bacon.

Gove, W., Hudges, M. and Galle, O. (1979). Overcrowding in the home: An empirical investigation of its possible pathological consequences. *American Sociological Review, 44*, 59-80.

Greenfield, R. and Lewis, J. (1969). An alternative to a density function definition of overcrowding. *Land Economics, 45*, 282-285.

Jain, U. (1978). Competition tolerance in high-low density, urban-rural areas. *Journal of Social Psychology. 105*, 297-298.

— (1987). *The Experiences and Consequences of Crowding.* New Delhi: Sage.

— (1997). *The Feeling of Crowding and Its Psychological Consequences.* New Delhi: Har-Anand publishers.

Kasl, S.V. (1974). Effects of housing on mental and physical health. *Man-Environment Systems, 4*, 207-226.

Kulkarni, K.M. (1984). *Geography of Crowding and Human Response.* New Delhi: Concept.

Lawton, M.P. (1975). *Planning and Managing Housing for the Elderly.* New York: John Wiley and Sons.

Nagar, D. (1985). *Experiences and Consequences of Crowding,* unpublished doctoral dissertation, University of Allahabad.

— (1998). *Human Reactions to Crowding.* Jaipur: Printwell Publishers.

— (1999). Environmental stress. In G. Mishra (Eds.), *Stress and Health*, New Delhi: Concept.

Nagar, D. and Paulus. P.B. (1997). Assessment and validation of crowding experience scale. *Community and Applied Social Psychology.*

Newman, O. (1972). *Defensible Space: Crime Prevention Through Urban Design.* New York: Macmillan.

Newman, O. and Franck, K.A. (1980). *Factors Influencing Crime and Instability in Urban Housing Developments.* Washington, DC: National Institute of Justice

Paulus, P.B. (1988). *Prison Crowding: A Psychological Perspective.* New York. NY: Springer-Verlag.

Paulus, P.B., Nagar, D. and Camacho, M. (1991). Environmental and psychological factors in reactions to apartments and mobile homes. *Journal of Environmental Psychology. 11.* 143-161.

Paulus, P.B., Nagar, D., Larey, T.S. and Camacho, M. (1996). Environmental, lifestyle, and psychological factors in the health and well-being of military families. *Journal of Applied Social Psychology, 26*, 2053-2075.

Rainwater, L. (1970). *Behind Ghetto Walls: Black Families in a Federal Slum.* Chicago: Aldine.

Rapoport, A. (1985). Thinking about home environment: A conceptual framework. In I. Altman and C.M. Wernet (Eds.), *Home Environments* (pp.255-280). New York, NY: Plenum.

Ruback, B. and Pandey, J. (1991). Crowding perceived control and relative power: An analysis of households in India. *Journal of Applied Social Psychology, 21*, 345-374.

Sarason, S.B. (1974). *The Psychological Sense of Community: Prospects for a Community Psychology.* San Francisco: Jossey-Bass.

Schaeffer, M.A., Baum, A., Paulus, P.B. and Gaes, G.G. (1988). Architecturally mediated Effects of social density in prison. *Environment and Behaviour, 20*, 3-19.

Shaly, A.B. (1985). Castles in the sky: Measuring housing and neighborhood ideology. *Environment and Behaviour, 17*, 593-626.

Sharma, A. (1996). Transformational and developmental analysis of open spaces in Bhopal. Project report submitted to the Indo-Dutch Government HSNLHUDCO, New Delhi.

Stutlles, A.L. (1976). *Images of the American City.* New Brunswick, N.J.: Transaction Books.

Tripathi, H.G. (1988). Cognitive and affective consequences of crowding stress. Doctoral Dissertation in Psychology, Barkatullah University, Bhopal.

Wandersman, A., Florin, P., Chavis, D., Rich, R. and Prestby, J. (1985). Getting together and getting things done. *Psychology Today*, pp. 64-71.

V

Community Health and Intervention

17

Health and Environment in Changing Times: Some Observations from the Eastern Himalayan Populations

BARUN MUKHOPADHYAY

Health and environment are two important issues that are inextricably linked with human survival in time and space dimensions. Health and environment are complex phenomena with several interrelated components. Health of human populations is linked with various features and components of the environment, viz., physical, biological and socio-cultural, in which they live. Further, changes in any features of the environment may lead to changes in health profile. Again, health can be ascribed to be a dynamic equilibrium, outcome of which is determined by a wide variety of biological, socio-cultural, economic, political and physical environmental factors. Measurement of health has not been an easy task and consequently health has been measured in many different ways. A widely accepted approach for evaluating health status of a community has been to evaluate the extent of ill-health, i.e., morbidity and mortality in the community, as well as to evaluate the means of combatting the ill-health, i.e., the health care practices, and the details of various health services available in the community. Again, morbidity measures can be classified as either observed or self-perceived. While observed morbidity consists of reports from clinicians or other investigators about illnesses they have observed in the people, self-perceived morbidity consists of reports from people about their own illnesses (Murray *et al.*, 1992).

The eastern Himalayas, comprising a long terrain, cover the range eastward of Garhwal mountain, the Nepal Himalaya, the Sikkim-Darjeeling Himalaya, Bhutan Himalaya and Assam Himalaya as well. The geographical area of the eastern Himalayas is uniquely endowed with considerable natural resources that have sustained varied human groups for long. A wide range of bio-cultural diversity exists in the eastern Himalayas with a multi-ethnic, multi-lingual and multi-religious mosaic. The fact remains that the socio-political history of this particular area is rich, and both the monarchy and democracy as political systems occur presently in different nation-states that are located here. As a consequence of global changes, this area is also exposed to the factors of modernization relating to socio-political, economic and socio-cultural domains of life. Needless to say, effects of these changes vary over a variety of social groups and sub-groups. Additionally, several ecological changes are also occurring owing to a plethora of factors – economic, demographic, and so on. Health of the social groups/sub-groups inhabiting this largely mountainous/hilly area remains an important aspect of life that needs a considerable attention in terms of overall development of the region.

Under this backdrop, the present paper attempts to (a) assess the major health problems as revealed through morbidity profile, (b) examine the possible effects of socio-cultural environmental factors on several health traits, (c) delineate health care practices and available health care resources, and (d) identify newly emerging community health care issues for the eastern Himalayan populations. Specifically though, it considers mostly populations inhabiting Sikkim Himalaya in general and some tribal populations, viz., the Lepchas and Bhutias of Sikkim and/or Darjeeling Himalayas in particular. Both large-scale and small-scale study findings have been utilized in this paper.

Major Health Problems

Considering the large-scale country studies as well as specific surveys conducted at the state level (WHO, 2002; AIIH&PH and GoS,

1989; Pulger *et al.*, 1992; GoS, 1998), the major health problems in the eastern Himalayas centre around the diseases, such as tuberculosis, gastro-intestinal tract infections that include diarrhoea, dysentery, gastro-enteritis, acute respiratory infections that include pneumonia, asthma, skin diseases, such as scabies, intestinal parasitic infestations, pyrexia of unknown origin, iron deficiency anaemia, protein-energy malnutrition and iodine-deficiency disorders. As a matter of fact, these diseases have ranked at the higher level in the eastern Himalayan region for quite some time. Certainly, there is a possibility of inter- and intra-community variations for these diseases in time and space dimensions, but the nature and extent of such variations for individual diseases cannot possibly be evaluated presently because of paucity of information.

It is beyond doubt that *in-situ* modernization is taking place in many different areas of the eastern Himalayas and changes in traditional lifestyles are becoming a reality. Consequently, appearance of diseases, especially the chronic and degenerative ones, such as hypertension, diabetes, gall bladder disease, gout and mental disorders, is presently conspicuous. Social disharmony, economic conflicts and political turmoil have also become evident in this region, which possibly have led to health problems emerging out of drug abuse, alcoholism and so on. STDs, including HIV infections, pose another important health problem that warrants serious attention. It seems that double load of both infectious, along with chronic and degenerative diseases, is needed to be handled simultaneously. In order to be able to assess the relative contribution of different biological, ecological and socio-cultural factors responsible for such a scenario, epidemiological and medical anthropological information will be necessary for each disease condition, which hitherto is almost lacking for the eastern Himalayan populations.

Environmental Correlates of Diseases/Conditions: Some Examples

Some examples are provided below that examined the environmental correlates, mostly socio-cultural ones, on several diseases/conditions considering survey reports and epidemiological investigations among the general populations and specific tribal communities of Sikkim and Darjeeling Himalayas.

Communicable diseases constitute definitely one major group of diseases in the eastern Himalayan region. The available data on the reported cases of communicable diseases in the health institutions of Sikkim in 1990 suggest that acute diarrhoeal diseases (excluding cholera), acute respiratory infections, pneumonia, pulmonary tuberculosis and measles ranked high in that order. More than half of the total cases reported belong to communicable disease category (Table 1). The table also shows that after six years, that is, in 1996, more or less similar trend exists with minor exceptions. It appears that after a gap of six years viral hepatitis becomes an important disease to consider. Further, reported cases of gonococcal infection increase to a considerable extent (GoS, 1998).

Table 1

Reported Communicable Diseases in Sikkim (1990-1996)

Diseases	*Reported cases*	
	1990	*1996*
Acute diarrhoeal diseases (excluding cholera)	42177 (16.08)	54124 (18.15)
Whooping cough	90 (0.03)	3 (0.001)
Measles	391 (0.15)	859 (0.29)
Acute respiratory infection	48500 (18.50)	40618 (13.62)
Pneumonia	2432 (0.93)	2099 (0.7)
Viral hepatitis	576 (0.22)	630 (0.21)
Gonococcal infection	1 (0.0004)	22 (0.007)
Tuberculosis (pulmonary)	2019 (0.77)	957 (0.32)
Others	166023 (63.32)	198862 (66.32)
Total	262209 (100.0)	298178 (100.0)

Note: Figures in parentheses indicate percentages.

Source: Government of Sikkim, 1998.

Among the communicable diseases, diarrhoeal diseases get considerable importance and seasonal variations in these diseases have been found to occur. In Sikkim, monsoon months of July and August are the ones when most cases are reported, while in winter months of November and December least cases are reported (Table 2). This observation is possibly valid for other areas of the eastern Himalayas, too.

Table 2

Diarrhoeal Diseases in Sikkim by Months of Most and Least Reported Cases

Cases (1992)		*Cases (1996)*	
Least (November)	Most (July)	Least (December)	Most (August)
3718 (6.76)	5717 (10.40)	3713 (6.86)	5516 (10.18)

Note: Figures in parentheses are percentages.

Source: Government of Sikkim, 1998.

Iodine deficiency disorders (IDD) are one of the major public health problems in practically the entire eastern Himalayan region. Available data from Sikkim (Pulger *et al.*, 1992) suggest that prevalence of goitre is increasing over the time. While in 1976, it was 37.81 percent, it reached 54.03 percent in 1989-91, considering all age and sex groups. Table 3 shows that in Sikkim, endemic goitre is highly prevalent in all the four districts. The East district is the worst sufferer (60.9%) while North district is the least (45.84%), considering all age and sex groups. The table further reveals that endemic cretinism exists in all the four districts showing a similar trend. The inter-district variation in goitre prevalence is possibly due to biological as well as micro-environmental differences which need be assessed. Intuitively, it can be suggested that the highest level of iodized salt intake in the North district, compared to other three districts (AIIH&PH and GoS, 1989), could be one of the probable reasons for the least IDD problems in the North district of Sikkim.

Table 3

Prevalence of Endemic Goitre and Cretinism by Districts in Sikkim

State/District	*Endemic goitre (%)*	*Endemic cretinism (%)*	*Number examined*
Sikkim	54.03	3.46	17,837
East	60.92	4.93	4,588
West	51.32	2.83	5,407
North	45.84	1.67	2,522
South	54.72	3.68	5,320

Source: Pulger *et al.*, 1992.

Iron deficiency anaemia is a well-known health problem among many populations in India and other neighbouring countries. A micro-level investigation among the Lepchas, a tribal population of Kalimpong in the district of Darjeeling, West Bengal, inhabiting both urban and rural villages and following both Buddhism and Christianity, reveals that as high as 75.34 percent of females and 54.41 percent of males have been anaemic as measured by WHO suggested haemoglobin level (Table 4). Urban-rural differences significantly exist in anaemic status among the Lepchas, irrespective of gender and religious affiliation (Mukhopadhyay *et al.*, 1996).

Table 4

Residence Status and Anaemia among Lepchas of Kalimpong

Study group	*Anaemic*		*Non-anaemic*		*Total*	
	Male Hb (g/dl) < 13	*Female Hb (g/dl) < 12*	*Male Hb (g/dl) ≥13*	*Female Hb (g/dl) ≥12*	*Male*	*Female*
Urban Buddhist	15 (53.27)	33 (71.74)	13 (46.43)	13 (28.26)	28 (100.0)	46 (100.0)
Rural Buddhist	33 (26.61)	57 (46.72)	91 (73.39)	65 (53.28)	124 (100.0)	122 (100.0)
Urban Christian	37 (54.41)	55 (75.34)	31 (45.59)	18 (24.66)	68 (100.0)	73 (100.0)
Rural Christian	34 (33.33)	34 (34.69)	68 (66.67)	64 (65.31)	102 (100.0)	98 (100.0)

Note: Figures in parentheses indicate percentages.

Source: Mukhopadhyay *et al.*, 1996

Table 5

Self-reported Illness Episodes among Lepchas of Kalimpong

Religious groups	*Total no. of persons*	*Persons reportedly ill*	*No. of illness episodes*	*Prevalence of reported illness episodes*
Buddhist				
Adults	260	114	203	0.44
Children	193	65	149	0.34
Christian				
Adults	258	123	244	0.48
Children	207	76	139	0.37

Note: Adult-children differences are significant in both the religious groups.

Source: Mukhopadhyay, 1997.

Table 6

Type of Treatment for Illness Episodes Reported by Religious Group and Age Group

Religious and age groups	*Type of treatment*						*No. of illness episodes treated*		*No. of illness episodes not treated*		*Total no. of illness episodes*	
	Allopathic		*Homeopathic*		*Traditional*							
	No.	%	No.	%	No.	%	No.	%	No.	%	No.	%
Buddhist												
Adults	114	56.2	6	2.9	16	7.9	136	67.0	67	33.0	203	100.0
Children	116	77.9	3	2.0	6	4.0	125	83.9	24	16.1	149	100.0
Christian												
Adults	134	54.9	20	8.2	21	8.6	175	71.7	69	28.3	244	100.0
Children	108	77.7	13	9.3	4	2.9	125	89.9	14	10.1	139	100.0

Source: Mukhopadhyay, 1997.

A common form of morbidity data pertains to perception and reporting of symptoms or impairments by individuals. An investigation on the self-perceived and self-reported morbidity profile among the Kalimpong Lepchas by Mukhopadhyay (1997) observed higher prevalence of reported illness episodes among the adults, compared to children in both the religious groups, Buddhists and Christians (Table 5). Table 6, on the other hand, shows that for most of such reported illness episodes, the Lepchas of Kalimpong took treatment from modern allopathic doctors. Taking help of any specific treatment regimen was much more conspicuous for illness episodes experienced by children. A study by Madan (1981) in an Indian city observed essentially similar trends.

Turning to the conditions that are considered to be the risk factors for cardiovascular diseases, such as essential hypertension, obesity, high blood sugar, some epidemiological investigations on blood pressures and blood glucose among the two tribal populations, viz., Lepchas and Bhutias of Sikkim were conducted. For example, Mukhopadhyay and Mukhopadhyay (2001) observed that both rural and urban Lepchas have high prevalence of essential hypertension and as expected, urban Lepchas showed higher prevalence of hypertension as well as higher number of borderline cases compared to their rural counterparts (Table 7). Urban Lepchas show higher mean values of both systolic and diastolic blood pressures (Table 8).

Table 7

Essential Hypertension among Lepchas of Sikkim

Type	*Rural*	*Urban*
Hypertensive	60 (28.85)	41 (29.71)
Borderline cases	24 (11.54)	26 (18.84)
Normotensive	124 (59.61)	71 (51.45)
Total	208 (100.0)	138 (100.0)

Note: Figures in parentheses indicate percentages.

Source: Mukhopadhyay and Mukhopadhyay, 2001.

Table 8

Blood Pressure among Lepchas of Sikkim by Residence Status

	Sample size	*Systolic*		*Diastolic*	
		Mean	*Standard error*	*Mean*	*Standard error*
Rural	208	127.91	1.01	85.46	1.01
Urban	138	131.33	1.01	90.68	1.01

Source: Mukhopadhyay and Mukhopadhyay, 2001.

In a recent study (Sarkar and Mukhopadhyay, 2003) of the Bhutias, inhabiting the town of Gangtok and its neighbourhood, high prevalence of both systolic and diastolic hypertension has been found (Table 9). Further, prevalence of obesity, as measured by Body Mass Index (BMI) value, has been found to be 34 percent and 39 percent among the females and males, respectively (Table 10). In the same study population, 40 percent of adult individuals, combining both sexes, showed high fasting blood glucose values, above the reference range for normality (Table 11). The above data sets show evidences suggesting the fact that in the Sikkim Himalaya, urban tribal populations are adversely affected by cardiovascular risk factors.

Table 9

Prevalence of Essential Hypertension among Urban Bhutias of Sikkim

	Male	*Female*	*Total*
Systolic (>140mm/Hg)	31 (31)	25 (25)	56 (28)
Diastolic (>90 mm/Hg)	39 (39)	28 (28)	67 (33.5)
Systolic and diastolic	28 (28)	22 (22)	50 (50)

Note: Figures in parentheses indicate percentages.

Source: Sarkar and Mukhopadhyay, 2003.

Table 10

Prevalence of Obesity among Urban Bhutias of Sikkim

BMI (kg/m²) value	*Male*	*Female*
≤ 18.49	3 (3)	1 (1)
18.50 - 24.99	52 (52)	52 (52)
25.00 - 29.99	39 (39)	34 (34)
30.00 - 39.99	6 (6)	13 (13)
Total	100 (100)	100 (100)

Notes: Obesity measured by BMI value. Figures in parentheses indicate percentages.
Source: Sarkar and Mukhopadhyay, 2003

Table 11

Prevalence of Hyperglycemia among Urban Bhutias of Sikkim

Male	*Female*	*Total*
44 (48.5)	28 (31.1)	72 (40.0)

Notes: Fasting blood glucose value above reference range (60-100 mg%). Figures in parentheses indicate percentages.

Source: Sarkar and Mukhopadhyay, 2003.

Health Care Practices and Available Health Care Resources

Observations on the health care practices undertaken by the populations of Sikkim-Darjeeling Himalayas will be largely considered here. It is a regular practice for each community to adopt pluralistic health care regimens in combatting illness episodes. An interesting mix of both traditional and modern medical practices is found to be followed for different kinds of diseases. Different culture-specific traditional medical practices arising out of traditional beliefs remain intertwined with the practice of modern medicine. Generally, government-run health institutions provide modern allopathic medicines almost exclusively. However, homeopathic medicine in some of the health institutions in Darjeeling, and Tibetan medicine in the central referral hospital in Gangtok, Sikkim, are also provided.

An example from amongst the Lepchas of Dzongu area of North district of Sikkim will be of interest to take note of the utilization pattern of traditional *vis-à-vis* modern medicine. For a vast majority of illness episodes, utilization of traditional medicine by way of taking plant and/or animal products happens to be the first option. If the condition is not cured within a specific period, it is believed that 'evil eye' is the cause. This will certainly pave the way for the *Bongthing* (the traditional Lepcha priest) to worship evil spirits and again watch for some days. If then also illness is not cured, utilization of modern medicine by visiting the Primary Health Centre (PHC)/sub-centre is opted for. It is also observed that simultaneous use of modern and traditional medicines is sometimes attempted. This particular scenario is prevalent among many populations in the eastern Himalayas as well as in other locales (Lieban, 1973). It is obvious that educated and modern segments of the populations have undergone cultural changes and are becoming more inclined to utilization of modern medicinal practices. But, even then, worship of evil spirits and other deities is a common practice for preventive health achievements and attainment of general well-being.

The fact remains that the nature and extent of availability of health care resources in a locality influence its population's capacity to utilize such resources. Of course, there are many factors that will determine how and when these resources will be utilized or underutilized by the local communities. In Sikkim, the network of health institutions has been continually developed since its merger with the Indian Union. From primary to tertiary level, much progress has been achieved in several aspects of health infrastructure development and implementation of health programmes (Chuttani and Gyatso, 1993; Lahiri *et al.*, 2001). Generally, disease eradication programmes of the Central Ministry of Health and Family Welfare are implemented through health institutions and national norms for health infrastructure aspects are accomplished already. For instance, the national norm of establishing one PHC for 20,000 population and one sub-centre for 3,000 people has been possible. Staff pattern and supply of medicines in the health institutions are also presently satisfactory (Lama, 2001). Additionally, Indian system of medicines, i.e., ayurveda, and homeopathy are also serving some sections of urban populations. Tibetan medicine is also popularly practised in the state, which is patronized by the state government as well as private enterprise of the Tibetan establishment of Dharamsala, Himachal Pradesh. In the rural areas, however, clinics providing treatment by the Tibetan system of medicine are presently absent. Barring the ethno-medicine specialists of several tribal and caste populations, no private registered medical practitioners are found to operate in rural areas of Sikkim. In Darjeeling hills, on the contrary, in many rural interior areas, health care resources are presently not that satisfactory. Population density is relatively high compared to Sikkim and the network of health centres is relatively weak. It is often found that in many remote areas of Darjeeling hills, some common allopathic medicines generally used for relief from headache, backache, fever, etc., are sold by the local vendors of bakery products. Remoteness of the geographical location often acts as a barrier in implementing plans for health infrastructure development and particular health programmes. Ethno-medicinal practices are therefore very common there. However, in many remote places of the hill sub-divisions of West Bengal, the medical establishments of the Christian missionaries are providing primary health care services of considerably good quality.

Community Health Care Issues: Newly Emerging Dimensions

It is but obvious that the goal of any health care strategy is to devise mechanisms by which health goals are achieved by reducing the disease/morbidity load experienced by the community. Surely, it is not always an easy task. Since health is a complex phenomenon and depends on a wide variety of factors, health care planning needs consideration of many factors relevant at the local level. Scientific judgement, administrative prudence, economic inputs, and above all, political commitment, are all important considerations for such a planning.

Keeping the above considerations in mind, some examples are provided on newly emerging community health care issues that need to be addressed. And, some suggestions are made that can be of help for community health planning in the Sikkim-Darjeeling Himalayan region in general and for the Sikkim Himalaya in particular. Although variations exist in respect of several components of health care practices and health care resource utilization patterns between populations of Sikkim and Darjeeling hills, because of the cultural and lifestyle similarities to a large extent, it makes a case for adopting broadly similar measures for health care.

It is to be noted that for a considerable majority of rural populations in the area in question, rural health institutions cater to the health needs of the local people. Major activities for these institutions pertain to services on family welfare or specifically ante-natal care to the deserving/willing mothers, immunization for mother and children, and treating common ailments for those who visit these institutions for help. It will be necessary to evaluate the strengths and weaknesses of these institutions in order to be able to assess the functional efficiency of these institutions. In the changing times, many additional health problems that arise out of social stresses and lifestyle changes in many peri-urban and rural areas are to be tackled locally. An analysis of the local problems that impinge upon health scenario will be necessary. Alcoholism, drug abuse and mental health issues have attained importance. Preventive measures for such ailments need urgent attention. Community participation and involvement of social, cultural and political institutions at the local level in an effective manner will be helpful in this regard. Further, it is evident that for many health problems, such as hypertension, liver diseases, obstetric and gynecological ailments, and so on, seeking help for medical care is minimal in the rural areas. As a consequence, morbidity load for the communities is not often properly evaluated. An example from Sikkim, in respect of essential hypertension, can be cited here to explain such a scenario. While prevalence of hypertension, as measured by blood pressure values following the WHO suggested cut-off, was found to be 29 percent in an epidemiological study in the Dzongu area of North Sikkim in 1993 (Mukhopadhyay *et al.*, 1996), extremely low (0.26%) rate of new cases for hypertension was reported in the Dzongu PHC, around the same time (Mukhopadhyay, 1998). It possibly indicates the necessity of regular population-based observed morbidity assessments for the local communities.

Another significant aspect of health problem that needs continuous attention is the high prevalence of iodine deficiency disorders (IDD) such as goitre as well as cretinism in the area. The local primary health institutions need to collaborate with local *panchayat* and/or local community institutions on a permanent basis for mitigating the problem of evaporation of iodine from the iodized salt, which occurs in many rural households owing to faulty storing methods of salt. Lama (2001) observes that the effectiveness of IDD prevention programme in Sikkim depends largely on the retention of adequate iodine content, particularly in the rural settings.

That persistence of tuberculosis (TB) in the eastern Himalayan region happens to be one of the major health concerns is clearly evident. Even after a relatively well-attended government programme in Sikkim for TB control, TB cases and deaths are on the increase. A steady growth of multiple drug resistant (MDR) tuberculosis is observed in the state. Lama (2001) rightly mentions that in Sikkim "the challenge of TB needs to be addressed on a priority basis, through both improved awareness and patient literacy as also greater resource allocation".

It is beyond doubt that urbanization and modernization are increasingly evident in the Sikkim-Darjeeling Himalaya. Because of population growth in the urban areas and also because of the fact that some of the urban areas have become popular tourist destinations, environmental pollution has made inroads. No assessment has yet been made on the health implications of environmental pollution in these urban areas. Such assessments in populations inhabiting the towns of Gangtok and Darjeeling will be necessary.

For providing better health care for the region, urgent attention will be needed to explore possibilities to recognize and bring the traditional medicine men into the formal health care arena. This is a complex issue but it will be a positive step towards better utilization of scarcely available health care resources.

Finally, it is rather apparent that health information generated by the governmental institutions does not capture disease profiles of the populations in its entirety. Assessments on the achievements of national disease eradication programmes are generally recorded. Some special health surveys are occasionally done, though not of much use. However, prevalence estimates based on population surveys of many diseases that are appearing as important ones in the changing socio-cultural environmental scenario are virtually lacking. Furthermore, understanding the determinants of such diseases will be necessary in order to be able to adopt appropriate health care planning. Conducting well-designed epidemiological investigations as well as medical anthropological studies on many chronic and degenerative diseases, gynecological morbidity, liver diseases, alcoholism and the like will be helpful in making a better and realistic health care strategy for the Sikkim-Darjeeling Himalaya.

Concluding Remarks

It can be surmised that there are evidences of changing socio-cultural environmental milieu in the eastern Himalayas, specifically in the Sikkim-Darjeeling Himalayan region that bring forth changing community health profile. The changing scenario of health needs to be addressed through appropriate health care delivery systems, for which reorientation of primary health care strategy may be necessary. Generation of varied types of health information, appropriate for the health care planning, should be given priority. On the basis of such information, innovative and location-specific health care programmes will have to be undertaken.

References

All India Institute of Hygiene and Public Health, Department of Health and Family Welfare, and Government of Sikkim (1989). *A Survey Report on the Nutritional Status in the State of Sikkim*. Gangtok: AIIH&PH, Calcutta and GoS.

Chuttani, C.S. and Gyatso, T.R. (1993). *Health Status of Women and Children in Sikkim.* New Delhi: UNICEF.

Government of Sikkim (1998). *Health Information Bulletin.* Department of Health and Family Welfare, Gangtok: Government of Sikkim.

Lahiri, A., Chattopadhyay, S., Bhasin, A., Premchand, A. and Roy, S. (2001). *Sikkim: The People's Vision*. New Delhi: Government of Sikkim in association with Indus Publishing Company.

Lama, M.P. (2001). *Sikkim Human Development Report 2001*. Government of Sikkim, New Delhi: Gangtok and Social Science Press.

Lieban, R.W. (1973). Medical anthropology. In J.J. Honigmann (Ed.), *Handbook of Social and Cultural Anthropology*. Chicago: Rand McNally.

Madan, T.N. (1981). Who chooses modern medicine and why. In G.R. Gupta (Ed.), *Main Currents in Indian Sociology*, Vol. IV: *The Social and Cultural Context of Medicine in India*. New Delhi: Vikas Publishing House Pvt. Ltd.

Mukhopadhyay, B. (1998). Health scenario in Sikkim: An assessment. In S.C. Rai, R.C. Subdriyal and E. Sharma (Eds.), *Sikkim: Perspectives for Planning and Development*. Gangtok: Sikkim Science Society and Dehradun: Bishen Singh and Mahendra Pal Singh.

— (1997). Morbidity experience and health care use among the Lepchas: A micro-level study of two religious groups. In S. Sengupta (Ed.), *Studies in Anthropology: Recent Perspectives*. New Delhi: Inter-India Publications.

Mukhopadhyay, B., Gupta, R. and Bhattacharya, S. (1996). Haematological traits, religion and rural/urban residence among the Lepchas of Kalimpong subdivision, Darjeeling district, West Bengal (India). *Anthropologischer Anzeiger, 54*, 35-43.

Mukhopadhyay, B. and Mukhopadhyay, S. (2001). Blood pressure and its biocultural correlates among the Lepchas of Sikkim, India: A micro-level epidemiological study. *Collegium Antropologicum, 25*, 97-110.

Mukhopadhyay, B., Mukhopadhyay, S. and Majumder, P.P. (1996). Blood pressure profile of Lepchas of the Sikkim Himalayas: Epidemiological Study. *Human Biology, 68*, 131-145.

Murray, C.J.L., Feachem, R.G.A., Phillips, M.A. and Willis, C. (1992). Adult morbidity: Limited data and methodological uncertainty. In R.G.A. Feachem, T. Kjellstrom, C.J.L. Murray, M. Over and M.A. Phillips (Eds.), *The Health of Adults in the Developing World*. Oxford: Oxford University Press.

Pulger,T., Sankar, R., Rai, B. and Rai, B.M. (1992). *Iodine Deficiency Disorders: Sikkim*. South Sikkim: Thyroid Centre, Government General Hospital, Namchi.

Sarkar, S.S. and Mukhopadhyay, B. (2003). Unpublished manuscript: 'Urban lifestyle and health among the Bhutias of Sikkim'.

World Health Organization (2002). *Health Situation in the South-east Asian Region, 1998-2000*. New Delhi: WHO Regional Office for South-East Asia.

18

Morbidity vis-à-vis Health Behaviour among the Tea Labourers in Assam

R.K. KAR

The Government of India, for the first time, could work out a National Health Policy (NHP) only in 1983. The policy document recognized the health problems and priorities of the rural masses, upholding in the background, the philosophy of the Alma Ata Declaration of Health for All by 2000 A.D., made in 1978. Accordingly, our government seems to have been making utmost efforts to reduce the massive burden of preventable ill-health through extension of health services to the masses. But, as we indulge in a stock-taking exercise, what do we really observe? Though considerable progress has been registered in raising the health status of the people, the fact remains that India is still among the countries having the lowest health status in the world. This raises some fundamental questions. Has the conceptualization of the policy within the divergent socio-cultural background been appropriately conceived? Has there been a matching commitment to operationalize the NHP, in the given socio-cultural, political and administrative milieux?

We know that every culture, irrespective of its simplicity and complexity, has its own notion regarding health and health-seeking behaviour. It is an integral component of the overall culture of the community, particularly of a simpler one. The health of a community, by and large, is a function of the interaction between socio-cultural and biological factors – the genetic attributes and the environmental conditions.

While writing on the ecology of human diseases and adaptation to diseases by human groups, Alland (1970) provides a useful summary of the major dimensions involved, and places these subjects in an anthropological perspective. Among the many factors in human disease ecology, besides sanitation and conditions of living, Alland notes the size, density, mobility of human populations, the organism's environment outside the human host, mode of infection, viability and type of vectors and carriers, immunity symptoms, incubation period, nutrition and stress. He also provides a useful model of adaptation analyzed as "behaviour strategies developed in response to pathology", and shows how these strategies on the part of human groups may succeed or fail as they provide the group with capability to deal with these factors: acute versus chronic disease, complexity of the route of infection, reservoir versus non-reservoir, degree of severity, endemic versus epidemic, degree of prevalence and incidence, discreteness of symptomology and degree of contagion.

There are a good number of other similar works dealing with the adaptive aspects of diseases and stress (e.g., Burnet, 1963; Paul, 1964; Dubos, 1965; Hobson, 1965; Burnet and White, 1972; Mauser and Bahn, 1974; Burton and Smith, 1975; Kar, 2000).

That society is more likely to survive, which is capable of designing cultural techniques, or behaviour strategies in Alland's conception, for preventing infections of its members, healing members once they are infected, and minimizing the possibilities for contagion. Dubos (1965) rightly observes that the prevalence and severity of microbial diseases are conditioned more by the ways of life of the afflicted persons than by the virulence and other properties of the etiological agents. Hence, there is a need to learn more of man and his societies in order to try to make sense of the patterns of his diseases. Of course, it is imperative that all ecological factors from house types to the methods of preparing food, from systems of social control to medical systems, are critical items in determining the health status of a group with regard to disease (infectious and non-infectious, acute and chronic). Likewise, it is the socio-cultural life of a community that generally determines the health care services that they can have the access to, and also the ones they should prefer to avail of.

Keeping all these facts, observations and ideas in mind, in the present paper, an attempt has been made to have an understanding of some aspects of health behaviour among the tea labourers in Assam with special reference to morbidity scenario.

Primary and secondary data incorporated in the study have been generated by the author himself as well as by other researchers from a number of tea plantations in Assam during 1970s, 1980s and 1990s. While generating primary data, standard anthropological techniques like observation, interview and questionnaire/schedule have been used in the field.

Tea Labourers in Assam

The tea and ex-tea labourers in Assam are a migrant population and are heterogeneous in composition. In the early 19th century, during the formative days of Assam plantations, the labour scarcity was a constant hindrance to the expansion of tea cultivation in Assam (Kar and Barua, 1997). At the initial stage, however, the local people like the Kacharis, the Mataks, the Kukis, the Nagas, the Singphos and the Apatanis could be employed with the active assistance of the chiefs of the respective groups (cf Chakravarty, 1973; Gait, 1926; Harlalka, 1975; Roy Burman, 1968; Sharma, 1987). But, these arrangements did not prove to be very successful. Prior to 1860, the local labourers in most of the plantations indulged in a number of protests and revolts (Kar, 1995).

Around 1855, with gradual expansion of the industry, the problem of labour became very acute. It was not only that the local people of Assam were unwilling to work in the tea gardens, but there was also an acute shortage of adult population in Assam to work in the tea gardens. Assam at that time was still experiencing the effect of the Moamaria rebellion (1770-75), the Burmese invasion (1819-24) and the raids of the hill tribes (cf Chakravarty, 1973; Dahotia, 1981; Gait, 1926).

Under the circumstances, the planters started procuring labour from other states of India. The labourers were recruited from various cultural, linguistic and ethnic heritages, mainly from Bengal, Bihar, Orissa, Madhya Pradesh, Andhra Pradesh and Tamil Nadu. Desperate poverty and land alienation on the countryside in those areas and the false promises of "less work and high wages" probably made this huge labour group available for transportation to Assam.

A good number of these labourers initially suffered from maladjustment: some of them died, others went back home after the expiry of the contracted period, and still others fled away before the expiry of that period. A major section of the migrants, however, survived that stage and gradually made up their mind to make a permanent settlement in the new habitat, in a new economy, and far away from their original homes (Kar, 1986).

Abundance of uncultivated land in Assam provided an opportunity to the recruits to have some land for cultivation while working in a plantation, and again after retirement, to have some for their settlement. This prospect of having some usufractuary right on cultivable land was probably an important factor that accelerated the rate of recruitment of labourers, as well as probably contributed to the settlement of the migrant labour/folk in Assam.

Sharma (1990) observes that the process of settlement of these labourers in rural areas began as early as in 1868. This section of the labourers is called ex-tea garden labourers despite the fact that most of them have already passed 3-4 generations since they left the tea gardens. They constitute a sizeable section of the rural population in the tea-growing districts of Assam. The tea labourers are now-a-days popularly known as *Baganiya*, *Bonua* or *Mazdoor*, and the ex-tea labourers as *Bongali*. Many of the members of the ex-tea labour families, who do not have some alternative sources of sustainable income, have been working in the neighbouring tea plantations, either as permanent or casual workers.

Regarding their degree of heterogeneity, it may be noted here that there are more than one hundred tribe and caste groups that compose the tea labour population in Assam. Crawford (1924) has discussed the details of the different groups along with their native homes.

The exact numerical strength of the tea and ex-tea labour population, presently residing in Assam, is not available. It has, however, been estimated that approximately 20 percent of the total population of the state is constituted by this section. The tentative figure, as reported by Kurmi (2000), may stand at around 70 lakh.

The tea industry, it may relevantly be noted here, has exerted some unique influences on the life of the people. They have been exposed to a different but common type of economy, administration, housing and ecology. As observed by a number of authors (e.g., Bhuyan, 1960; Barua, 1963; Gohain, 1974; Ghatowar, 1975; Kar, 1975; Kurmi, 1977; Kar and Baruah, 1979; Phukan, 1984; Karmakar, 1985; Das, 1988), for the purpose of the present discussion, the people have been considered as members of a single community (tea labour) subscribing, by and large, to a common socio-cultural life, notwithstanding some differences observed at micro level.

Diseases among the Tea Labourers

Human diseases have been defined in different forms such as sickness, illness and morbidity (Fasu, 1981). All these are appropriately defined human disorders that disturb normal physical as well as social functioning (Sarkar 1986). Again, Dash (1986) maintains that the occurrence of disease may refer to certain biological conditions of the body which are responsible for causing abnormal or disturbed functions of the parts of system in the body. This may be manifested in different forms in various systems. Moreover, besides the biological or physical causes, illness is also believed to be caused by the aberration of mental, moral or spiritual orders of the individuals.

The tea labourers in Assam seem to possess reasonably sound health. Both men and women work in the tea bed and agricultural field throughout the day, apparently without any physical constraints. The womenfolk, in addition, attend to their domestic chores as well as reproductive obligations. But, as a matter of fact, they have been found to suffer from a good number of diseases/ailments. Records from plantation hospitals (e.g., Kar, 1986; Dowerah, 1995; Barua, 2000) reveal that they suffer from at least 26 frequently occurring diseases. The more common ones include cold and fever, gastroenteritis including worm and other bowel troubles, anaemia, dysentery and diarrhoea, skin diseases including ring worm, eye diseases, rheumatism, ulcer and respiratory problems. The other relatively less frequent diseases are boil, toothache, urinary infection, tuberculosis, measles, dog bite, snake bite, insect bite, tonsilitis, jaundice, cancer, pneumonia, malaria and pox. Morbidity data obtained from the records of four plantation hospitals in different calendar years are presented in Table 1.

Table 1

Percentile Incidence of Major Diseases among the Tea Labourers from Four Different Plantations

Disease	P_1 N= 4,491 (1994)	P_2 N=387 (1991)	P_3 N=2,687 (1981)	P_4 N=13,420 (1979)	*Total* N=20,985
Cold and fever	17.55	17.95	15.98	15.98	16.70
Gastroenteritis including other bowel diseases (including worm)	14.71	13.90	15.58	16.90	15.27
Anaemia	12.75	11.85	11.93	8.15	11.17
Skin diseases (including ring worm)	9.80	9.11	9.97	8.79	9.42
Dysentery	10.29	9.57	9.15	5.07	8.52
Diarrhoea (including bacillary dysentery)	6.95	6.38	8.07	6.59	7.00
Injury	5.39	6.83	5.80	9.97	7.00
Eye disease	7.35	5.69	6.32	5.65	6.25
Rehumatism	3.43	4.78	4.35	10.25	5.70
Respiratory trouble	2.45	4.56	5.62	6.56	4.80
Ulcer	2.55	3.69	2.49	2.42	2.78
Others	6.78	5.69	4.74	4.72	5.48
Total	100.00	100.00	100.00	100.00	100.00

Mancotta (P_1), Chalkhowa and Athabari (P_2) and Rajgarh (P_3) are situated in Dibrugarh district in upper Assam, whereas Monabari (P_4) is situated in Sonitpur district on the northern bank of the mighty Brahmaputra.

A cursory glance of the Table 1 makes it apparent that notwithstanding the minor quantitative differences, the distribution of the different frequently occurring diseases is largely the same in all the plantations except rheumatism, which is more frequent in plantation P_4 than any other plantations. Morbidity data on total population show that barring cold and fever that afflict about 17 percent of the patients, a good number of people (around 44%) suffer from gastroenteritis (15%), anaemia (11%), skin disease (9%) and dysentery (9%). The incidence of other frequent diseases in decreasing order is as follows: diarrhoea and injury (7% each), eye disease (6.25%), rheumatism (5.70%), respiratory diseases (4.80%) and ulcer (2.75%). The less frequent diseases together account for about 5 percent of the patients.

It has, however, been observed that there is a seasonal variation in the incidence of various diseases. Thus, for example, influenza leading to the infection of respiratory tract and acute bacillary dysentery (diarrhoea) are reported to be in higher frequency during monsoon.

It will also be interesting to note that the various diseases show an observable correlation with specific age and sex groups. Thus, for example, infancy (0-4 years) and childhood (4-17 years) seem to be characterized by the incidence of a relatively limited number of diseases/ailments like cold, cough and fever, worm infestation, skin diseases and injuries of various types. Majority of the infant deaths are caused by pneumonia, diarrhoea and nutritional deficiency. This happens partly because of their traditions. For example, in many groups, the mother is required to sleep on the floor and wash her clothes by herself during the confinement period; and mainly because of non-availability of timely medical attention; and also ignorance of the people.

The adults, on the other hand, appear to be more prone to all types of diseases in varying degrees. One of the possible explanations for this observation lies in the fact that during adulthood, the people overexert themselves in the tea beds as well as in their agricultural fields. But, most of them do not take food with requisite nutrient contents. Thus, malnutrition, coupled with their overall unhygienic living condition, poor sanitation and addiction to alcohol, may make them more prone to various diseases. As a matter of fact, they seem to have a relatively poor defence system, and also seem not to be very prompt in taking medicare services. It may, however, be noted here that skin disease and dysentery seem to cut across the age and sex parameters.

The women labourers very often get afflicted with anaemia and gynaecological disorders. Pre- and post-natal anaemia is quite frequent among the pregnant women and the mothers of the newly-born babies. This may be considered as one of the major health problems afflicting women of child-bearing age, contributing substantially towards maternal morbidity and mortality. It very often leads to stillbirth and low birth weight. In two different micro-studies, Kar (1990) observed that the stillbirth rate ranges from 56.14 to 111.11, whereas the infant mortality rate ranges from 60.66 to 123.07. One of the probable reasons for this observation may lie in the fact that during pregnancy a woman does not take any special diet that is necessary for both the mother and the foetus. Besides, though the garden hospitals are supposed to have provision for supplying iron and vitamin tablets to the pregnant women free of cost, in many cases, these are not available, and in many other situations people do not seem to volunteer themselves to avail of the benefit. It may relevantly be highlighted that in many cases, despite the availability of relatively improved medical facilities in the form of modern medicines and improved equipment, the people, by and large, still rely mainly on the *ojhas* and sorcerers, that is, their traditional medicine men. They believe that these medicine men have spiritual and magical expertise for curing diseases. Many people attribute disease and pre-mature death to evil spirits and the act of magicians or breach of taboos. They go to the traditional medicine man or the magician who discovers the causes of the ailment and prescribes appropriate sacrifices or counter-magic.

Health Behaviour and Morbidity

Most of the ethnic communities constituting tea labour population in Assam seem to have their own concepts of various ailments, disease causation and preventive and curative measures. Besides the natural causes, most of the groups believe that diseases occur under certain other conditions are like:

(1) Wrath of ancestral spirits for showing negligence or disrespect to them.
(2) Interference of some supernatural agency (their worshipping deity). It is considered to be the major cause, responsible for the incidence of most of the diseases. If any deity is dissatisfied for any act of omission or commission of a person, he/she or any member of his/her family may be inflicted with some disease by way of punishment.
(3) Aggressive intention of *jati* (community) mates or neighbours with magical potentiality to cause harm out of envy.
(4) Projection of morbid objects or substances.
(5) Abstraction of some organ from, or an organic component of the body.
(6) The action of a sorcerer on some part of the body or some objects, once associated with the body of a person. This concept of disease is based on the concept of supernaturalism and sorcery as an expression of contagious magic.
(7) Spirit intrusion.
(8) Individual act (deliberate or inadvertent) of breach of taboo.

For example, the Oraons believe that when a child weeps and laughs too much, it means *Kandi Devi* or *Rati Devi* and *Hashani Devi* (some malevolent spirits) have entered into the body of the child to cause the disease. To appease the responsible spirit, the *ojha* offers *pujas*. Similarly, for an expectant mother, the society prescribes a series of restrictions/taboos, the breach of which may cause a number of diseases among the children. Thus, after the fifth month of conception, an expectant mother is forbidden to take pork and indulge in sexual cohabitation. It is believed that if she takes pork during the period, the new-born baby may have deformities in the body. In case, she sleeps with her husband during the period, there may be eczema on the head of the baby. For such eczema, the local medicine man himself prepares herbal medicine for external application.

Though the people believe that a woman conceives only by the blessings of God, pregnancy is considered to be a natural phenomenon. They do not seem to consider it necessary to have regular medical check-up and to administer medicine during pregnancy. Only a very few educated and the baptised families go for the same in the plantation hospital.

Generally, the delivery of a baby takes place at home (labour quarters), being attended by women only. No male member, including the husband, is allowed to be present at the delivery spot. The expectant mother is helped in the delivery by the old and experienced women, usually a kinswoman (mother-in-law) or a neighbour. The members of the medical staff, as a convention, never attend a patient in the labour quarters. Data collected from a number of plantations in this regard reveal that not more than 15 percent of the deliveries take place in the hospital. In many groups, the traditional belief is that the placenta is to be disposed of by some specific kin member within the household compound. So, hospitalization of an expectant mother is, in many cases, the last resort.

The traditional curative measures preferred and highly valued by the tea labourers can broadly be classified into three categories, namely, (a) magical extraction and counter-magical endeavours, (b) sacrifices, offerings and prayer to the deity, and (c) administration of medicinal herb.

As preventive measures, in a number of diseases, some rituals are performed at regular intervals. For example, in *Gram Puja*, the Savaras and many other groups propitiate the village gods (*Gaon ka Malik*) to protect the villagers from any misfortune; *Thakuranima* (spirit, believed to be responsible for epidemic diseases like smallpox and cholera) is propitiated in *Mongol Puja*; *Kali* (spirit connected with the family welfare) gets a share of any sacrifice made in a family ritual, and so on. They believe that propitiations of these deities, spirits and family ancestors protect the families and the entire community from different unforeseen odds and hazards.

Sometimes (e.g., in case of cough, fever and dysentery) modern medical attention is sought immediately and is followed by traditional treatment and the two go side by side. Sometimes again, they attend hospital only to get medical leave sanctioned with full wages, as per the existing provisions of the Plantation Labour, P.L. Act, 1951.

Morbidity and Living Condition

Besides insufficient management of the health care services and the people's traditional beliefs and practices, it seems that a good number of other possible human factors do contribute towards the observed morbidity scenario among the people under investigation. Incidence of quite a good number of diseases can probably be explained in terms of environmental sanitation, food habits and the overall life style of the people.

The environmental sanitation in a tea labour settlement is by and large very poor. The P.L. Act, 1951, along with Plantation Labour (PL) Rules, 1956, has defined many conditions of labour employment in clear terms. Various social security benefits for them have also been provided in the Act (cf Barua, 2000). However, in reality, most of the provisions, especially those with regard to health, hygiene and sanitation (and also education), have not been found to be implemented properly in most of the plantations.

Thus, for example, under clause 8 of the P.L. Act, in every plantation, effective arrangements shall be made by the employer to provide and maintain a sufficient supply of wholesome drinking water for all the workers at convenient places in the plantation. According to clause 9(1), a sufficient number of latrines and urinals of prescribed types shall be provided separately for males and females in every plantation, so situated as to be convenient and accessible to the workers employed therein.

The standard of these facilities has been found to be quite good in some plantations. But, in other ones, the facilities are far from being satisfactory. Provision of drinking water, community bathrooms and drainage system is inadequate in many plantations. Besides the numerical insufficiency, in many cases, the tubewells have not been provided with any *pucca* platforms and drainage outlets from their basements. Absence of proper drainage arrangement sometimes converts many labour settlements into pigsties with the accumulation of filth and muck that provide a breeding ground for various organic disease agents. As a consequence, the people are afflicted with a number of diseases. The situation worsens during the rainy season.

According to clause 58 of the Act, at least 8 percent of the labour quarters should be made *pucca* annually. But, a huge number of *kaccha* quarters with thatched roof in a very dilapidated condition are seen in many plantations. Because of waterlogging, in many labour settlements during monsoon, these quarters become very damp and the inmates suffer from a number of ailments. Family latrines are also absent in most of the cases and the members respond to the nature's call in tea bushes, bamboo grooves or in some other convenient outdoor spots.

Observations on household and housing pattern make it apparent that the overall living condition of the people is responsible for a good number of diseases. As a matter of fact, gross lack of personal cleanliness, sanitation, potable water, minimum light and ventilation in the house are responsible for the incidence of a number of diseases. Thus, there seems to be positive association between diseases like tuberculosis and conjunctivitis and lack of light and ventilation in the house, infantile diarrhoea and impurity of water and lack of cleanliness, skin disease and lack of personal cleanliness, and unsanitary habits and occurrence of worm infestations. Poor lighting during night hours, absence of suitable exit arrangement of smoke, i.e., too much of smoke in crowded and ill-ventilated houses may be a cause (in addition to Vitamin A deficiency) for the high incidence of eye troubles (night-blindness). Non-availability of fresh air during night may be a contributing factor towards respiratory troubles.

Absence of any drainage system, as noted earlier, helps the germs of different bacterial diseases, e.g., diarrhoea, dysentery, typhoid and paratyphoid fever to multiply. Flies, which also breed in the accumulated sullage water, may carry different viruses from sewage to food during the monsoon, and this may be aggravated by the habit of defecation in the open. Improper disposal of night soil and human excreta may be responsible for (a) direct infection in man, (b) the contamination of soil, and (c) the possibility of disease transference to man through the agency of insects or animals.

The habit of defecating in the open is an important factor responsible for hookworm infestation. The eggs of hookworms pass out with faeces and are deposited on the soil. These may be scattered to nearby soil by rain and wind. In suitable environment, these eggs may develop into larvae. These larvae usually find their way back into the human body through the skin of the barefoot. The retention of wet soil or mud between the toes greatly favours the larvae's entry into the human body.

It has been stated earlier that the incidence of anaemia is quite high among the people. Hookworm infestation along with repeated pregnancy also results in anaemia. This may be a reason why anaemia is more frequent among women of reproductive age. Among the menfolk, one of the other contributing factors may be their regular habit of drinking alcohol. Gastritis generally follows the drinking of liquor which in turn prevents iron absorption that ultimately leads to anaemia.

All these, however, relate to the observed deficiencies and flaws in the preventive and promotive strategies with regard to the people's morbidity scenario.

With regard to the curative aspects, it may once again be highlighted that the medicare service facilities and the management of the same are not satisfactory in many cases, and in many other instances, the traditional beliefs and practices of the people deter them from timely acceptance of the available health care services.

Concluding Remarks

The foregoing discussion makes it clear that both the elements of culture in the form of health habits as well as the inadequate provision of requisite health care services made by the management, do make a significant contribution towards the observed morbidity scenario among the tea labourers in Assam.

Thus, it seems, the problem of health welfare and an overall development of the community needs a two-way approach for finding a probable solution. Alongside the provision for proper medical and sanitation facilities, the people need to be carefully motivated and educated, on the one hand, for undoing some of their habits (e.g., addiction to alcohol and outdoor defecation habit), and on the other hand, for availing of the available modern health facilities in time and in true spirit.

The following tentative strategies may be contemplated for the purpose:

(1) Efforts should be made for proper sanitation, personal hygiene, safe drinking water, and dispelling misbelieves, taboos, magico-religious practices, etc.
(2) Health services in the form of health education should be given more emphasis by developing effective communication strategies on health education and health care.
(3) Young boys and girls from the labour community should be given training in public health and mid-wifery respectively. They may regularly visit the labour settlements and advise the people on health, sanitation and the necessity of availing of the modern medical attention in time. In the meantime, the trained midwives may attend the expectant mothers in the labour settlements in need. This is expected to reduce the stillbirth and infant mortality rate among the people.
(4) Efforts should be made for an effective Family Welfare Programme among the people.
(5) Studies at micro level need to be conducted to evaluate the nutritional status and health.
(6) In view of the fact that the people have their traditional concept of ailment and health-seeking means, efforts should be made to have a negotiable synthesis between the two systems in order to avoid confrontation and enhance acceptability of the modern medicare system.
(7) An effective collaboration and coordination between the management and the NGOs may be a fruitful exercise in this direction.

References

Alland, A. (1970). *Adaptation in Cultural Evolution: An Approach to Medical Anthropology*. New York: Columbia University Press.

Barua, R. (1963). *Seuj Pator Kahini* (Assamese). Shillong: Chapala Sahitya Sadan.

Baruah, T. (2000). *Mundas in Tea Plantation: A Study in Their Health Behaviour*. Dibrugarh: N.L. Publisher.

Bhuyan, N.C. (1960). *Cha Bagichar Banua* (Assamese). Jorhat: Assam Sahitya Sabha.

Burnet, F.M. (1963). *The Integrity of the Body*. Cambridge, Mass: Harvard University Press.

Burnet, M. and White, D.O. (1972). *Natural History of Infectious Disease*. Cambridge: Cambridge University Press.

Burton, L.D. and Smith, H.H. (1975). *Public Health and Community Medicine for the Allied Medical Professions*. Baltimore: The William and Wilkins Co.

Chakravarty, L.N. (1973). *Glimpses of Early History of Arunachal*. Shillong: Research Department, Arunachal Pradesh Administration.

Crawford, T.O. (1924). *Handbook of Castes and Tribes Employed on the Tea Estates in North-East India*. Calcutta: Indian Tea Association.

Dahotia, S.K. (1981). *Maran Matak Mayamora*. Calcutta: Indian Studies, Past and Present.

Dash, J. (1986). The concept and treatment of disease in tribal Orissa. In Chaudhuri, B. (Ed.), *Tribal Health*. New Delhi: Inter-India Publications.

Das, P.K. (1988). *Cha-bagichar Ahomiya* (Assamese). *Prantik*, Vol.7, No.28.

Dowerah, B. (1995). *Health Behaviour of the Sobors of Mancotta Tea Plantation, Dibrugarh, Assam*. Unpublished M.Sc. Dissertation, Dibrugarh: Dibrugarh University.

Dubos, R. (1965). *Man Adapting*. New Haven: Yale University Press.

Fasu, G.B. (1981). Disease classification in rural Ghana: Framework and implications for health behaviour. *Social Science and Medicine, 115*, 474.

Gait, E. (1926). *A History of Assam* (Reprint, 1933). Calcutta: Thacker, Spink and Co.

Ghatowar, N. (1975). *Banuar Sanskritik Jiwanar Ebhumukhi* (Assamese). Jorhat: Assam Sahitya Sabha.

Gohain, R. (1974). *Karampuja aru Jhumur Geet* (Assamese). Jorhat: Assam Sahitya Sabha.

Harlalka, S.S. (1975). *Tea Garden Labour in Assam*. Dhubri: People's Publishing House.

Hobson, W. (1965). *The History and Practice of Public Health*. London: Oxford University Press.

Kar, R.K. (1975). Unity in diversity: A note on the process of adaptation of a tribe in tea industry. *Bulletin of the Department of Anthropology*, Dibrugarh University, *4*, 11-15.

— (1986). A note on health and sanitation among the tea labour in Assam. *Vanyajati*, *34*, 1-9.

— (1990). Health and sanitation versus culture: An appraisal of tea labour in Assam. In B. Chaudhuri (Ed.), *Cultural and Environmental Dimensions on Health*. New Delhi: Inter-India Publications.

— (1995). *Assamer cha-shramik ebong Orang upajati* (Bengali). *Nandan, 31*, 53-55.

— (2000). Ecology of health and culture: A case study among the tea labourers in Assam. In R. Khongsdier (Ed.), *Contemporary Research in Anthropology*. New Delhi: Commonwealth Publishers.

Kar, R.K. and Baruah, G. (1979). Tea labour: Preliminary appraisals of common identity in a multi-ethnic community: A case study in Assam. *Man in India*, *59*, 33-42.

Kar, R.K. and Baruah, T. (1997). Morbidity and health behaviour: A case study among the migrant Munda tea labourers. In F. A. Das and R.K. Kar (Eds.), *Health Studies in Anthropology*. Dibrugarh: Dibrugarh University.

Karmakar, M. (1985). Cha majdoor samaj aru sanskriti. In N. Ghatowar (Ed.), *Hansali* (Assamese). Dibrugarh: Asam Tea and Ex-Tea Garden Tribes Association.

Kurmi, G.C. (2000). Cha janajatir samajik unnayanar samasya (Assamese). *Amar Asom* (An Assamese Daily). Guwahati, 25 January, p.3.

Kurmi, S. (1977). *Tushu Geetor Majhe* (Assamese). Dibrugarh: Dibrugarh Cha Mazdoor Sapha.

Mauser, J.S. and Bahn, A.K. (1974). *Epidemiology: An Introductory Text*. Philadelphia: W.B. Sunders Co.

Paul, H. (1964). *The Control of Disease (Social and Communicable)*. Baltimore: The Williams and Wilkins Co.

Phukan, U. (1984). *The Ex-Tea Garden Labour Population in Assam*. Delhi: B.R. Publishing Co.

Roy Burman, B.K. (1968). *Socio-economic Process in Tea Plantation with special reference to Tribal Labourers*. Delhi: Census of India, 1961. Vol. 1. of VII-A.

Sarkar, P.C. (1986). Culture, disease and treatment system in rural Bangladesh. *Social Science International*, *2*, 22-30.

Sharma, J.L. (1987). *Tradition and Change Among the Migrant Oraons in Assam: A Case Study*. Unpublished Ph.D. Dissertation, Dibrugarh: Dibrugarh University.

Sharma, J.L. (1990). Ex-tea labour settlement in upper Assam: A case study. In S. Karotempral and B. Dutta Roy (Eds.), *Tea Garden Labourers in North-East India*. Shillong: Vendrame Institute.

19

Methodological Issues of Participatory Health Care Management: A Case Study of Maternal Anaemia among the Urban Poor of Tamil Nadu

V. SUDARSEN, S. SUMATHI AND P.I. PRABHAKAR

The prevalence of nutritional anaemia and its potentially deleterious effects on pregnant, lactating and menstruating women, as well as on growing children, is a major public health problem in India (Nair, 1999). Several studies carried out during the last 50 years have shown a high prevalence of maternal anaemia (WHO, 1982; 1992a; 1992b). The causes and consequences of maternal anaemia in the above mentioned groups are manifold (ICMR, 1989; Prema, 1981; Usha *et al.*, 1995). Nutritional deficiencies such as iron, folic acid and Vitamin B12 deficiency are the main causes of anaemia (Allen and Ahluwalia, 1997). Poor socio-economic conditions, poverty, illiteracy, contaminated environment and cultural beliefs are some contributing factors of anaemia.

Maternal anaemia is seen as a medical or technical problem, and narrow technical solutions are sought without understanding the essential causal factors such as powerlessness of the community. Unless the community is empowered through different strategies to utilize/comply with the programmes and services, the expected results will not be realized.

This being the background, an operation research project was planned to address the above issues of empowerment of field functionaries, and empowerment of women of the local community to determine whether the implementation of a suitable programme can reduce maternal anaemia. This project proposed to compare the existing government health delivery system with two alternative approaches. In the first approach, the field level functionaries are empowered to address and analyze the problem of maternal anaemia and decide the intervention and methods of implementation with support from the health care delivery system. In the second approach, the local community members, particularly women's groups, are empowered to assess and analyze the problem of maternal anaemia and decide on interventions and methods of implementation in partnership with the local field functionaries.

In this paper, an attempt is made to bring out the methodological issues and the inability of large multidisciplinary teams to come to grip with the ground realities. The intricacies of this process presented here will be useful in planning and implementing future projects of managing specific health problems.

This paper is presented in terms of phases of the project followed by an analysis at the end of each phase.

Preparatory Period (January-October '97)

(1) UNICEF (Madras office) took the initiative and brought together experts from several fields – epidemiology, urban studies, economics and anthropology – to discuss and formulate the project. A Programme Officer of UNICEF (Chennai office) introduced the framework paper which formed the basis for discussion.

(2) The major and primary objective of this project was to reduce the rate of anaemia, especially among the pregnant women among the urban poor.

(3) In order to achieve the primary objective, a single research question was formulated which the present project envisaged to answer at the end. It was:

Can empowerment of field-level functionaries of government programmes and empowerment of local communities improve implementation of identified set of interventions that will result in a demonstrable reduction in maternal anaemia?

(4) Keeping in view the primary objective and the research question, the methodology was determined:

(i) The study included all women in the age group of (15-45) years.

(ii) The study was conducted in the UBSP[1] (Urban Basic Infrastructure for the Poor) and non-UBSP areas of Dindigul and Tiruppur towns of Tamil Nadu.

(iii) Two models – "the community empowerment" and the "field functionary empowerment" – were envisaged to be tested.

(iv) The whole project was planned to be conducted in three main phases:

(a) Baseline survey

(b) Intervention phase

(c) Evaluation

(v) The whole intervention was planned to be carried out in a participatory and learning mode. In this phase, the local community, governmental agencies and the project personnel were supposed to work together as equal partners.

(vi) The impact of interventions and the relative efficacy of the two models was planned to be measured by gathering data on the proportion of women in the age group of 15–45 years with haemoglobin (Hb) levels < 11gm/dl in the first three months (baseline) and comparing it with similar data generated in the last three months (evaluation) in each town.

(vii) Similarly, the Anthropological Base Line Survey (BLS) was conducted to collect data on the levels of awareness, food habits, traditional practices of treatment pertaining to anaemia among the communities of the two towns. A similar study on the same communities in the last three months of the project was planned to be conducted to evaluate whether there is any change in the broad parameters as a result of interventions.

(viii) The original time-frame to complete the project was 24 months, of which three months from for BLS, 18 months for the intervention phase and three months for evaluation.

Analysis and Findings

- There was no clear understanding as to why this project has to be conducted in two towns.
- It is taken for granted that the UBSP structure/organization works as per the precept and the community is very vibrant and hence empowerment is a simple process.
- Similarly, it is also taken for granted that the field functionaries (FF) can carve out an 'autonomous' space for themselves in organizing and implementing the micro plans they draw.
- There was good amount of discussion and planning on the baseline survey phase on both epidemiological as well as anthropological parts. But, there was almost no discussion as to what constitutes intervention and no planning of intervention phase, except for the mention of Participatory Learning and Action (PLA) workshops.
- How are the plans of the field functionaries/local community going to be ploughed back into intervention activities? Rather, the question is how is the 'participatory learning' process going to be operationalized? This kind of a discussion was completely missing.
- Planning an 'evaluation' phase at the end of the project was to bring out the impact of eighteen months of interventions; by comparing the baseline data and the data generated in the last three months, one gets to assess the changes and also the relative efficacy of the two models. This certainly was very much true theoretically in epidemiological terms than anthropological. Cultural values and practices, even those impinging on anaemia, do not change in such a short time.

Now, a brief description of different phases of the project is presented below:

Phase I: Baseline Survey (November '97-May '98)

What was surveyed and why?

(1) The anthropological survey was started to generate data about the major communities living in the slums of UBSP and

non-UBSP areas, their distribution, sanitary conditions, the infrastructural facilities available, and so on.

(2) On the basis of the preliminary field reports, a careful selection of clusters of four to five representative slums in each town was made. Within each cluster, purposive sampling of households in terms of proportion of the major communities of the study was followed.

How was the survey conducted?

(1) Following three major techniques for data collection were utilized:
— Focus group method,
— Case study, and
— Household schedule.

(2) The basic information that was generated through the focus group method was on awareness, food system, treatment and risk factors. Focus groups were drawn from five different categories as under:
— Post-pubertal girls,
— Married women without children,
— Married women with children,
— Post-menopausal women, and
— Married men.

(3) Case studies consisting of interviews with individuals in the study area were conducted to fill the gaps in the information collected through the focus group methods.

(4) Household schedules were used to relate the socio-economic data to the levels of anaemia in the various communities. About 200 households were selected in each town for this purpose.

What did the baseline suggest?

The data generated through this survey were analyzed in terms of the four areas, viz., UBSP intervention, UBSP control, non-UBSP intervention and non-UBSP control areas. It was found that there was no significant difference between the four areas, whereas the differences in terms of communities, cutting across the four areas, have been significant. Hence, the analysis was continued in terms of the major communities.

Towns surveyed

Dindigul

(i) The four major communities among the urban poor in Dindigul are the Chakkiliyar (SC), Parayar (SC), Paramalai Kallar (OBC) and Muslims. The knowledge and awareness of the focus groups vary according to the age and experience. However, community-wise, the four major communities feel that maternal anaemia is a normal condition, which does not need any specific medical attention. The women groups use different linguistic terminology, which perhaps reflects their awareness of the problems of anaemia. Each community segregates the food items into "hot and cold" and "good and bad" in different trimester periods during pregnancy. Green vegetables are considered as good food to reduce anaemia. The household survey shows that majority of the households depend on public handpump for their source of drinking water and public toilets for their personal use. The household food expenditure shows that the majority of them live in poor conditions.

(ii) Community-wise observation indicates that Chakkiliyar is the most affected group in respect of poverty and lack of other facilities compared to Parayar, Paramalai Kallar and Muslim. Their perceptions about anaemia, however, have little variation while their food patterns and cultural practices vary considerably. The members of the Kallar community marry at young age. Muslims consider that non-vegetarian food is good, while other communities feel that vegetarian food is good during pregnancy.

Tiruppur

(i) Gounder, Chakkiliyar and Muslims are the main groups inhabiting the slums of Tiruppur.

(ii) The focus group members in Tirupur perceive industrial work as the major risk factor. However, some of them feel that anaemia occurs due to a 'pica habit' while others feel that it is due to body heat. All the members accepted vegetables as 'good food'. Members of the community feel that herbal treatment is the best one. But, the knowledge of 'good food' varies among the different communities. The married men of the group consider short birth interval, teenage pregnancy and heavy work burden as risk factors of anaemia.

(iii) Though the communities have good earning possibilities in Tirupur, their living conditions were poor. They depend on public facilities for their fulfilment of basic needs such as water and toilet. High percentage of food expenditure (73% of the households spend more than 55% on food alone) indicates that they are in poverty. This leaves very little amount for other essentials like health care and sanitation.

A Comparative Account of Dindigul and Tiruppur

(i) The average household size in Dindigul is 4.7 whereas in Tiruppur it is 4.4.

(ii) In both the towns majority of the people live in tiled houses. However, the frequency of tiled houses is more in Dindigul (58.5%) than in Tirupur (91%).

(iii) Similarly, a majority of the households surveyed in each town have access to a public tap. Again, the proportions vary between Dindigul (86.5%) and Tiruppur (56.5%).

(iv) Although a majority of households surveyed in both the towns have no toilets in the premises of the houses, the proportions vary between Dindigul (89.5%) and Tirupur (70%). It is significant to note that 24 percent of all the households surveyed in Tiruppur have access to flush toilets within the premises of their houses.

(v) The per capita income/expenditure is more in Tirupur than in Dindigul. But, when the expenditure on food as a percentage of total expenditure is considered, distinct trends are observed community-wise. It is seen that 24.3 percent of the Chakkiliyar households in Dindigul spend less than 55 percent of their total expenditure on food, while only 9.8 percent of the households of Chakkiliyar of Tirupur fall in this category. Thus, the Chakkiliyar in Tiruppur has relatively less to spend on other needs like health and education.

(vi) The Hb levels clearly show a distinct trend in Dindigul and Tiruppur – whether considered in general or community-wise. The Hb levels are higher in Tirupur than in Dindigul. This is a cumulative effect of higher per capita availability of food, greater access to individual tap water and access to flush toilets in the premises of the houses.

Analysis and Findings of Baseline Survey

- All the communities, both from Dindugal and Tirupur, and from whatever study area they come from, consider that maternal anaemia is common during pregnancy. In fact, some of them consider it inevitable. They do not think that it can be prevented. This fact is not tackled at the intervention phase at all.
- The awareness about anaemia is quite reasonably high, again, among all the communities. Some of them have potentially effective curative practices. However, there is a clear disjuncture between the awareness and actual practice. Almost everyone agrees that consumption of green leafy vegetables is good in general and for anaemic in particular, but in practice not even 10 percent of the households surveyed consume green vegetables on a regular basis.
- Although there is considerable data on consumption of food at the household level, the data on intra-household sharing of food is very limited.
- Use of iron vessels for cooking is very limited and used only for frying. The basic reason is the strong perception that iron vessels consume more fuel while cooking.
- The use of footwear (or the non-use, as often the case) follows a pattern. Almost none of the people use footwear within the house, except for a few, who are relatively better off. Most of the people do not use footwear when they are in their neighbourhood. Majority of the people who use footwear, use them when they go out of their neighbourhood to distant places. Most of the houses are single-room tenements and hence they do not normally come with footwear inside, and leave them on the threshold. Obviously, the concept of private/public

domain explains why the women do not use footwear while they are in their neighbourhood. As long as they are not wearing footwear, they are in their neighbourhood, and as long as they are in their neighbourhood, they are in the private domain. Stepping out with footwear means entering the public domain.

- In Dindugal, the database is exclusively community-oriented to the exclusion of field functionaries. To a large extent, this imbalance was overcome in Tirupur where field functionaries formed a part of the BLS.
- It would have served a better purpose had the community-centred data from UBSP intervention area and FF-centred data from non-UBSP intervention area been generated. Though these two sets of data are generated from Tirupur, they are not exclusively from the two study areas where the two models are to be tested.

Phase II: Interventions (June '98-May '99)

(1) The documentation part of this phase was the responsibility of the anthropology team. This team was not involved in any intervention activity directly.

(2) During the preparatory period, there was intensive discussion and minute planning for the baseline survey but not for the intervention phase. From the beginning it was the intention of the core group not to provide a rigid framework for intervention. Such an understanding was based on the bottom-up and participatory approach, which was being adopted for the intervention phase. As a part of this was the initiation of Participatory Learning and Action (PLA) workshops. However, it was agreed upon that such workshops should be conducted only after the BLS in Dindigul.

It was the understanding that the PLA workshops will be conducted at different levels; starting with the most wide – the trainers training workshop – and at the bottom will be the one at the level of the Neighbourhood Group (NhG). Once the PLA training is given, the community at the NhG level was expected to takeover and ultimately leading to planning for the reduction of maternal anaemia in their area. The intervention team was expected to facilitate this process and the anthropology team was vested with the responsibility of recording this process by using appropriate methods.

(3) The anthropology team started documenting the first round of meetings/training at the local level. At the end of the first round of the 'training' exercise, it was realized that there was not much of PLA in those exercises and there was absolutely no micro-planning at all. The PLA training was not standardized.

(4) The second major issue, which has emerged in this context, is that the PLA trainings are being organized in such a way that both community leaders and the field functionaries were participants in the same training session. From the standpoint of the methodology agreed upon, this leads to severe complications, as these two groups have to work out their own micro-plans.

(5) The anthropology team has further improvised the methodology for generating data for documentation and it was followed till the end of March 1999.

(6) It was at the Scientific Advisory Committee (SAC) that the seriousness of the matter was realized and it was decided to discuss these issues alone and to decide the future strategy.

Analysis of Interventions

- There was no integrated strategy for intervention phase. Through out this phase 'intervention' remained nebulous. Intervention phase started in Dindugal even before the BLS started in Tirupur. That situation could have been fruitfully used in Tirupur to avoid the shortcomings of intervention in Dindugal, but it did not happen.
- The intervention phase remained a hazy one, as the only activity that was discussed and was supposed to be implemented was the PLA workshop.
- At the ground level, these workshops took in the shape of meetings/trainings and the content of these was confined to talking to the participants about PLA techniques.
- Often, these meetings/trainings remained without any methodological purpose: what are the participants from local

community supposed to do with this knowledge? How are they going to translate this knowledge into something connected to maternal anaemia? More importantly, where is the participatory process in this exercise? These questions remained unanswered throughout this phase.

- Generally, the meetings were conducted as a part of a mechanical motion to complete the routine, rather than with a purpose and commitment. These meetings lasted less than an hour and the UBSP structure, which was supposed to be integrated into this intervention process, remained just on paper.
- No effort was made during this phase to create interventional situations that could pave the way for testing the two models.
- There was hardly any effort to use the participatory learning mode, with the result the community took it for granted that it is "another of those governmental meetings" for which they need some people. They were never involved so as to feel that it is their programme and planning that the project management is looking for.
- Essentially, what this project envisaged to accomplish – to empower the community – is swept away by the bureaucratic attitude of the project team itself. The project managers were not sensitized to understand the participatory learning role they need to play.

Change in Intervention Strategy

It was in the extended core group meeting held on 12th April, 1999 that some clarification was made on participatory research methods, grounded theory and linkages between the three main groups working in the project. It was agreed that the intervention should not be extractive but should be participatory and learning mode. The alternative strategy suggested was clustering method[2] for desirable outcomes to be taken up at household level.

(1) It was also decided that the anthropology team would find out the cognitive explanations for the clustering phenomena. It would also report back after meeting field functionaries whether or not to continue as the second arm of FF model.

(2) Three major parameters that would be considered for clustering were: (i) food and food habits, (ii) medicines and treatment, and (iii) sanitation. On the basis of these three, households in an NhG would be clustered. This process of clustering of households in an NhG would be conducted and recorded by the anthropology team. There was a considerable discussion on the logistics of clustering process. Since clustering of households cannot be done among all the NhGs of UBSP area, one NhG each from the 14 neighbourhood communities (NhCs) in Dindigul could be taken up for clustering. It was decided that when an NhG is being clustered, the Resident Community Volunteers (RCVs) of the rest of the NhGs of the same NhC would be observers of this process. Later, these RCVs would conduct the clustering process in their respective NhGs.

(3) At the field level, there was an immediate impediment. The anthropology team found that none of the NhGs have a clear-cut household affiliation and often many do not know their RCV.

(4) It took more than two months for the anthropology team to structure the NhGs in two NhCs with the result, the Focus Groups for clustering of households started only in June-July 1999.

(5) Clustering was done in the NhGs by visiting the households individually and eliciting the outcome information. The anthropology team has completed ten clustering case studies in other NhCs.

The outcomes utilized for clustering process are:

(a) Food consumption: green vegetables/dates/*kothavarangai*/ iron-rich food
(b) Deworming
(c) Wearing *chappals* (footwears)
(d) Cooking in iron vessels
(e) Consuming iron folic acid (IFA) tablets
(f) Avoiding consumption of tea

If green vegetables are consumed more than four days a week and other iron-rich foods are consumed in a household, then it is inferred as 'yes', if not 'no' with respect to a food consumption.

Having collected this information, the households in the NhG are segregated into 'bad', 'moderate' and 'good' households. It was decided to include those households with five or six positive practices as good, three or four as moderate and one or two as bad.

Azhagammal's NhG

Under the NhG of the RCV Azhagammal in Vinobhaji Nagar (Dindigul), there were 21 households at the time of initial survey. Later, seven of them had left the locality and two others have come to reside here making it a 16-household NhG. The clustering outcome was as follows:

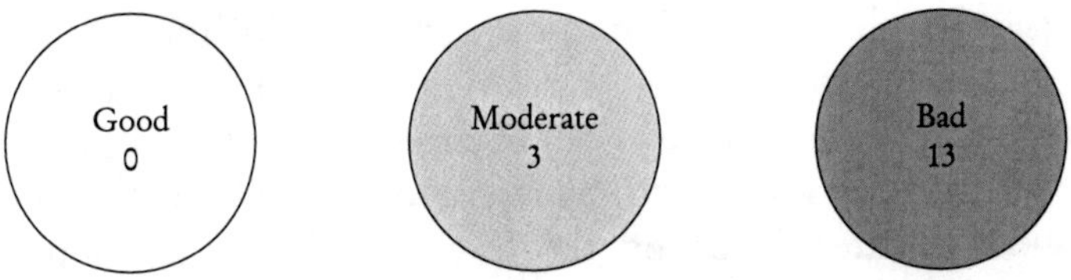

In the backdrop of the information from the individual households on specific outcomes, more information was also collected. For example, only one woman in this NhG uses iron vessel for cooking. She had been doing it since she was advised in a meeting to do so; also she had made inquiries whether it is good for diabetics. When many of them told her that it is good, then only she started using it. Whereas, the same woman does not consume green vegetables often, for many in her house do not like it, and she herself mostly subsists on tea. Similarly, each household has their own reasons for certain practices.

Analysis and Findings of Changed Intervention

- This phase brought into focus the deficiencies of the UBSP structure. The structure existed in terms of the 'leaders' but not at the level of the people. One can find conveners of NhCs and RCVs in-charge of NhGs, but the crucial factor is that the NhGs each consisting of about 20 households is never formed. The RCVs do not know which 20 odd households they represent nor the households know which specific NhG they belong to. This was the reason why it took two months for the anthropologists to structure the NhGs in two NhCs. Without such a structuring, the clustering exercise would have been meaningless.

- For the first time, there was a possibility of participatory method being used in earnest. But, the core group felt that there is no need to spend a lot of time with the community as the job could be done in a short period.
- During the process of group discussions, it was realized that the priorities of the community are different and health problems occupy at best the third priority after education and employment. Even, within the sphere of health, anaemia occupies a lower position in the order of priority.
- Clustering process would have meaning if it is repeated at regular intervals. What should be the length of the interval and how many times it has to be repeated is a question which needs wider debate guided by the level to which the community reaches in terms of the clustering behaviour.
- A major task was to analyze the possible causes for the clustering behaviour. This needs more time and more cycles of clustering process and gathering more case studies.
- This changed strategy also meant that there is no separate 'evaluation phase'. At the end of each round of clustering, there is going to be a decrease in the rate of occurrence of maternal anaemia. Tracing the process of this decrease and the explanation thereon would have met the primary goal of this study. But that did not happen.

Sum up

At the end of two years, what emerged is the following:

(1) Participatory methodology, to achieve reduction in the rate of maternal anaemia among the urban poor of Tamil Nadu was agreed upon as the main objective of this project. But, the project managers, which include experts from epidemiology, economics, anthropology and urban planning, themselves were not sensitive to the needs of participatory methodology. The local community was also not given adequate time and provided knowledge that could have given them an

opportunity to participate and plan for managing the problem of maternal anaemia.

(2) The basic outcomes of BLS – of both epidemiology and anthropology – were not ploughed back to the people so that they could take part in the planning sufficiently informed about the problem.

(3) The intervention phase of the project was the weakest link. This phase included several *lessaize-faire* activities such as speeches, advocacy, rallies, and so on. The main aim was to present intervention in terms of quantifiable numbers – a modified target approach – without much of a concern for what that particular activity is meant for and what it means in terms of participation of local communities.

(4) The attempts to understand the role of, and the autonomous space required for, the field functionaries was a complete failure. That aspect has never been tested nor discussed.

(5) The modified approach – the clustering approach – for the first time opened up a new avenue for practising participatory approach. At the same time, the local community owns this programme. This also avoids a separate 'evaluation phase'.

But, as the first round of clustering was in progress, the project management decided to terminate the project itself.

The clustering approach was also restricted to the UBSP areas and completely left out the non-UBSP areas where the field functionary model was supposed to be tested.

(6) Largely, if this project is considered a failure, it is not because the people failed, but the managers failed. Participatory method cannot be considered a failure, as it was never practised. This project is an object lesson in how a participatory project should not be managed.

Lessons Learnt

- In a multidisciplinary research situation a clear understanding on the methods and objectives – that is, means and goals – by all the researchers is absolutely important. Terminological clarity and frequent discussions/exchange of notes between all the researchers is the minimal requirement if the overall goals are to be achieved.

- In a project with participatory learning mode as the methodology, all efforts should be made to create enabling conditions for all the stakeholders to participate – this includes all the researchers, agencies and the local communities.
- All the researchers/agencies involved in the project should be sensitized to the requirements of a participatory mode, i.e., accepting all the stakeholders as equal, respect for the knowledge of all the stakeholders and prepared to learn from all the stakeholders.
- More importantly, there is an absolute need to create conditions for the local communities to participate as equal partners, know their priorities and evolve solutions.
- In such multidisciplinary and participatory projects, there is a need to monitor and progress, through process documentation, and review the process and goals at each stage with mid-course correction, if necessary.

Notes

1. The Scheme Urban Basic Infrastructure for Poor (UBSP), which is in operation in Dindigul since 1994, is basically a community participation programme. To ensure the participation of local community, there is a bottom-up structure for UBSP working. At the bottom is the Neighbourhood Group (NhG) consisting of 20 households. There is a Resident Community Volunteer (RCV), representing each NhG, who is a resident of one of the 20 households.

   The Neighbourhood Community (NhC) is formed by around 20 NhG in a locality. If the locality has less than 20 NhGs, those constitute an NhC. There is a convener who represents an NhC.

   All the NhCs come together to form the local community, the community organizer from the municipality looks after the activities of the local community.
2. This method involves segregating the basic units of the universe of study in terms of desired outcomes (say, into good, moderate, bad). This method is very useful in understanding the process of achieving the goals of the study through several cycles of segregation over a period of time.

References

Allen, L.H. and Ahluwalia, N. (1997). Improving iron status through diet: The application of knowledge concerning dietary iron bioavailability in human population (Internet: OMNI_Project@jsi.com).

ICMR (1989). *Evaluation of the National Nutritional Anaemia Prophylaxis Programme*. New Delhi: ICMR.

Nair, M.K. (1999). Iron absorption and its implications in the control of iron deficiency anaemia. *Nutrition News, 20,* 1.

Prema, K., Neelakumari, S. and Ramalakshmi, B.A. (1981). Anaemia and adverse obstetric outcome. *Nutrition Reports Interventions, 23,* 637.

Rajaratnam, A., Rajaratnam, J. and Kamaladass, T. (1997). Maternal and child health practices and nutritional status of Malto tribals in Bihar. *Man in India, 1,* 29-32.

Usha, K., *et al.* (Eds.) (1995). *Anaemia: The Weak Gets Weaker. Safe Motherhood (Issue II)*. Bangalore: Astra-IDPL Ltd.

WHO (1982). *The Prevalence of Nutritional Anaemia in Women in Developing Countries: A Critical Review of Available Information*. Geneva: WHO.

— (1992a). *National Strategies for Overcoming Micronutrient Malnutrition*. Geneva: WHO (Document A45/17/1992).

— (1992b). *The Prevalence of Anaemia in Women: A Tabulation of Available Information (Maternal Health and Safe Motherhood Programme)*, 2nd edition. Geneva: WHO.

20

Going Beyond Tertiary Prevention of Cervical Cancer: Expanding the Role of Behavioural Scientists

NEENA KOHLI

Cervical cancer is a major women's health problem, which affects over four lakh women all over the world each year and causes three lakh deaths, making it the second most common form of cancer found in women after breast cancer; is also widespread in India. In much of the developing world, it is the leading cause of death in women between the ages of 40 and 60 years. In India, this disease has been the main form of malignancy in women with about one lakh new cases reported annually. The rate is 4-5 times higher as compared to women globally. In more than 90 percent of these cases, the lesions are in an advanced stage by the time the patient seeks medical care (NIP, 2003). An important reason for the sharply higher cervical cancer incidence in developing countries is the lack of effective screening programmes aimed at detecting pre-cancerous conditions (dysplasia) and treating them before they progress to invasive cancer and failure on part of the women to avail screening services.

Causation of Cancer

Unlike the identification of bacteria and viruses as causal agents of infection, scientific research has only rarely been able to identify single, sufficient and necessary causes of cancer. Typically, the scientific evidence used to determine causality in cancer is largely circumstantial, although nonetheless convincing (Doll and Peto, 1981). Laboratory experiments can measure in vitro effects of dietary, chemical and hormonal factors in carcinogenesis. Epidemiological studies seek to confirm the influence of these factors in populations of humans using increased probabilities of risk to infer a causal association. Examples include the accepted causal association of cigarette smoking and lung cancer. Three quarters of cancer deaths are due to environmental factors, many of which can be modified and potentially controlled (Tomatis, 1990).

Human papillomavirus (HPV) – a sexually transmitted agent that infects the cells of the cervix probably – is the cause of almost all cervical cancers worldwide (Bosch, 1995; Schiffman, 1995; Pisani, 1997; Hernandez-Avila, 1997). A recent study estimates worldwide HPV prevalence in cervical carcinoma at 99.7 percent (Walboomers, 1999).

However, human papilloma virus (HPV) slowly causes cellular changes (dysplasia) that can result in cancer. These changes can be relatively mild ones. Mild dysplasia almost always regresses spontaneously and most moderate dysplasias also regress (Holowaty, 1999; Critchlow and Kiviat, 1999). Larger deeper lesions (severe dysplasia) are more likely to progress to cancer. Women generally are infected with HPV in their teens, twenties or thirties, although the disease can take upto 20 years after HPV infection to develop. Studies also suggest that persistence of HPV infection is related to the development of cancer (Moscicki *et al.*, 2001; Wallin, 1999; Burk, 1999).

Biswas (1997) investigated the role of sexual risk factors in cervical cancer among rural women with a low rate of sexual promiscuity. Results from multiple logistic regression analysis showed that cervical cancer is associated with early age at first coitus, extra-marital sexual partners and the time interval since first exposure.

Certain sexually transmitted infections (STIs), such as chlamydia trachomatis and herpes simplex virus also may be associated with an increased risk of developing cervical cancer (Anttila, 2001; Zenilman, 2001; Moscicki *et al.*, 2001).

Salient Findings of a Study Conducted with Indian Cervical Cancer Patients

A study was conducted on 132 stage III female cervical cancer patients, undergoing treatment at a local hospital in Allahabad. The modality of treatment for all the patients was radiotherapy. In radiotherapy, the area to be irradiated is marked and patients are required to maintain the marking. Wiping away the marks increases the risk of the unaffected area also being irradiated. The patients had no understanding of the salience of marking. At times patients wiped off the marking unintentionally due to ignorance and low level of education. About 95 percent of the women were illiterate and the remaining 5 percent could hardly read and write. Such a low level of education acted as a hindrance in understanding the disease and its ramifications.

The findings showed that patients on an average waited for 43 weeks before reporting for treatment. This time lag further worsened the situation. Some cancers progress at a rapid pace and the earlier the detection, the better the prognosis. The lag of 43 weeks diminished the chance of recovery. With early detection of cervical cancer, the chances of recovery increase to 80 percent. Also, 90 percent of the sample came from a rural background. For some patients, visit to the hospital was an unusual experience. The hospital environment frightened them. The medical jargons of the doctor could not be understood by the patients and the local dialect of the patients was hard for the doctors to understand. This led to poor doctor-patient communication. There was lack of appreciation of each other's language. These findings serve as a base for expanding the role of behavioural scientists. Also, the fact that all the rural women get married early in life, have their first coitus before the age of 18, have multiple pregnancies and fail to adopt family planning methods, increases the domain where the behavioural scientists can intervene and contribute towards reducing the incidence of the disease.

Preventive Approach to Cancer Control

Cancer control can be achieved in three ways: primary prevention – reducing the incidence of the disease, secondary prevention – detecting and treating the disease early, and tertiary prevention – relating to minimizing the impact of established disease.

Traditionally, behavioural scientists have adapted an individual and curative focus to disease such as cancer, working with patients who are receiving treatment or who have a terminal disease (Leventhal, 1983). However, it can be argued that the most productive task for behavioural scientists in the cancer field is to find ways of modifying relevant health-risk behaviours of whole populations rather than of selected individuals. To date, behavioural scientists have largely been involved in tertiary prevention.

Tertiary Prevention

Psychosocial interventions available during different phases of the cancer experience usually fall into one or more of four common forms, including education, behavioural training, group supportive therapy and individual supportive therapy (Fawzy *et al.*, 1997).

Reviews of studies of psychosocial interventions with cancer patients by Andersen (1992), Trijsburg *et al.* (1992) have revealed mostly positive effects on indices of psychosocial adjustment using procedures that involve cognitive behavioural stress management (CBSM). Comprehensive cancer centres in the United States mostly use CBSM interventions (Coluzzi *et al.*, 1995) and these interventions have had a major impact in the area of pain relief, controlling aversive reactions to chemotherapy (e.g., nausea) and enhancing quality of life (Jacobsen and Haan, 1998). Issues of personal control coping and hopelessness are central to the phenomenology of cancer patients. The CBSM interventions show promise in dealing with these issues.

Another type of psychosocial intervention, known as existential/experiential group therapy or supportive expressive therapy (SET), is designed to help individuals express and work through anxieties (e.g., death anxieties) (Spiegel *et al.*, 1981) and ventilate negative feelings. The interventions provide opportunities for group members to share their strategies for dealing with stressors common to cancer patients, the chance for members to help one another and a sense of universality (Spiegel *et al.*, 1981). Fawzy and Fawzy (1998) suggest that it is plausible for patients with early stage disease (and a good prognosis) to benefit more from a CBSM intervention, whereas those with advanced metastasis disease may benefit more from SET group programmes that focus on pain management and existential issues. Behavioural scientists can continue contributing to tertiary prevention but along with tertiary prevention behavioural scientists can also expand their role to primary and secondary prevention.

The following section will highlight the role of the behavioural scientist in a preventive, population-oriented approach to cancer control, especially cervical cancer.

Primary Prevention

Although primary prevention of HPV infection would greatly reduce cervical cancer mortality, the prevention of HPV transmission presents greater challenges than most STIs. HPV generally is symptomatic and easily transmitted. It is not entirely clear that barrier methods of protection against STIs are effective in protecting women from cervical cancer. A number of studies have found barrier methods to be protective (Grimes and Economy, 1995; Coker, 1992; Thomas, 1996; Wen, 1999). Other studies have not found a significant association between use of barrier methods and cervical cancer prevention (Hildesheim, 1990). Researchers also are beginning to focus on the possible role of men who may be acquiring high-risk HPV from frequent contact with prostitutes and transmitting the infection to their wives (Thomas, 2001). Result from pooled data from IARC's seven case-control studies shows a strong association between circumcision and a reduced risk of penile HPV and subsequent cervical cancer in female partners (Castellsague, 2002). Other suggestions of primary prevention strategies for cervical cancer are based on risk associations in case-control studies and include maintaining a high dietary intake of Vitamin C (Grimes and Economy, 1995). Both the World Health Organization (WHO) and the National Institutes of Health (NIH) also recommend sex education and efforts to change sexual behaviour as part of their primary prevention strategies (WHO, 1985; Shepherd, 1999). The role of the behavioural scientist lies in making people understand that cervical cancer is preventable and males can play a major role in protecting their wives from becoming a victim of cervical cancer.

Secondary Prevention

The role of behavioural scientists in enhancing the use of tests or measures used to identify (screen) persons who have already developed cancer risk factors, or who have pre-clinical or clinically apparent disease, is also important. The objective of such screening is to allow treatment of those identified so as to reduce cancer morbidity and/or mortality.

In industrialized countries, cervical cancer incidence and mortality have been reduced significantly through screening. The challenge for the behavioural scientists is to promote screening programme in India where cervical cancer affects rural women the most but which can be greatly reduced with timely intervention.

Before promoting cervical cancer screening programme, it is necessary to briefly review the criteria of what constitutes an appropriate screening programme. These criteria were initially developed by the Canadian Task Force on the Periodic Health Examination (1979) and further refined by the US Preventive Services Task Force (1989). These groups have argued that a screening test should have demonstrable accuracy. It should also have a high sensitivity. That is, the test should identify a high proportion of persons with the condition. A test with poor sensitivity will miss those individuals who have the condition and produce a large proportion of false negative results, that is, true cases will be told incorrectly that they are free of the disease and consequently will be inappropriately reassured. The test should have a high specificity, that is, a high proportion of persons without the condition will correctly be tested as not having the disease. A test with poor specificity will result in a large proportion of healthy people being told they have the condition (false positives) resulting in anxiety and unnecessary further testing. For the sensitivity and specificity of screening tests to be assessed, it is necessary to have an accepted reference or gold standard which provides an accurate distinction between those with and those without the condition.

Apart from having acceptable levels of sensitivity and specificity, the screening test must also possess reliability. Poor reliability might arise as a result of difference in judgement between different individuals or laboratories (inter-observation variation), or by differences within the same individual or laboratory (intra-observer variation).

When evaluating whether early detection is effective, it is also necessary to consider whether or not an individual has simply been diagnosed at an earlier stage of the disease, thereby appearing to lengthen survival, when in fact it only increases the amount of time for which a patient knows that he has cancer. This phenomenon is known as lead-time bias. Another problem of particular relevance for cancer screening is the notion of length bias. This refers to tendency to detect a disproportionate number of cases of a slowly progressing disease and to miss those cases of a disease where there is a rapid progression of the condition. In this situation, people with the more aggressive malignancies may be underestimated in the number of cases detected by screening, with those that are detected having a better prognosis even if the screening itself does not influence outcome. Such a bias may lead to the assumption that screening is more effective than it really is.

Traditional Approach to Prevention

Cervical cancer prevention worldwide has focussed on screening women at risk using Pap smears and treating pre-cancerous lesions. Where screening quality and coverage has been high, these efforts have reduced invasive cervical cancer by as much as 90 percent. Most developing countries, however, have been unable to implement comprehensive Pap smear screening-based programmes. In countries where Pap smear screening is available, it often is accessible only to a relatively small proportion of women attending private sector health providers, or is offered primarily to young women through maternal/child health or family planning clinics where the population that is screened is not generally at high risk. These approaches have had little effect on morbidity and mortality and are not cost-effective.

Emerging Approaches to Prevention

Several alternative approaches to cervical cancer screening have been proposed along with Pap test. These include: (a) visual screening, (b) human papilloma virus DNA tests, and (c) cryotherapy and LEEP.

Visual Screening

For low-resource settings there is particular interest in the accuracy and acceptability of visual screening as a means of detecting cervical dysplasia and/or cancer (Megevand, 1996). This type of screening may reduce the cost and complexity of Pap smear screening and holds the potential for screening and treatment in the same visit.

Nene (1996) conducted a population-based study in rural India. The objectives of this study was to evaluate the use of unaided visual inspection. The visual inspection (VI) refers to methods of examining the cervix for obvious lesions by trained paramedical workers (PWs) in detecting cervical cancer in low-resource settings. In all, 1,954 women from the Maharashtra (India) were examined by two PWs followed by gynaecologists. PWs score on sensitivity and specificity was similar to values obtained by the gynaecologists. However, the author concludes that unaided visual inspection probably is not a useful procedure for cervical cancer control. The cost savings achieved by 40 to 50 percent of visually normal women not requiring cytology examinations will be offset by those needing repeat examinations, colposopy and biopsy.

Another study by Varghese (2000) compared unaided VI (also known as 'down staging') and Pap smear results in two populations in South India. The findings show that VI had low sensitivity and specificity in detecting cervix dysplasias. Although VI is an appropriate tool for low-resource settings, to do VI properly, the setting should have facilities privacy, water and electricity – all of which may be lacking in many sites. Both diagnostic and treatment services are limited in many sites, and many women fail to comply with referral subsequent to VI. If VI is to be used for cervical control, behavioural scientists can contribute immensely towards motivating potential risk group to adhere to screening and subsequent referrals.

A more promising visual screening approach – visual inspection with acetic acid (VIA) – is used to describe examination of the cervix after treatment with acetic acid to identify acetowhite lesions. Evidence shows moderate to substantial inter-rater reliability for clinicians' assessment of the cervix using the acetic acid wash. Sankaranarayan *et al.* (1998) conducted a study in Kerala (India) to compare visual inspection of the cervix after the application of acetic acid (VIA) with cytology as methods for detecting cervical cancer and its precursors. The findings reveal that VIA worked as well as Pap smears. In another study (Sankaranarayan *et al.*, 1999), VIA used by nurses detected 95.8 percent of dysplasias and cancers, whereas cytology detected 62 percent (VIA detected more mild and moderate dysplasias than cytology). The effectiveness of VIA in detecting pre-cancerous lesions as well as the immediacy of VIA results) makes it a potentially attractive case findings tool in developing country settings.

HPV DNA Tests

Research is ongoing to determine acceptable protocols for testing for the human papilloma virus (HPV) as part of cervical screening and treatment strategies. Proposed uses of HPV testing in cervical cancer prevention programmes include (1) where Pap smear screening is the norm, as a triage for women with Pap smear findings of atypical cells of unknown significance (cells that are atypical but not definitely dysplasia); women who test positive for high-risk HPV type would be monitored closely or referred for colposocpy; (2) as a means of surveillance of women after treatment for high-grade lesions or micro-invasive cancer; those who test positive for high-risk HPV types would be monitored more closely than those who test negative; and (3) as a primary screening method for high-grade lesions among women aged 30 to 35 or older; those who test positive for high-risk HPV would undergo diagnosis via colposcopy or another visualization technique (Cuzick, 2000).

Upto 99.8 percent of cervical cancers are associated with HPV. The DNA probe would provide assurance to millions of women that they are at low risk for the disease. The Pap smear currently misses about 50 percent of patients with significant precursors for cervical cancer and is less than a perfect lest. Demographic studies in various countries including India show that considerable percentage of women who test abnormal on Pap test stand the greatest risk of progressing to cervical cancer with very little prognostic outcomes indicated at the time of testing when followed up from two to five years. On the contrary, if tested once for HPV DNA, which is a single most critical causative factor for cervical cancer, these women could be diagnosed 5-15 years before their cancer can be clinically identified.

Cryotherapy and LEEP

Two outpatient dysplasia treatment approaches have demonstrated particular utility in low-resource settings (Bishop, 1996). These are cryotherapy (freezing of diseased tissues through application of refrigerated probe) and the loop electrosurgical excision procedure (LEEP), which uses a thin electrified wire to excise cervical lesions. These methods have been found to have comparable rates of successes and complications (Mitchell, 1998). Cryotherapy is a simple, inexpensive procedure and does require electricity. Twelve months after treatment, cryotherapy has been associated with cure rates of approximately 80 to 90 percent (Andersen and Husth, 1992; Olatumbosun, 1992). Cryotherapy generally produces a lower cure rate for larger lesions and/or lesion that extend into the cervical canal. Complications associated with cryotherapy are minimal, suggesting that offering cryotherapy in settings where women may not have access to follow-up medical care may be a rational approach. LEEP has been associated with cure rates of about 80 to 93 percent (Flannelly, 1997; Hulman, 1998; Keijser, 1992), and may be the preferred method for treating larger, deeper lesions. Compared to cryotherapy, LEEP has been associated with slightly higher rates of complications and side-effects such as post-operative bleeding and preoperative pain (Mitchell, 1998). The likelihood of cure for both methods decreases with higher-grade lesions and larger lesions. Older age also may be associated with lower cure rates (Mitchell, 1998; Paraskevaidis, 2000), possibly because older women are more likely to have persistent, higher-grade lesions.

Role of Behavioural Scientists

The important task for the behavioural scientist is to identify the barriers to screening and to make efforts to reduce them. Many studies have shown that women in developing countries and other underserved populations lack information on cervical cancer and available services. Ajayi and Adewolfe (1998) investigated Nigerian women's knowledge about cervical cancer, their source of information, and their general attitude about cancer. Out of a sample of 254 women, only 15 percent had heard of cancer of the cervix. Over half of the respondents had no knowledge of the description of cervical cancer, clinical presentation, or causes. Kohli (1995) found that women afflicted with cervical cancer had no understanding of the illness. Additional barriers to screening are lack of knowledge about cervical cancer aetiology, lack of knowledge of the Pap test, the perception that it is an inevitably fatal disease, problems in client-provider relationship, competing priorities due to extreme poverty and culturally biased altitudes towards cancer (Lazcano-Ponce, 1999; Masood, 1999).

Other factors reducing women's participation in cervical cancer screening programmes include poor awareness of the indications and benefits of the cervical smear test, fear of embarrassment pain or cancer, anxiety caused by receiving an abnormal cervical smear result, poor understanding of cervical screening procedures and unavailability of female screeners (Fylan, 1998) and anxiety about a lack of confidentiality and perceived relationship between cervical smears and sexual activity.

Overcoming Barriers

Educating women and increasing awareness is key to eliminating barriers. In India, majority of rural women do not know about cervical cancer or that detecting and treating pre-cancerous lesion can prevent the disease; this lack of awareness is a major barrier to seeking screening services. In order for women to seek cervical cancer screening services, they must be informed about the disease and have access to services that are sensitive and responsive to their needs. Involving women at risk of cervical cancer (particularly women in their thirties and forties) in the development of educational messages and programmes is the key. Participatory qualitative research methods, such as focus group discussions, in-depth interviews, or community mapping with women of various ages and their partners, can provide insights into their needs and concerns. An advisory team consisting of women at risk can be established. These activities can help ensure that services are provided in an acceptable manner, thereby increasing women's willingness to seek screening and necessary follow-up care.

The key challenge for a screening programme is to encourage women at highest risk for treatable pre-cancerous lesions – often women in their 30s and 40s – to seek services. The important task for behavioural scientists is to motivate women, and to increase their readiness for screening. Many women in this age group have completed childbearing age and therefore are not likely to access family planning or maternal health services. Therefore, special efforts are required to inform them of the need for and availability of screening. The best approaches for increasing awareness among women in their post-reproductive years will vary from place to place and can be best developed with inputs from women themselves. Possible approaches include reaching women through their community or a voluntary counsellor who is known to these women, linking screening to an important event in an older women's life, such as becoming a grandmother, or linking screening to other mid-life health needs, such as contraceptive sterilization. The role of the behavioural scientist would lie in encouraging the promoters to use multiple communication strategies, to make screening more successful.

In India, the risk of developing cervical cancer is amplified by poverty and isolation. Strategies such as special 'screening days' in remote villages can be initiated using media, loudspeakers and calls from religious congregations to encourage hard-to-reach women to attend screening. Women normally gather for religious purposes and it is easy to tap the risk group at such sites. Overall, it is essential to ensure good quality care at screening sites, treating women with respect and paying attention to their concerns. Women will not attend preventive care services if they believe that they will be treated poorly.

The success of the programme largely depends upon (i), assisting service providers in adopting a public health-oriented approach to screening and treatment, and (ii) training them in the skills necessary to counsel clients and provide high quality services that respect women's concerns and needs. Experience from cervical cancer control efforts worldwide suggests that some policies in low-resource settings call for inappropriate service delivery approaches; for instance, screening women as frequently as every six months, focusing screening on younger women, and focusing treatment on advanced cancers. Widespread use of such practices prevents programmes from achieving a significant health impact by draining programme resources. Both pre-service and in-service provider trainings can address this issue by presenting clear information about the public health rationale for focussing on broad coverage of older women in their thirties and forties and emphasizing treatment of pre-cancerous conditions.

Service providers also need appropriate training on key clinical and counselling issues related to cervical cancer prevention, along with ongoing supervisory support and assistance in establishing and maintaining referral links. Particularly important is ensuring the quality of screening programme. For example, if visual screening approaches are used, the providers must be trained to properly identify abnormal tissue and know what action to take. Appropriate counselling is also critical. Providers must also be trained to establish a respectful rapport with women and address their fears and concerns; only then will women be motivated for screening. Thus, by expanding their roles, behavioural scientists can go a long way in reducing cervical cancer incidence and mortality and improving women's health.

References

Ajayi, I.O. and Adewolfe, I.F. (1998). Knowledge and attitude of general outpatient attendants in Nigeria to cervical cancer control. *African Journal of Medicine, 44,* 41-43.

Andersen, B.L. (1992). Psychological interventions for cancer patients to enhance the quality of life. *Journal Consulting Clinical Psychology, 60,* 552-568.

Andersen, E.S. and Husth, M. (1992). Cryosurgery for cervical intraepithelial neoplasia: 10 year follow up. *Gynaecologic Oncology, 45,* 240-242.

Anttila, T. (2001). Epidemiology and natural history of cervical cancer: Stereotypes of Chlamydia trachomatis and risk for development of cervical squamous call carcinoma. *JAMA, 285,* 47-51.

Bishop, A. (1996). Cervical dysplasia treatment: Key issues for developing countries. *Bulletin of PAHO, 30,* 378-386.

Biswas, L.N. (1997). Sexual risk factors for cervical cancer among rural Indian women: A case control study. *International Journal of Epidemiology, 26,* 491-495.

Bosch, F.X. (1995). Prevalence of human papilloma virus in cervical cancer: A world wide perspective. *Journal of the National Cancer Institute, 87,* 796-802.

Burk, R.D. (1999). Pernicious papilloma virus infection (editorial), *The New England Journal of Medicine, 341,* 1687-1688.

Canadian Task Force on the Periodic Health Examination (1979). The periodic health examination. *Canadian Medical Association Journal, 121,* 1194-1254.

Coker, A.L. (1992). Primary prevention of cervical cancer. Barrier methods of Contraception and cervical intraepithelial neoplasia. *Contraception, 45,* 1-10.

Coluzzi, P.H., Grant, M., Doroshow, J.H., Rlliner, M. and Ferrell, B. (1995). Survey of the provision of supportive care services at National Cancer Institute-designated cancer centres. *Journal Clinical Oncology, 13,* 756-764.

Critchlow, C.W. and Kiviat, N.B. (1999). Old and new issues in cervical cancer control (editorial). *Journal of the National Cancer Institute, 91,* 200-201.

Cuzick, J. (2000). Human papilloma virus testing for primary cervical cancer screening. *JAMA, 283,* 108-109.

Doll, R. and Peto, R. (1981). *The Causes of Cancer: Quantitative Estimates of Avoidance Risks of Cancer in the U.S. Today.* Oxford: Oxford University Press.

Fawzy, F.I. and Fawzy, N.W. (1998). Psychoeducational interventions. In J. Holland (Ed.), *Textbook of Psycho-oncology*. New York; Oxford University Press, 676-693.

Fawzy, F.L., Fawzy, N., Hyun, C. and Wheeler, J. (1997). Brief coping-oriented therapy for patients with malignant melanoma. In J. Spria (Ed), *Group Therapy for Medically Ill Patients.* New York: Guilford, 133-164.

Flannelly, G. (1997). A study of the treatment failures following large loop excision of the transformation zone for the treatment of cervical intraepithelial neoplasia. *British Journal of Obstetrics and Gynaecology, 104,* 718-722.

Fylan, F. (1998). Screening for cervical cancer: a review of women's attitudes Knowledge, and behaviour. *British Journal of General Practice, 48,* 1509-1514.

Grimes, D.A. and Economy, K.E. (1995). Primary prevention of gynaecologic cancers. *American Journal of Obstetrics and Gynaecology, 172,* 227-235.

Hernandez-Avila, M. (1997). Human papilloma virus 16-18 infection and cervical cancer in Mexico: A case control study. *Archives of Medical Research, 28*, 256-271.

Hildesheim, A. (1990). Barrier and spermicidal contraceptive methods and risks of invasive cervical cancer. *Epidemiology, 1*, 226-272.

Holowaty, P. (1999). Natural history of dysplasia of the uterine cervix. *Journal of the National Cancer Institute, 91*, 252-258.

Hulman, G. (1998). Frequency of cervical intraepithelial neoplasia following large loop excision of the transformation zone. *Journal of Clinical Pathology, 51*, 375-377.

Jacobsen, P.B. and Hann, D.M. (1998). Cognitive behavioural interventions. In J. Holland (Ed.), *Textbook of Psycho-oncology*. New York: Oxford Press, 717-729.

Keijser, K. (1992). Diathermy loop excision in the management of cervical intraepithelial neoplasia diagnosis and treatment in one procedure. *American Journal of Obstetrics and Gynaecology, 166*, 1281-1287.

Kohli, N. (1995). *Coping with Tragic Life Events: A Study of Cancer Patients*. Unpublished doctoral dissertation, University of Allahabad, Allahabad.

Lazcano-Ponce, E.C. (1999). Barriers to early detection of cervical uterine cancer in Mexico. *Journal of Women's Health, 8*, 399-408.

Leventhal, H. (1983). Behavioural medicine: Psychology in health care. In D. Mechanic (Ed.), *Handbook of Health, Health Care, and the Health Professions*. New York: Free Press, 709-744.

Masood, S. (1999). A plea for worldwide volunteer cervical cancer education and awareness program. A proposal from the International Academy of Cytology Committee on Cancer detection for medically underserved women. *Journal of Clinical Cytology and Cytopathology, 43*, 539-543.

Megevand, E. (1996). Acetic acid visualization of the cervix: An alternative to cytologic screening. *Obstetrics and Gynaecology, 88*, 383-386.

Mitchell, M.F. (1998). A randomised clinical trial of cryotherapy, laser vaporization and loop electrosurgical excision for treatment of squamous intraepithelial lesions of the cervix. *Obstetrics and Gynaecology, 92*, 737-744.

Moscicki, A., Hills, N. and Shiboski, S. (2001). Risks for incident human papilloma virus infection and low-grade squamous intraepithelial lesion development in young females. *JAMA, 285*, 2995-3002.

Nene, B.M. (1996). Early detection of cervical cancer by visual inspection: a population based study in rural India. *International Journal of Cancer, 68*, 770-773.

Northern India Patrika (2003). DNA test and prognosis of cervical cancer, August 29, Allahabad.

Olatunbosun, O.A. (1992). Outcome of cryosurgery for cervical intraepithelial neoplasia in a developing country. *International Journal of Gynaecology and Obstetrics, 38*, 305-310.

Paraskevaidis, E. (2000). Cervical intraepithelial neoplasia outcomes after large loop excision with clear margins. *Obstetrics and Gynaecology, 95*, 828-831.

Pisani, P. (1997). Cancer and infection: Estimates of the attributable fraction in 1990. *Cancer Epidemiology, Biomarkers and Prevention, 1*, 387-400.

Sankaranarayanan, R., Budukh, A.M. and Rajkumar, R. (1999). Visual inspection with acetic acid in the early detection of cervical cancer and precursors. *International Journal of Cancer, 80*, 161-163.

Sankaranarayanan, R., Budukh, A.M. and Rajkumar, R. (1998). Visual inspection of the uterine cervix after the application of acetic acid in the detection of cervical carcinoma and its precursors. *American Cancer Society, 83*, 2150-2156.

Schiffman, M.H. (1995). New epidemiology of human papilloma virus infection and cervical neoplasia. *Journal of the National Cancer Institute,* 87, 1345-1347.

Shepherd, J. (1999). Interventions for encouraging sexual lifestyles and behaviours intended to prevent cervical cancer (Cochrane Review), In the *Cochrane Library*, Issue 3, Oxford.

Spiegel, D., Bloom, J. and Yalom, I. (1981). Group support for patients with metastatic cancer: A randomised prospective outcome study. *Archives General Psychology, 38*, 527-533.

Thomas, D.B. (2001). Human papilloma virus and cervical cancer in Bangkok: The role of husbands and commercial sex workers. *American Journal of Epidemiology, 153*, 740-748.

— (1996). Prostitution, condom use, and invasive squamons cell cervical cancer in Thailand. *American Journal of Epidemiology, 143*, 779-786.

Tomatis, L. (1990). *Cancer: Causes, Occurrence and Control.* Lyon. International Agency for Research on Cancer.

Trijsburg, R.W., Van Knippenberg, F.C.E. and Rijpma, S.E. (1992). Effects of psychological treatment on cancer patients: A critical review: *Psychosomatic Medicine, 54*, 489-517.

U.S. Preventive Services Task Force (1989). *Guide to Clinical Preventive Services*. Baltimore: Williams and Wilkins.

Varghese, C. (2000). Cervical cancer control in developing countries: Beyond visual inspection. *Journal of Cytology, 17*, 97-101.

Walboomers, J.M.M. (1999). Human papilloma virus is a necessary cause of invasive cervical cancer worldwide. *Journal of Pathology, 189*, 12-19.

Wallin, K.L. (1999). Type-specific persistence of human papilloma virus DNA before the development of invasive cervical cancer. *The New England Journal of Medicine, 341*, 1633-1638.

Wen, L.M. (1999). Risk factors for the acquisition of genital warts: Are condoms protective? *Sexually Transmitted Infections, 75*, 312-316.

World Health Organization (1985). *Primary Prevention of Cervical Cancer.* CAN/85, 1. Geneva. WHO.

Zenilman, J.M. (2001). Chlamydia and cervical cancer: A real association? *JAMA, 285*, 81-83.

Author Index

Subject Index